Exam Preparatory Manual for Undergraduates
OPHTHALMOLOGY

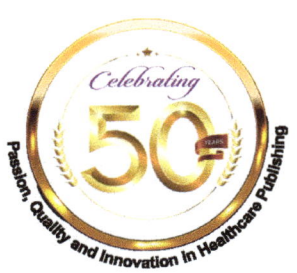

Exam Preparatory Manual for Undergraduates
OPHTHALMOLOGY

SECOND EDITION

K Mohan Raj MS DO
Retired Professor and Head, Ophthalmology
Sree Balaji Medical College and Hospital
Chromepet, Chennai, Tamil Nadu, India

Formerly
Director and Superintendent
Regional Institute of Ophthalmology
Government Ophthalmic Hospital
Chennai, Tamil Nadu, India

Foreword
P Kumaravel

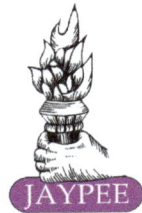

JAYPEE BROTHERS MEDICAL PUBLISHERS
The Health Sciences Publisher
New Delhi | London

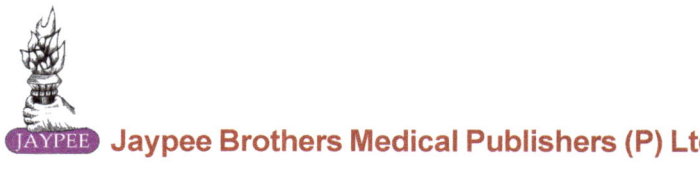

Jaypee Brothers Medical Publishers (P) Ltd

Headquarters
Jaypee Brothers Medical Publishers (P) Ltd
EMCA House, 23/23-B
Ansari Road, Daryaganj
New Delhi 110 002, India
Landline: +91-11-23272143, +91-11-23272703
+91-11-23282021, +91-11-23245672
Email: jaypee@jaypeebrothers.com

Corporate Office
Jaypee Brothers Medical Publishers (P) Ltd
4838/24, Ansari Road, Daryaganj
New Delhi 110 002, India
Phone: +91-11-43574357
Fax: +91-11-43574314
Email: jaypee@jaypeebrothers.com

Overseas Office
J.P. Medical Ltd
83 Victoria Street, London
SW1H 0HW (UK)
Phone: +44 20 3170 8910
Fax: +44 (0)20 3008 6180
Email: info@jpmedpub.com

Website: www.jaypeebrothers.com
Website: www.jaypeedigital.com

© 2021, Jaypee Brothers Medical Publishers

The views and opinions expressed in this book are solely those of the original contributor(s)/author(s) and do not necessarily represent those of editor(s) of the book.

All rights reserved. No part of this publication may be reproduced, stored or transmitted in any form or by any means, electronic, mechanical, photocopying, recording or otherwise, without the prior permission in writing of the publishers.

All brand names and product names used in this book are trade names, service marks, trademarks or registered trademarks of their respective owners. The publisher is not associated with any product or vendor mentioned in this book.

Medical knowledge and practice change constantly. This book is designed to provide accurate, authoritative information about the subject matter in question. However, readers are advised to check the most current information available on procedures included and check information from the manufacturer of each product to be administered, to verify the recommended dose, formula, method and duration of administration, adverse effects and contraindications. It is the responsibility of the practitioner to take all appropriate safety precautions. Neither the publisher nor the author(s)/editor(s) assume any liability for any injury and/or damage to persons or property arising from or related to use of material in this book.

This book is sold on the understanding that the publisher is not engaged in providing professional medical services. If such advice or services are required, the services of a competent medical professional should be sought.

Every effort has been made where necessary to contact holders of copyright to obtain permission to reproduce copyright material. If any have been inadvertently overlooked, the publisher will be pleased to make the necessary arrangements at the first opportunity. The **CD/DVD-ROM** (if any) provided in the sealed envelope with this book is complimentary and free of cost. **Not meant for sale**.

Inquiries for bulk sales may be solicited at: jaypee@jaypeebrothers.com

Exam Preparatory Manual for Undergraduates—Ophthalmology

First Edition: 2016
Second Edition: **2021**
ISBN: 978-81-948028-6-0

To
*Almighty, my parents, and students
who were my source of inspiration*

Foreword

It is indeed an honor for me to write the Foreword for *Exam Preparatory Manual for Undergraduates—Ophthalmology* written by Dr K Mohan Raj. The author has provided comprehensive knowledge by the way of questions and answers which is needed for MBBS students. This book is a sure success formula for the students to face the examination with confidence. Even though many textbooks are available, this manual is very apt for the quick revision before exams. The author has put in great efforts to bring in such useful manual using his vast experience as a teacher as well as an examiner. This book provides all materials necessary for theory, clinical and viva voce examinations. I am confident that the students can secure very good marks by using this manual.

P Kumaravel MS DO
Professor and Head, Ophthalmology
Sri Muthukumaran Medical College Hospital and Research Institute
Chikkarayapuram, Chennai, Tamil Nadu, India

Former Professor and Head, Ophthalmology
Government Stanley Medical College and Hospital
Chennai, Tamil Nadu, India

Preface to the Second Edition

Four years have been elapsed since the publication of the first edition. The contents of this edition has been updated as per the latest competency-based undergraduate curriculum of National Medical Council of India. Each chapter has been enriched with colorful diagrams, tables and flowcharts wherever necessary. Annexure has been included for quick reference to the clinical cases described in the book. The main aim of the book is to simplify the difficult topics and give students a practical and concise summary for better understanding which can help them to perform better in the exam. This book will facilitate the students in covering theory, practical and viva requirements for the final year MBBS examination. It can also be used as a reference book for optometry students. Postgraduates can use this book for better revision of important points of various topics in ophthalmology.

K Mohan Raj

Preface to the First Edition

Eye is the window of the world. It is the most important sensory organ. As our longevity has increased, we have to take care of our eyes till our death to make our lives worth living. Hence, ophthalmology is one of the most important specialties about which, every MBBS doctor should have adequate knowledge.

During the final year of MBBS, students are posted in various departments and they do not have enough time to prepare for part I examinations. Studying this book three months before the examinations will amount to a comprehensive study of different textbooks.

Numerous textbooks have come out but the students find it difficult to answer the questions relevant to the theory, clinical and oral examinations. This manual is aimed to help the student in facing the examinations with confidence.

This book is mainly from my PowerPoint lectures given to the students. Each and every effort has been made to include the answers what the examiners expect. Even though this book is mainly for undergraduates, it will also be useful for the postgraduates and residents in ophthalmology in order to learn the basic aspects of the subject. Recent concepts have been included in all chapters. For further improvements in future, I welcome suggestions from the readers to my email id, mohanrajdr@yahoo.com.

K Mohan Raj

Acknowledgments

I would like to thank my students Dr Jeyadharshini, Dr Ramya and associate professor Dr L Subha of Balaji Medical College and Hospital, Chennai, Tamil Nadu, India in helping to prepare this manual. I would like to thank my wife Uma and my daughters Nisanti and Vandhana for their encouragement and support. I also appreciate the inquisitiveness of my grandchildren Ayana, Rohan, Sean and Tara during the preparation of this book.

I am highly thankful to Shri Jitendar P Vij (Group Chairman), Mr Ankit Vij (Managing Director), Mr MS Mani (Group President), Dr Madhu Choudhary (Publishing Head–Education), Ms Pooja Bhandari (Production Head), Ms Sunita Katla (Executive Assistant to Group Chairman and Publishing Manager), Ms Samina Khan (Executive Assistant to Publishing Head–Education), Dr Akanksha Singh (Development Editor), Mr Rajesh Sharma (Production Coordinator), Ms Seema Dogra (Cover Visualizer), Mr Narsingh Kumar (Proofreader), Mr Omprakash Mishra (Typesetter), Mr Ankush Sharma (Graphic Designer), Mr Sabyasachi Hazra (Commissioning Editor, Kolkata Branch) and the whole team of M/s Jaypee Brothers Medical Publishers (P) Ltd, New Delhi, India. Without their cooperation, I could not have completed this project.

Contents

1. Anatomy of the Eye 1
2. Physiology of the Eye 7
3. Neurology of Vision 11
4. Ocular Pharmacology 19
5. Errors of Refraction 23
6. Conjunctiva 33
7. Cornea 44
8. Sclera 60
9. Uvea 63
10. Lens 77
11. Glaucoma 86
12. Vitreous 98
13. Retina 100
14. Intraocular Tumors 121
15. Lids 125
16. Lacrimal Apparatus 133
17. Injuries to the Eye 140
18. Orbit 146
19. Neuro-ophthalmology 153
20. Squint 162
21. Ocular Manifestations of Systemic Diseases 170
22. Community Ophthalmology 172
23. Clinical Examination 178
24. Instruments and Lenses 184
25. Miscellaneous 191

Annexure *197*
Index *199*

CHAPTER 1

Anatomy of the Eye

INTRODUCTION

The eyeball is an organ of vision. It is suspended in the orbit by extraocular muscles and their fascial sheaths. Eyeball is not typically spherical but an oblate spheroid.

1. What are the dimensions of adult eyeball?
- Anteroposterior diameter: 24 mm
- Circumference: 75 mm
- Volume: 6.5–7 cc
- Weight: 7 g.

2. Name the coats of eyeball.
- Cornea forms 1/6th of the outer protective coat and sclera forms the 5/6th
- Middle vascular coat is the uveal tract viz iris, ciliary body, and choroid
- Retina forms the inner nervous coat.

3. What constitutes the anterior segment?
Anterior segment consists of conjunctiva, cornea, iris, anterior sclera, aqueous humor, lens, and anterior and posterior chambers.

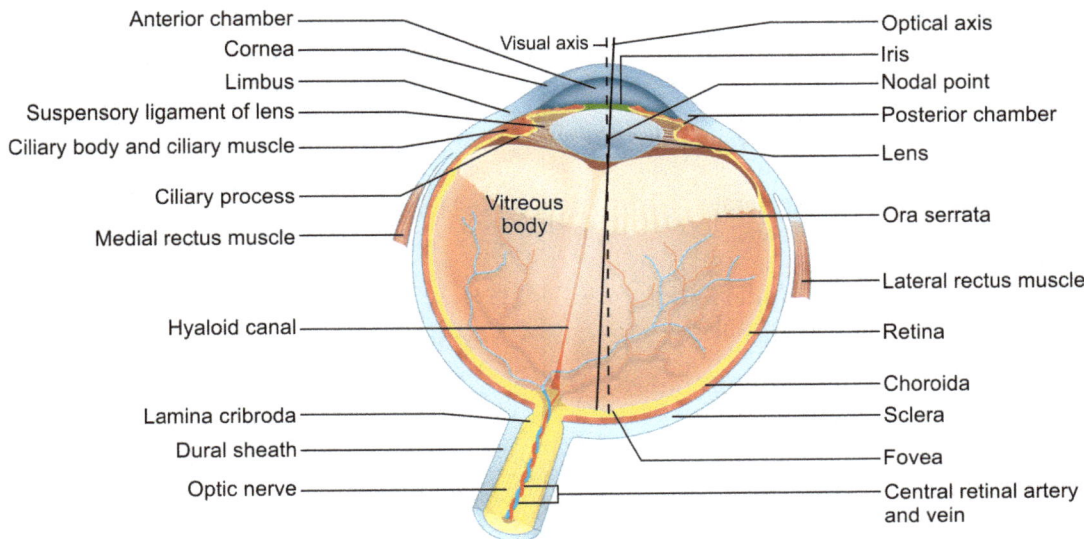

Fig. 1.1: Anatomy of eye with cut section.

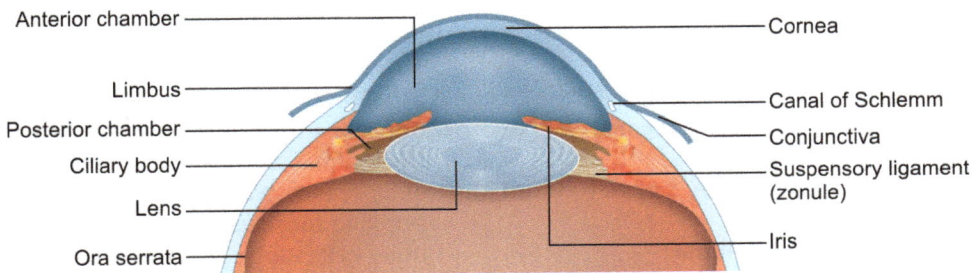

Fig. 1.2: Anterior segment.

Anterior chamber is the space filled with aqueous humor bounded in front by back of the cornea and behind by iris and lens. In peripheral recess lies the angle of anterior chamber. Its depth is 2.5 mm and the volume is 0.25 mL.

Posterior chamber is the triangular space bounded in front by back of iris and behind by lens and ciliary zonules, laterally by ciliary body. Its volume is 0.06 cc.

4. What is posterior segment?

Posterior segment is formed by structures posterior to lens. They are vitreous humor, retina, choroid and optic disk and pars plana of ciliary body.

5. Name the structures forming angle of anterior chamber.

Angles of anterior chamber from anterior to posterior are:
- Schwalbe's line
- Trabecular meshwork
- Scleral spur
- Band of ciliary body
- Root of iris.

6. What are the dimensions of adult cornea?

- Vertical diameter: 11 mm
- Horizontal diameter: 12 mm
- Radius of curvature: Anterior 7.8 mm; posterior 6.5 mm
- Thickness: In center—0.52 mm; in periphery—1 mm
- Refractive index: 1.37; power: + 43D to + 45D.

7. List the layers of cornea.

- Epithelium-stratified squamous type—replaces every 7 days
- Bowman's membrane—does not regenerate
- Stroma—90% thickness—collagen fibers
- Pre-Descemet's layer or Dua's layer
- Descemet's membrane—regenerates after injury
- Endothelium—adult 2,800–3,000 cells/mm^2.

8. What are the features of corneal endothelium?

- It consists of single layer of polygonal cells
- Once damaged, it does not regenerate
- Corneal decompensation occurs if it falls < 500 cells/mm^2
- They contain active pump mechanism.

9. What is the blood supply of cornea?

Cornea is an avascular structure. Small loops from the anterior conjunctival vessels invade the peripheral cornea.

10. What are the causes for corneal transparency?

- Arrangement of corneal lamellae (lattice theory)
- Avascularity
- Relative dehydration maintained by epithelial and endothelial barriers
- Active bicarbonate pump of endothelium.

11. What is the nerve supply of cornea?

It is supplied by nasociliary nerve which is a branch of ophthalmic division of trigeminal nerve.

12. What is the thickness of sclera?

- At posterior pole: 1 mm (thickest)
- At insertion of muscles: 0.3 mm (thinnest)
- At the equator: 0.5 mm.

Lamina cribrosa is the thinnest sieve like sclera through which optic nerve fiber passes.

13. What are the dimensions of lens?

- Diameter: 9 mm
- Thickness of lens
  - At birth: 3.5 mm
  - Adult lens: 4 mm
  - Above 60 years: 5 mm
- Weight of the lens varies from 135 mg (0–9 years) to 260 mg (> 60 years).
- Refractive power: + 16D
- Radius of curvature: Anterior—10 mm; posterior—6 mm
- Refractive index: 1.42.

14. Describe the structure of lens.

- Thickness of lens capsule—at posterior pole—4 μ; at pre-equatorial region—14 μ
- The capsule encloses outer cortex and inner nucleus
- Central part of lens consists of older fibers.
- **It consists of different zones:**
  - Embryonic nucleus—innermost and formed at 1–3 months of gestation
  - Fetal nucleus—formed at 3 months to birth
  - Infantile nucleus—formed from birth to puberty
  - Adult nucleus—corresponds to lens in early adult life.

15. How lens transparency is maintained?

- Avascularity
- Tightly packed lens fibers
- Semipermeable lens capsule
- Active pump mechanism in lens fibers
- Auto-oxidation and high concentration of reduced glutathione.

16. Describe the structure of iris.

Anterior surface of iris is divided into a ciliary zone and a pupillary zone by the collarette (a zigzag line). It is thinnest at the root.

The iris consists of four layers, from anterior to posterior it is as follows:
  i. Anterior endothelial layer—single layer of cells.
  ii. Iris stroma—forms the main bulk of stroma. It consists of loose collagenous network, sphincter pupillae, dilator pupillae muscles, vessels, nerves, pigmented cells and other cells such as lymphocytes, macrophage cells, etc.

Anatomy of the Eye

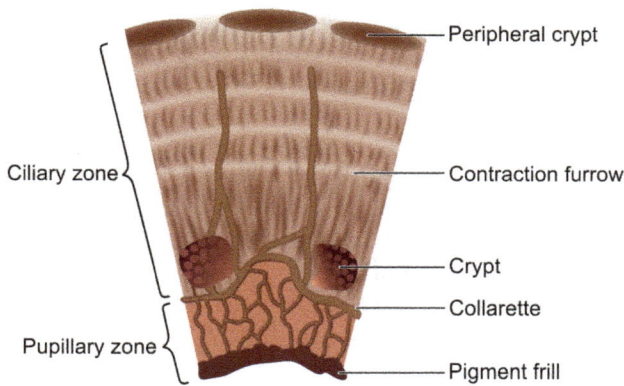

Fig. 1.3: Anterior surface of iris.

iii. Anterior pigmented epithelium.
iv. Posterior pigmented epithelium.

17. Describe ciliary body. What are its functions?

Ciliary body is the middle part of the uveal tract. Anterior 2 mm is called pars plicata and posterior 4 mm is called pars plana. About 70-80 ciliary processes project inward from the pars plicata. Ciliary muscle supplied by parasympathetic (through short ciliary nerves) forms the main bulk of ciliary stroma. It has three parts with a common origin circumferentially at the sclera spur:
  i. Meridional—fibers running anteroposteriorly inserted at the suprachoroid
 ii. Circular—concentric fibers
iii. Radial.

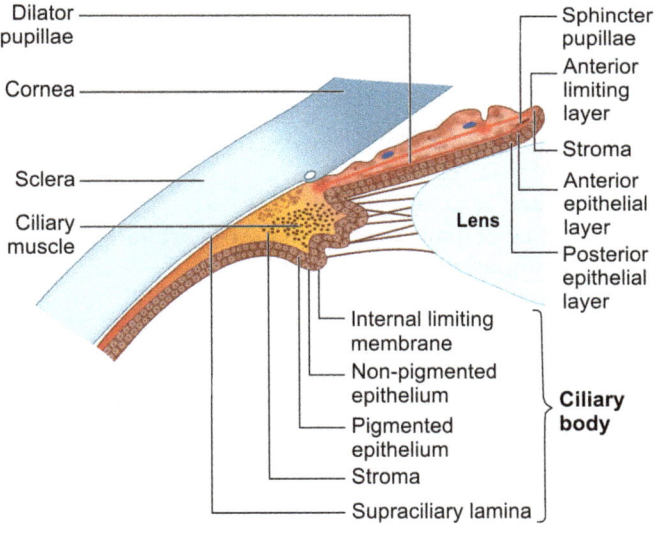

Fig. 1.4: Iris and ciliary body.

Functions
  i. Important role in accommodation
 ii. Ciliary processes are the site of aqueous production
iii. Play a role in drainage of aqueous (uveoscleral).

18. Enumerate the layers of choroid. What are its functions?

Layers of Choroid
- Suprachoroidal lamina
- Stroma of choroid. Its main bulk is formed by vessels which are arranged in following three layers:
  - Layer of large vessels (Haller's layer)
  - Layer of medium size vessels (Sattler's layer)
  - Choriocapillaris
- Layers of vessels—from outer to inner, vessels decrease in size
- Basal lamina or Bruch's membrane.

Function
Choroid nourishes the macular area of the retina and outer layers of rest of the retina.

19. Describe the structure of retina.

Retina
- Optic disk—1.5 mm
- Macula lutea (posterior pole)—5.5 mm in diameter, rich in cones and temporal to disk.
- Fovea—central 1.5 mm of macula—two disk diameters temporal to optic disk (1 disk diameter = 1.5 mm)
- Foveola—central depression of 0.35 mm in diameter which lies 1 mm below the horizontal meridian. Seen as foveal reflex which is a bright spot of light due to reflection of light from the walls of foveal depression.

Structure of retina.	
Layers	Features
Retinal pigment epithelium	A single layer of cuboidal cells
Layer of rods and cones	Comprises photoreceptors outer segments
Outer limiting membrane	It is not a true membrane but a zone of adhesion between the photoreceptors and Muller's cells, forming a boundary
Outer nuclear layer	Comprises photoreceptors cell nuclei
Outer plexiform layer	Layer of synapse between the photoreceptors, bipolar cells and horizontal cells
Inner nuclear layer	Comprises nuclei of bipolar cells, horizontal cells, amacrine cells and Muller's cells
Inner plexiform layer	Layer of synapse between the bipolar cells, ganglion cells and amacrine cells
Ganglion cell layer	Comprises ganglion cell nuclei
Nerve fiber layer	Comprises ganglion cell axons
Inner limiting membrane	Muller's cells terminations

- Layers—10
- Thickness—near optic disk—0.5 mm
  - Equator—0.2 mm
  - Anterior—0.1 mm
  - Rods—120 million; cones—6 million.

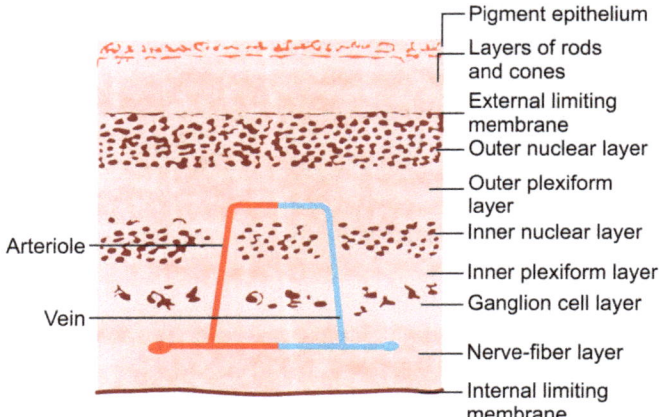

Fig. 1.5: Structure of retina (from outer to inner).

20. What are the dimensions of optic nerve?
- Axons of 1 million ganglion cells
- Total length: 47–50 mm
- Intraocular (optic disk): 1 mm
- Intraorbital: 30 mm
- Intracanalicular: 6–9 mm
- Intracranial: 10 mm.

21. What structures constitute the visual pathway?
Visual pathway consists of optic nerve, optic chiasma, optic tract, lateral geniculate body (LGB), optic radiations and visual cortex.

22. Enumerate the neurons in visual pathway.
- First-order neurons—bipolar cells of retina
- Second-order neurons—ganglion cells of retina (from bipolar cells to lateral geniculate body)
- Third-order neurons—optic radiations—from lateral geniculate body to occipital cortex.

23. Write short notes on extraocular muscles.
Six Muscles

Origin
- The four rectus muscles arise from the common tendinous ring (annulus of Zinn) at the apex of orbit.

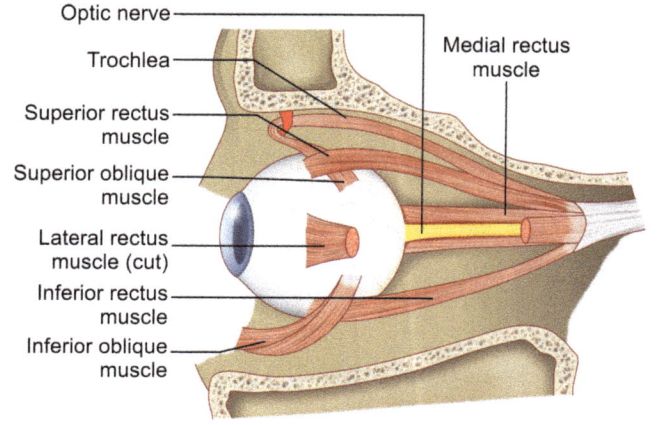

Fig. 1.6: Anatomy of extraocular muscles.

- The superior oblique arises from the apex of the orbit.
- The inferior oblique arises from the floor of the orbit.
- Insertion: Insertion distance from limbus
    - Superior rectus—7.7 mm
    - Lateral rectus—6.9 mm
    - Inferior rectus—6.5 mm
    - Medial rectus—5.5 mm (Mnemonic: SLIM)
    - Inferior oblique (shortest) —inserts into lower and outer quadrant of eyeball
    - Superior oblique (longest)—inserts into upper and outer quadrant of eyeball.

Nerve Supply
- 3rd cranial nerve—superior rectus, medial rectus, inferior rectus and inferior oblique
- 4th cranial nerve—superior oblique (SO_4)
- 6th cranial nerve—lateral rectus (LR_6).

Actions of extraocular muscles.			
Muscle	Primary	Secondary	Tertiary
Medial rectus	Adduction	–	–
Lateral rectus	Abduction	–	–
Superior rectus	Elevation	Intorsion	Adduction
Inferior rectus	Depression	Extorsion	Adduction
Superior oblique	Intorsion	Depression	Abduction
Inferior oblique	Extorsion	Elevation	Abduction

24. Enumerate the layers of eyelid.
From Anterior to Posterior
- Skin
- Subcutaneous areolar tissue
- Layer of striated muscle
- Submuscular areolar tissue
- Fibrous layer made of tarsal plate and orbital septum
- Layer of nonstriated muscle fibers
- Conjunctiva.

25. Name the glands of eyelid.
- Meibomian glands (modified sebaceous gland)
- Glands of Zeis (modified sebaceous gland) which open into follicles of eyelashes
- Glands of Moll (modified sweat gland) open into hair follicles
- Accessory lacrimal glands of Wolfring are present near the superior border of upper tarsus. Krause's glands are in upper and lower fornix—42 in upper and 6–8 in lower fornix.

26. Write short notes on anatomy of orbit.
- Volume of the orbit—30 cc
- Each orbit is formed by seven bones namely (1) frontal, (2) ethmoid, (3) lacrimal, (4) palatine, (5) maxillary, (6) zygomatic and (7) sphenoid
- Medial wall of the orbit is thinnest and lateral is thickest.

There are four Surgical Spaces in the Orbit (Fig. 18.2 on Page 147)

i. Subperiosteal space—between bone and periorbita
ii. Peripheral space—between periorbita and extraocular muscles
iii. Central space—enclosed by four muscles
iv. Tenon's space—between sclera and Tenon's capsule.

Orbital Foramina

i. Superior orbital foramen—between roof and lateral wall
ii. Inferior orbital foramen—between floor and lateral wall
iv. Optic foramen—lies at the apex of orbit through which optic nerve passes.

27. Describe the blood supply to the eye.

Arterial Supply

Branches of ophthalmic artery which is a branch of internal carotid:
- Short ciliary—20
- Long ciliary—2
- Central retinal artery.

Venous Drainage: Order of Drainage
- Short ciliary
- Anterior ciliary
- Four vortex veins:
  - Central retinal vein
  - Superior ophthalmic vein
  - Inferior ophthalmic vein
  - Cavernous sinus.

28. Describe the nerve supply of the eye.

Three Types

i. Motor
ii. Sensory
iii. Autonomic

Motor Nerves
- Trochlear—superior oblique
- Abducens—lateral rectus
- Facial nerve—orbicularis oculi.

Sensory Nerve

Trigeminal nerve.

Autonomic Nerves
- Sympathetic nerve supply
- Parasympathetic nerve supply.

Sympathetic Nerve Supply
- Cervical sympathetic fibers
- It supplies dilator pupillae, ciliary body, Muller's muscle in the lids
- Lacrimal gland.

Parasympathetic Nerve Supply
- Originates from nuclei in the midbrain
- It supplies sphincter pupillae, ciliary body and lacrimal gland.

29. Describe the development of the eye.

Central nervous system develops from neural tube which runs longitudinally down the dorsal surface of the front of embryo. Eye forms from an outpouching of the embryonic forebrain (neuroectoderm) with contributions from neural crest cells, surface ectoderm and to a lesser extent mesoderm.

Thickening (optic plate) appears on either side of the neural tube in its anterior part. Optic plate grows toward the surface to form the optic vesicle.
- Optic vesicle invaginates to form the optic cup
- Line of opening remains open for sometime as embryonic fissure
- Hyaloid artery enters through fissure to provide nutrition
- Later it atrophies and disappears
- Surface ectoderm invaginates, separates to form the lens
- Inner layer of cup forms the retina
- Outer layer develops into pigment epithelium
- Neural ectoderm secretes jelly-like structure the vitreous
- Ciliary body and iris formed from anterior portion of cup and mesoderm

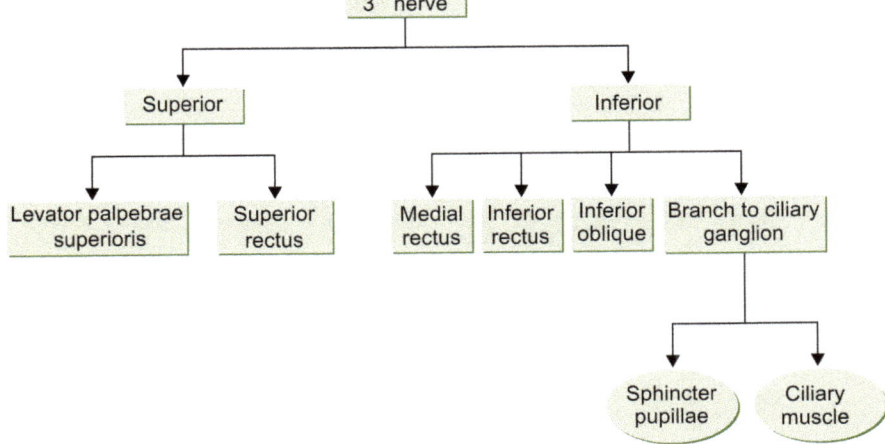

Flowchart 1.1: Branches of third cranial nerve (oculomotor nerve).

Anatomy of the Eye

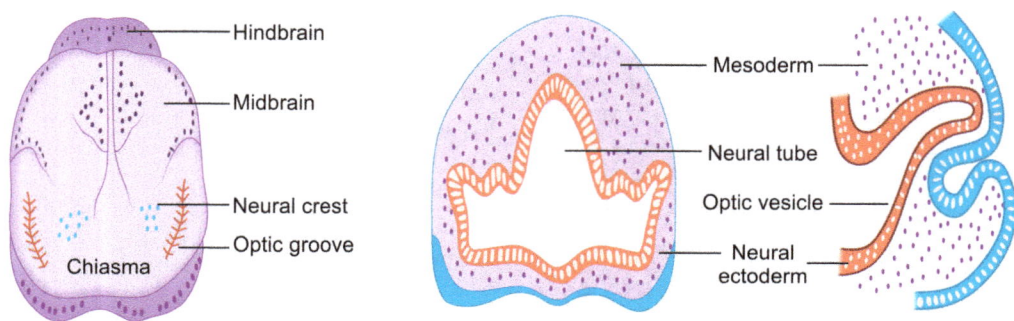

Fig. 1.7: Formation of optic groove, neural tube and optic vesicle.

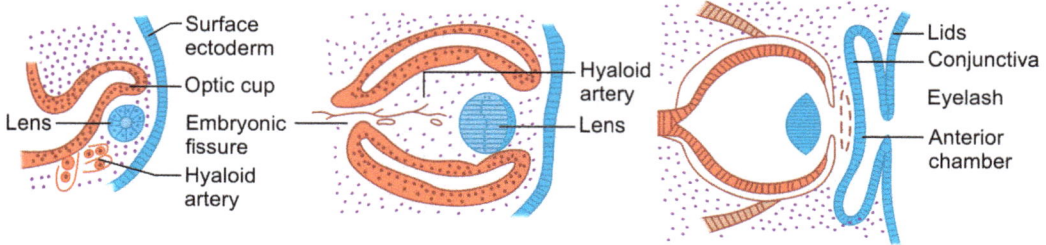

Fig. 1.8: Formation of optic cup and lens.

- Mesoderm around the cup forms coats of eye, orbit, angle of anterior chamber (AC) and stroma of the cornea
- Surface ectoderm forms cornea and conjunctival epithelium
- Mesoderm in front of cornea forms the lids.

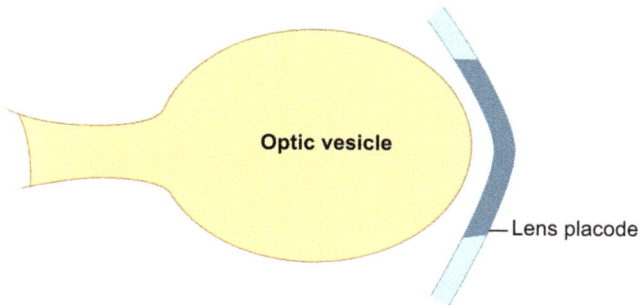

Fig. 1.9: Formation of optic vesicle and invagination of surface ectoderm (lens placode) to form lens.

Structures from the Surface Ectoderm
- Crystalline lens
- Epithelium of cornea and conjunctiva
- Lacrimal gland
- Epidermis of lids and its derivatives
- Epithelium of lacrimal apparatus.

Structures from Neural Ectoderm
- Retina
- Epithelial layer of iris and ciliary body
- Sphincter and dilator pupillae
- Definitive vitreous and ciliary zonules
- Fibers of optic nerve.

Structures from Mesoderm
- Extraocular muscles
- Corneal stroma
- Sclera
- Iris
- Choroid.

CHAPTER 2

Physiology of the Eye

1. Describe the optical system of the normal eye.

- Comprises of four refractive media
- **Refractive indices:**
  - Cornea: 1.37
  - Lens: 1.42
  - Aqueous humor: 1.33
  - Vitreous humor: 1.33
- **Refractive power:**
  - Cornea: + 43 to + 45 D
  - Lens: + 16 to + 18 D
  - Total power: + 60 D.

Distance Viewing

When normal eye is at rest, parallel rays from distant objects (6 m and beyond) are focused on retina. Image is real and inverted and it is reinverted in brain.

Near Viewing

When we view from less than 6 m, divergent rays are emitted and we converge and focus on the retina by increasing the refractive power of the eye by accommodation of the lens.

2. Write short notes on accommodation.

Accommodation is the power of changing the focus by which near object is seen clearly. Radius of curvature of anterior surface of the lens is 10 mm and posterior surface of the lens is 6 mm. In accommodation, anterior surface becomes 6 mm and lens becomes spherical.

Convergence is increased as per viewing distance. Contraction of ciliary muscle relieves the tension of zonules on the lens.

Amplitude of accommodation decreases with age due to hardening of the lens.

Presbyopia is physiological insufficiency of accommodation leading to progressive fall in near vision. There is receding of near point. In 7 years, it is 7 cm but in 40 years, it is 25 cm.

Anomalies of accommodation are insufficiency, paralysis and spasm.

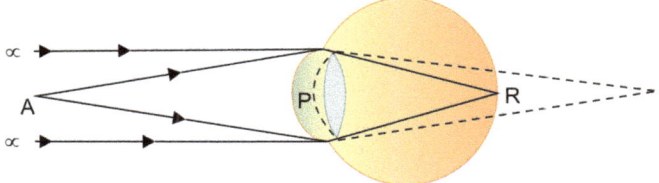

Fig. 2.1: Mechanism of accommodation.

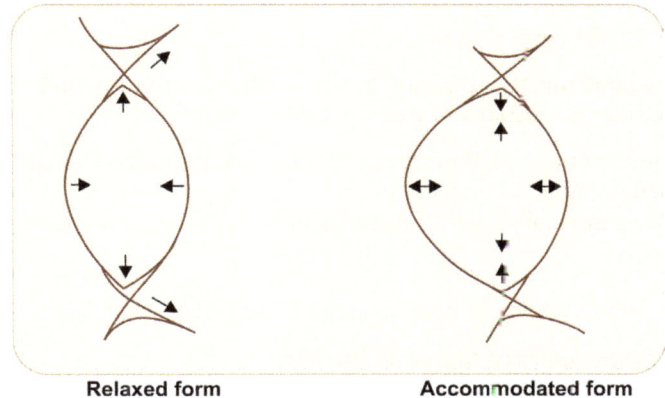

Relaxed form Accommodated form

Fig. 2.2: Bulging of anterior surface of lens in accommodation.

3. What is visual acuity?

- Recorded by Snellen chart test
- Largest letter can be read at 60 m
- Each letter subtends 5 minutes angle at nodal point
- Normal distant visual acuity is 6/6
- Other Tests:
  - Illiterate "E" chart
  - Landolts "C" chart
  - Picture chart.

Near Vision

- Tested at 30 cm or 14 inches
- Reading N6 on the chart is normal.

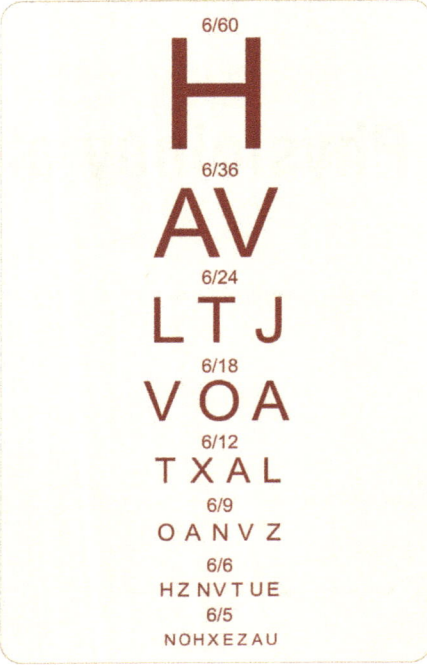

Fig. 2.3: Snellen distant visual acuity chart.

Snellen Distant Visual Acuity Chart
- If the patient can read the top most letter from a distance of 6 m, his vision is 6/60
- If he can read second line, his vision is 6/36
- If he can read third line, his vision is 6/24
- If he can read fourth line, his vision is 6/18
- If he can read fifth line, his vision is 6/12
- If he can read sixth line, his vision is 6/9
- If he can read seventh line, his vision is 6/6
- If he can read the eighth line, his vision is 6/5.

4. What does 6/60 mean?

Numerator: It is constant. It denotes the distance at which the patient is normally examined, which is 6 m(meters).

Denominator: Letters designed for 60 m distance can be read at 6 m only.
What normal person can read at 60 m can be read at 6 meters only.

5. What are the components of aqueous humor?

Components of Aqueous Humor
- Water: 98.75%
- Solids: 1.25%
  - Proteins
  - Glucose
  - Ascorbic acid
  - Lactic acid and electrolytes.

6. How is aqueous formed?

It is secreted by ciliary epithelium of ciliary body.

Two Mechanisms
  i. Secretions—80%. Active metabolic process
  ii. Ultrafiltration—20%. Influenced by level of blood pressure in the ciliary epithelium, plasma osmotic pressure and intraocular pressure (IOP).

7. What are the functions of aqueous?
- Provides nutrition
- Removes metabolic products
- Maintains the optical clarity of the eye
- Regulates IOP.

8. What is blood aqueous barrier?

Ciliary epithelium and walls of capillaries of iris are the blood-aqueous barriers. It does not allow large molecules to pass through the barrier. It is altered in inflammation and trauma.
Aqueous becomes plasmoid decreasing the optical clarity and decreasing the vision.

9. What is the pathway for aqueous outflow?
- Angle of anterior chamber—80% (conventional route)
- Uveoscleral outflow—20%.

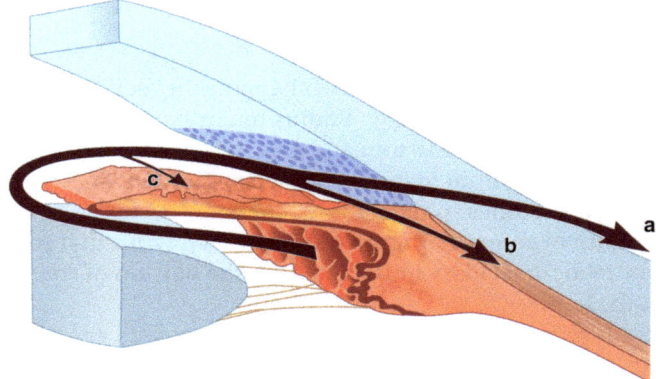

Fig. 2.4: Pathway for aqueous outflow through: a. Through trabecular meshwork, b. Uveoscleral outflow, c. Through iris.

Angle of Anterior Chamber
(Grade 4 wide open, Grade 0 closed).

Conventional route
The aqueous flows from ciliary region to posterior chamber. Through pupil it enters anterior chamber. Then it enters

trabecular meshwork in the angle of anterior chamber. From there through aqueous veins it enters episcleral veins. The flow is increased by miotics, parasympathomimetics, laser trabeculoplasty and trabeculectomy.

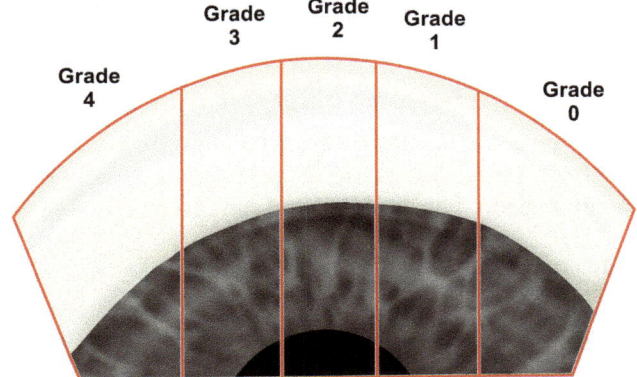

Fig. 2.5: Angle of anterior chamber.

Uveoscleral Outflow

- From ciliary body to suprachoroidal space
  - Choroid
  - Episcleral veins.
- Uveoscleral outflow increased by sympathomimetics, atropine, brimonidine and latanoprost.
- Decreased by miotics.

10. Describe the factors which maintain normal intraocular pressure.

- Formation of aqueous
- Outflow of aqueous
- Pressure in episcleral veins.

Secretion of Aqueous

- Atrophy of ciliary process decreases IOP
- Increased permeability of capillaries of ciliary process which results in plasmoid aqueous causes increased IOP.

Resistance to Outflow: Three Factors

i. Sclerosis of trabeculum—in primary open angle glaucoma
ii. Exudates blocking the angle—in inflammation
iii. Narrow or closed angle—in primary angle closure glaucoma.

Orbital tumors increase pressure in episcleral veins which in turn increases IOP.

11. Describe how light is perceived (physiology of vision).

Light reflected from objects is focused onto retina. It depends on refraction of light rays by accommodation of eyes. Focused light creates reactions on the retina.

Refraction of Light Rays

Light from distance object needs least refraction. Close objects need more refraction. To increase refractive power, ciliary muscles contract releasing pull on suspensory ligament. Anterior surface of lens bulges forward.

To decrease refractive power, ciliary muscle relaxes, increasing pull on suspensory ligaments which makes the lens thinner. Looking at near objects tires the eyes due to ciliary muscle contraction.

Light rays from objects enter into the eye at different angles. For sharp vision, corresponding areas of retina must be stimulated. Extraocular muscles rotate the eyes for that. This activity is under autonomic nervous system control. If convergence is not complete, diplopia or suppression may occur.

Reactions of Light on the Retina

- Photochemical changes
- Electrical response.

Photochemical Change

Change in the pigments of rods and cones.

Light breaks rod pigment—rhodopsin which is 11-cis-retinal (aldehyde) to all-trans retinal (alcohol) form and then to colorless vitamin A. This reaction is reversible in dark. This is called Wald's visual cycle.

Electrical Response

Photochemical reactions induce electrical potential. This is transmitted through bipolar cells to ganglion cells and then to brain through optic nerve. Visual perception occurs. This can be recorded by electroretinogram (ERG).

12. Write short notes on visual perceptions.

- Light sense
- Sense of contrast
- Form sense
- Color sense.

Light Sense

Permits to perceive light at all gradations of intensity even the light minimum which is the minimum amount of light energy which induces light sensation. Rods are more sensitive to low illumination which are concerned with scotopic vision. Defect in rods results in night blindness. Dark adaptation is also affected. Cones are concerned with bright illumination which is called photopic vision.

Sense of Contrast: Contrast Sensitivity

Ability to perceive slight changes in luminance between two regions which are not separated by a demarcation line. As we get older, contrast sensitivity decreases. This is recorded by Pelli Robson chart. This is reduced in optic neuritis, age-related macular degeneration, amblyopia, cataract and after LASIK.

Form Sense

This enables to perceive shape of objects. Cones play a dominant role. This sense is most acute at fovea where cones are closely set. Visual acuity is a record of form sense.

Color Sense

Ability to differentiate between different colors with varying shades. This is better appreciated by cones in photopic vision.

Primary colors are red, green and blue. When they are mixed, produce white color.

13. Describe color vision tests.

- **Edridge-Green lantern test:** Depending on the number of mistakes, the patient makes in naming the colors, a rough estimate is made.
- **Holmgren's wool test:** The patient is asked to make a series of color matches from a heap of colored wools. A color deficient person will choose wools of confusing colors.
- **Ishihara pseudoisochromatic plate test:** Bold numbers are shown in dots of various tints. These dots are made up of primary colors printed on a background of similar dots of confusing colors. Red-green defect is identified from the number of mistakes he does.
- **Farnsworth-Munsell 100 hue test:** Color blindness is identified by the number of mistakes the patient makes in rearranging the caps in the order of each of the four racks.
- **City University test:** It contains 10 plates. Each plate contains one central color and four peripheral colors. The subject is asked to select one of the peripheral colors which closely matches the central color.

14. Write short notes on color blindness.

It can be congenital or acquired. Congenital is more common. The causes of acquired are due to diseases of macula and optic nerve namely macular degeneration, optic neuritis and toxic amblyopia (e.g. ethambutol). It can be partial or total. In partial type, one of the colors cannot be recognized. In total color blindness, everything appears gray.

- **Achromatic:** Unable to appreciate any primary color
- **Monochromatic:** Able to appreciate only one primary color
- **Dichromatic:** Able to appreciate two primary colors
- **Trichromatic:** Able to appreciate three primary colors but defective to one of the colors
- **Protanomalous:** Defective red color appreciation
- **Deutranomalous:** Defective green color appreciation
- **Tritanomalous:** Defective blue color appreciation
- **Protanopia:** Complete red color defect
- **Deuteranopia:** Complete green color defect
- **Tritanopia:** Complete blue color defect.

15. Write short notes on binocular vision.

Each eye sees slightly differently. Images are fused in cerebrum. Only one image is perceived. This is called binocular vision. This is also called stereoscopic vision.

Grades of Binocular Vision

- Simultaneous macular perception
- Fusion
- Stereopsis.

Tests for Binocular Vision

- Worth 4-dot test
- Lang's two-pencil test
- Bagolini striated glasses test
- Titmus fly test
- TNO random dot test
- Frisby stereo test.

Impaired binocular vision results in strabismus, suppression or diplopia.

16. Write short notes on metabolism of lens.

Metabolic activity of the lens is largely limited to epithelium and cortex. Nucleus is relatively inert. 80% of glucose is metabolized anaerobically by the glycolytic pathway. 15% is metabolized by hexose monophosphate pathway and a small portion by Krebs cycle. Sorbitol pathway plays a role in diabetic cataract. Lens has a free radical scavenging system regulated by ascorbate and reduced glutathione.

CHAPTER 3
Neurology of Vision

1. Describe the visual pathway, type of lesions and visual field defects.

Visual pathway consists of:
- Optic nerve
- Optic chiasma
- Optic tract
- Lateral geniculate body (LGB)
- Optic radiations
- Occipital cortex.

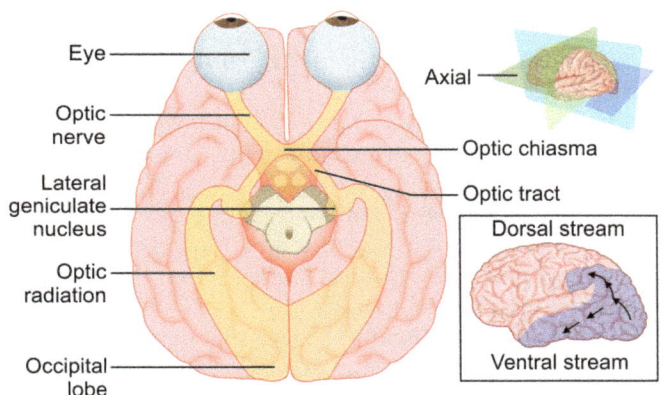

Fig. 3.1: Visual system.

Optic Nerve Lesions versus Retinal Vascular Lesions
- Optic nerve lesions produce field loss with apex at fixation
- Retinal vascular lesions produce field loss with apex at blind spot.

Visual Field and Retinal Fibers
- Have inverted and reverse relationship
- Upper visual field falls on inferior retina
- Lower visual field falls on superior retina
- Nasal visual field on temporal retina
- Temporal visual field on nasal retina.

Crossing in Chiasma
- Optic nerves join the chiasma at anterolateral part, nasal fibers cross in chiasma, joins uncrossed temporal fibers of contralateral eye.
- Lower retinal fibers lie in lateral part of the optic tract.
- Upper retinal fibers lie in medial part of optic tract.
- Inferonasal fibers decussate in chiasma travel anteriorly in contralateral optic nerve before passing into optic tract—von Willebrand's knee.

Optic Tract
- Originate from posterolateral angle of chiasma
- Cylindrical bands running out and posteriorly to LGB
- Consist of temporal fibers of the same side and nasal fibers of the opposite side.

Lateral Geniculate Body
- Lateral geniculate bodies are oval structures at posterior end of optic tracts
- New fibers of optic radiation originate from them
- These fibers proceed backward and medially to end in visual cortex of occipital lobe.

Three Neurons of Visual Pathway
- Neurons of first order are bipolar cells of retina. Rods and cones are sensory end organs.
- Neurons of second order are ganglion cells of retina. They end in LGB.
- Neurons of third order are optic radiations which take impulses to the visual center in occipital cortex.

Types of Lesion

Lesions of Visual Pathway
- Optic nerve—ipsilateral blindness
- Proximal part of optic nerve
  - Ipsilateral blindness with contralateral quadrantanopia (or hemianopia).

Neurology of Vision

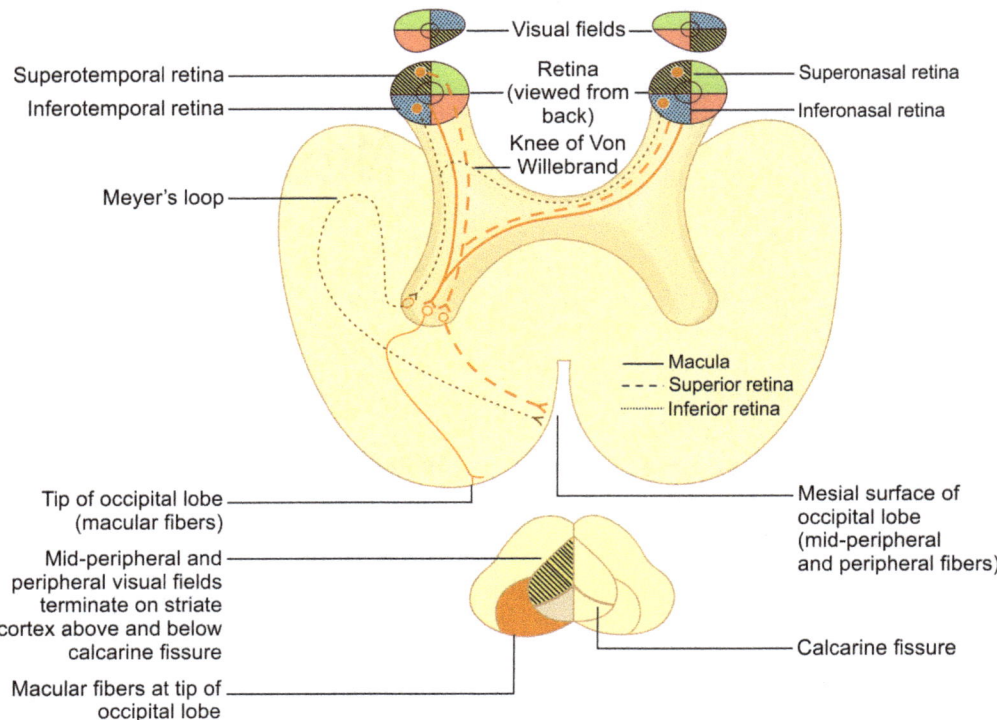

Fig. 3.2: Fiber arrangement in optic nerve and chiasma.

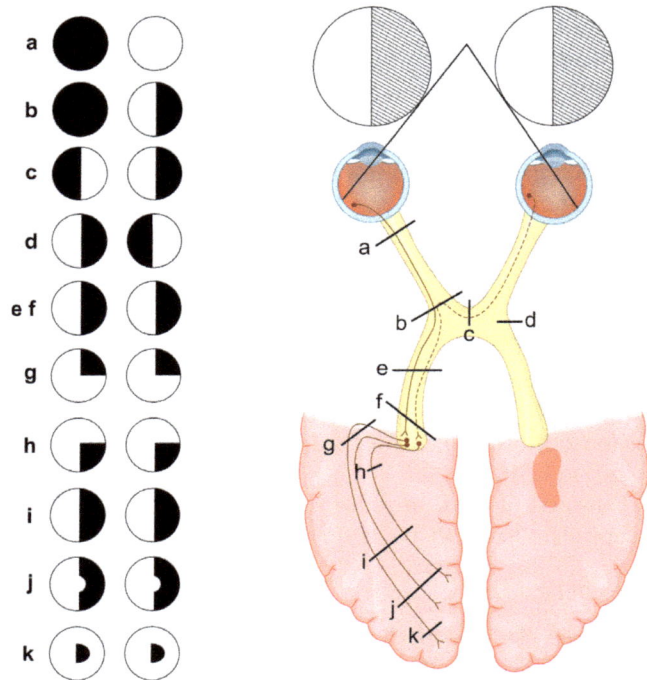

Fig. 3.3: Field defects at various levels of visual pathway. (a) Optic nerve, (b) proximal part of optic nerve, (c) central chiasma, (d) lateral chiasma (both sides), (e) optic tract, (f) geniculate body, (g) part of optic radiations in temporal lobe, (h) part of optic radiations in parietal lobe, (i) optic radiations, (j) visual cortex sparing the macula, (k) visual cortex involving macula only.

- Median chiasma lesion—bitemporal hemianopia (c).
- Lateral chiasmal lesion—binasal hemianopia (d).
- Optic tract—markedly incongruous homonymous hemianopia (e).
- Proximal part of optic tract—LGB or lower part of optic radiation—clear-cut homonymous hemianopia with macular sparing (f).
- Anterior loop of optic radiation (temporal lobe—Meyer's loop)—incongruous superior quadrantanopia (g).
- Upper part of optic radiation (parietal lobe)—incongruous inferior quadrantanopia (h).
- Middle of optic radiation—slightly incongruous homonymous hemianopia without macular sparing (j).
- Posterior part of optic radiation—congruous homonymous hemianopia
  - Anterior part of calcarine sulcus—contralateral blindness in temporal crescent
  - Middle part of calcarine cortex—congruous homonymous hemianopia with macular sparing and contralateral sparing of temporal crescent
  - Posterior part of occipital lobe—congruous homonymous hemianopic central scotoma (k).

Causes of Lesions in the Visual Pathway

- Optic nerve—absent direct and consensual light reflex
- Traumatic avulsion of optic nerve
- Acute optic neuritis.

Proximal Part of Optic Nerve

- Pupillary reaction—absent direct and consensual light reflex
- Causes—traumatic avulsion of the optic nerve or acute optic neuritis.

Median Chiasmal Lesions
- Suprasellar aneurysm
- Pituitary tumors
- Craniopharyngioma
- Glioma of the 3rd ventricle.

Lateral Chiasmal Lesions
- Pupillary paralysis
- Causes—distention of the 3rd ventricle
- Atheroma of posterior communicating artery.

Optic Tract Lesion
Wernicke's hemianopic pupillary response is seen—light reflex is absent when light is thrown on temporal half of retina of affected side and nasal half of retina of opposite side.
- Normal in intact hemianopic field
- Minimal in abnormal hemianopic field.

Lateral Geniculate Body Lesion
Causes:
- Syphilitic meningitis
- Tuberculosis and tumors of the optic thalamus
- Pupil-spared.

Temporal Lobe Lesions
- Anterior loop of optic radiation—pie in the sky
- Pupillary reflexes—normal.

Upper Part of Optic Radiation
Anterior parietal lobe lesions.

Middle Part of Optic Radiation to Occipital Cortex
- Vascular occlusions
- Primary and secondary tumors
- Trauma.

2. What are the methods of field testing?
- Confrontation: Manual testing by fingers
- Tangent screen: Central field testing (kinetic)
- Lister perimeter: Kinetic perimeter
- Automated perimetry: Static perimeter

3. Define field of vision.

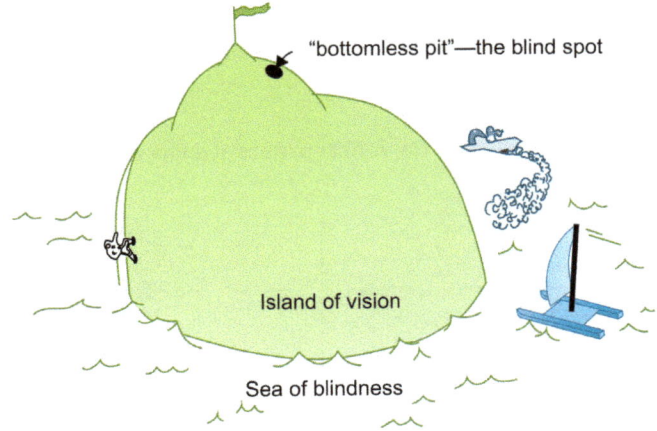

Fig. 3.4: Island of vision in sea of blindness.

The field of vision is a total area in which objects can be seen while fixing straight ahead. According to Traquair, it is island of vision in sea of blindness. The peak of the island represents the point of highest acuity, the fovea, while the bottomless pit represents the blind spot, the optic disk.

4. What are the types of fields?
- Central—30°
- Peripheral—beyond 30°.

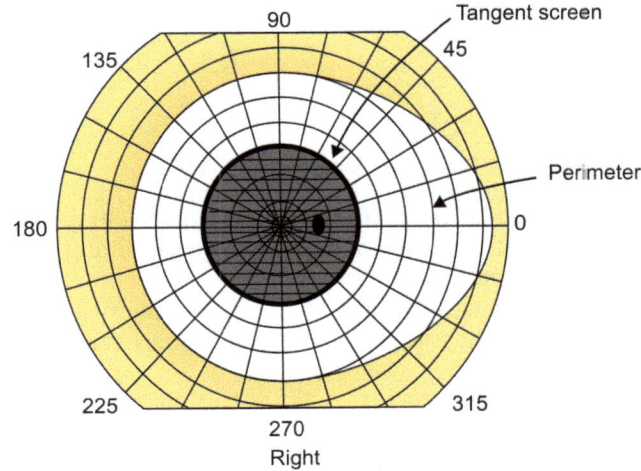

Fig. 3.5: Central (striped) tested with Bjerrum's screen and peripheral field (beyond 30°) tested with perimeter.

5. What is the extent of normal visual field?
- Superior—60°
- Inferior—70°
- Nasal—60°
- Temporal—90°.

6. What is blind spot?
This corresponds to optic nerve head. Since there are no photoreceptors in this area, the stimulus is not seen.

7. What is an isopter?
An isopter is a peripheral limit of given stimulus of the same intensity.

8. What is threshold?
Threshold at a given retinal point is the intensity of a stimulus that is perceived 50% of the time. It is measured in decibels (dB).

9. What is kinetic and static perimetry?
In kinetic perimetry, the target is moved from an area where it is not seen to an area where it is just seen. Target size and color determines the different cross-section or isopter. Goldmann perimetry is used.

In static perimetry, a stationary stimulus is presented at various locations. The intensity of stimulus is increased until it is seen. Humphrey or Octopus perimetry is used.

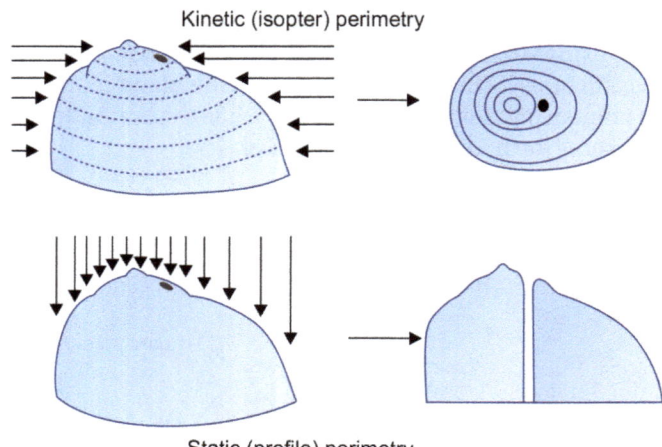

Fig. 3.6: Field testing methods.

- Top picture in Figure 3.6—kinetic perimetry—mapping of contours of the island at different levels resulting in one isopter for each level tested.
- Bottom picture in Figure 3.6—static perimetry—vertical contours of the island along a selected meridian.

10. Describe various types of scotomas.

Scotoma is blindness in a part of field of vision. It is a localized defect in the visual field.

Central Scotoma

- Positive
- Negative
- Absolute
- Relative
- Translucid
- Specific.

Positive Scotoma

Seeing a blind spot in front of eye corresponding to retinal lesion. Pericentral or paracentral scotoma—involvement of macula.

Causes of Positive Scotoma

- Central choroiditis
- Macular retinal detachment
- Disciform degeneration of macula
- Macular hemorrhage in high myopia
- Macular hole
- Lead poisoning.

Negative Scotoma

- Patient does not complain of field defect
- Black spot in visual filed similar to blind spot
- Brought out only on field testing.
    Normal Blind Spot
    - Vertically oval 7.5° × 5.5°
    - 15° temporal to fixation spot
    - 1.5° below horizontal median
    - Blind spot enlargement
    - Blind spot larger than 7.5° × 9.5° with test object 5/1,000 is significant.

Blind Spot Enlargement
- Papilledema
- High myopia
- Opaque nerve fibers
- Coloboma of the optic disk.

Absolute Scotoma

- Extent of scotoma is similar both for white and color objects
- Defect persists even with maximal stimuli
- Causes—toxic amblyopias in late stages, lead, tobacco and methyl alcohol
- Optic neuritis
- Leber's optic atrophy
- Central retinal lesions.

Relative Scotoma

- Scotoma for color only—not for white
- Defect seen with weak stimuli

Cause: Above lesions in early stages.

Translucid Scotoma

- Partial—seen as though he is seeing through a mist.

Cause: Central serous retinopathy.

Specific Scotomas

- Central
- Cecocentral
- Seidel's scotoma
- Paracentral
- Bjerrum's scotoma
- Junctional scotomas
- Central bitemporal scotoma.

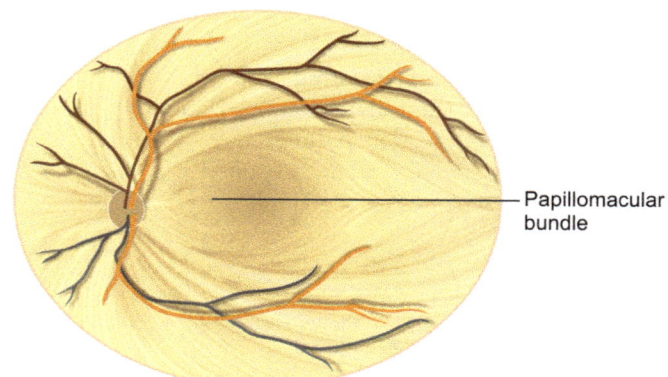

Fig. 3.7: Nerve fiber pattern of retina.

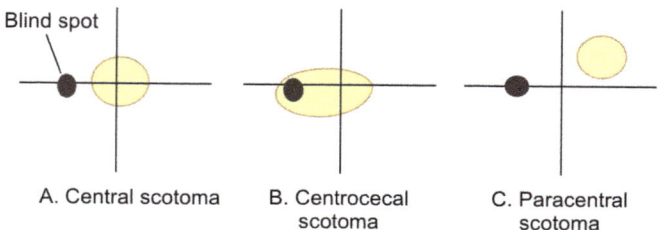

A. Central scotoma B. Centrocecal scotoma C. Paracentral scotoma

Figs. 3.8A to C: Types of scotomas in central field—field defects are due to interruption of the papillomacular bundle.

Central Scotoma: Defect covering central fixation—seen in lesions of macula.

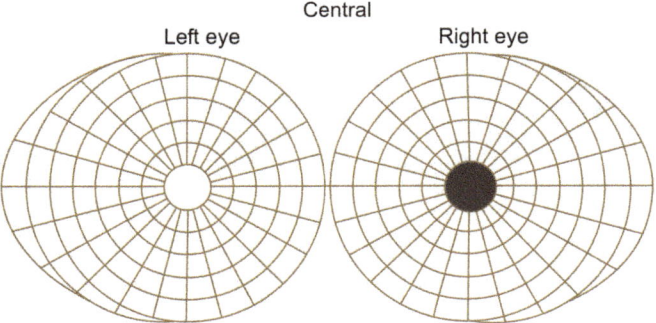

Fig. 3.9: Central scotoma in right eye.

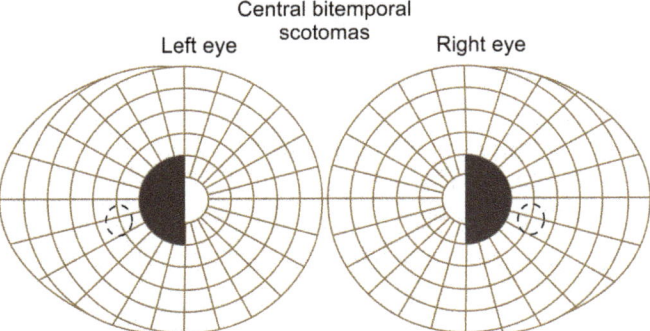

Fig. 3.10: Central bitemporal scotoma.

Cecocentral scotoma: Central scotoma connected to the blind spot.

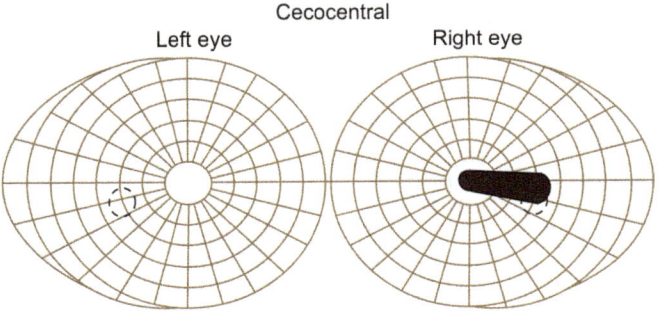

Fig. 3.11: Cecocentral scotoma in right eye.

Seidel's scotoma: In glaucoma, as the disease progresses the paracentral scotoma joins with the blind spot to form a sickle-shaped scotoma known as Seidel's scotoma.

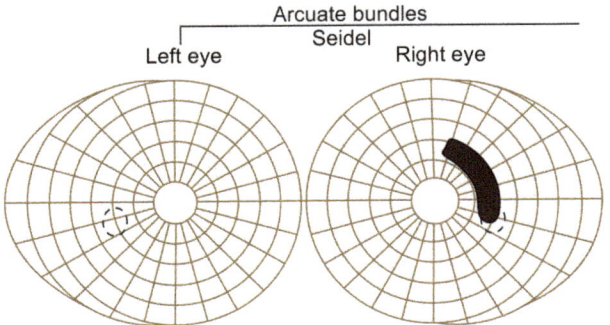

Fig. 3.12: Seidel's scotoma.

Paracentral scotoma: A defect of some of the fibers of the papillomacular bundle, lying next to central fixation.

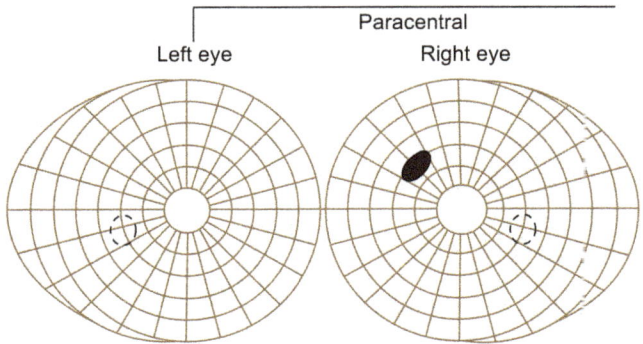

Fig. 3.13: Paracentral scotoma in right eye.

Bjerrum's scotoma: It is an arcuate scotoma extending above and below the blind spot between 10° and 20° of fixation point (Bjerrum's area). Visual loss in glaucoma commonly occurs within this arcuate area, especially in the superior half.

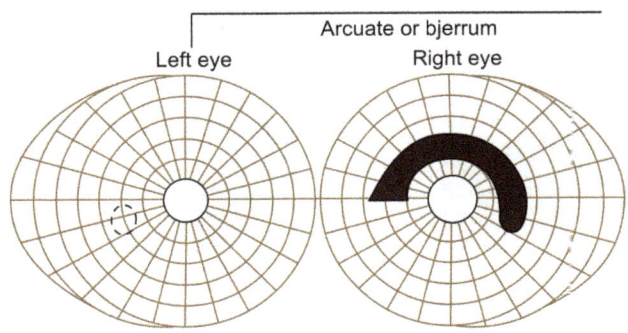

Fig. 3.14: Bjerrum's scotoma in right eye.

Junctional scotoma: It is central scotoma in one eye with a superotemporal defect in the fellow eye indicating a lesion at the junction of the optic nerve and chiasma.

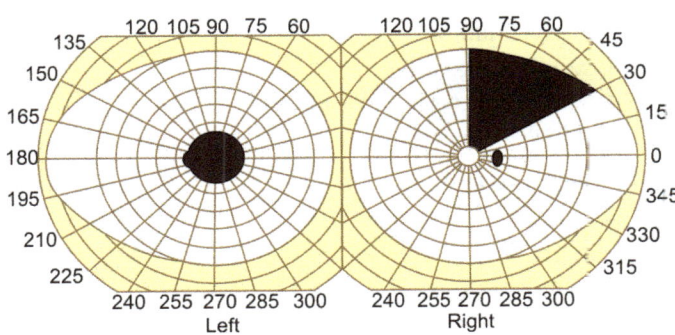

Fig. 3.15: Junctional scotoma in left eye.

Central scotoma in one eye with a superotemporal defect in the fellow eye.

Central bitemporal scotoma: When decussating nasal fibers are affected in the chiasma, central bitemporal scotoma (or hemianopia) results.

11. Define hemianopia. Describe the types of hemianopias.

Hemianopia
Field defect bounded by horizontal or vertical radii.

Types
- Homonymous
- Heteronymous
- Altitudinal
- Quadrantic.

Homonymous Hemianopia
- Loss of visual field to the same side in both eyes
- Site of lesion—postchiasmal on opposite side from tract to occipital lobe.

Causes
- In old patients
- In young patients.

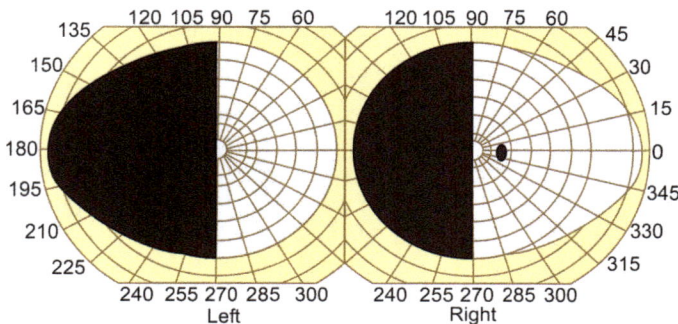

Fig. 3.16: Left homonymous hemianopia with macular splitting.

Causes in old patients
- Arteriosclerotic vascular disease in posterior cerebral artery distribution
- Cardiac source from atrial fibrillation
- Tumor: Trauma
- Demyelination.

Causes in young patients
- Mitral valve emboli: Vasculitis
- Migraine.

Tract Hemianopia
- Uncommon
- Incongruous
- Vision reduced
- Wernicke's hemianopic pupil.

Causes: Tumors or aneurysms acting as mass lesions.

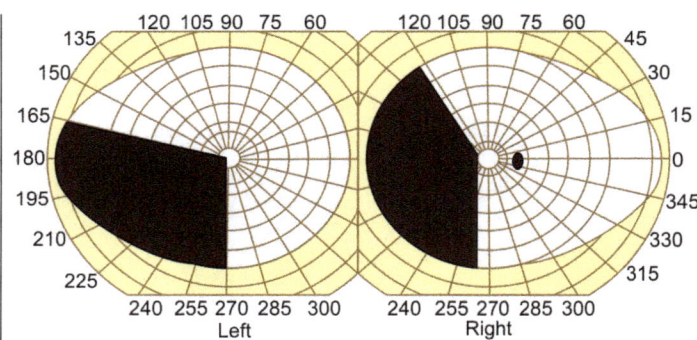

Fig. 3.17: Incongruous left homonymous hemianopia.

Geniculate Hemianopia
- Rare
- Sparing of wedge of field just above and below horizontal meridian.

Optic Radiation Hemianopia
- Congruous
- Superior wedge-shaped quadrantanopia
- Pie in the sky
- Temporal lobe affected.

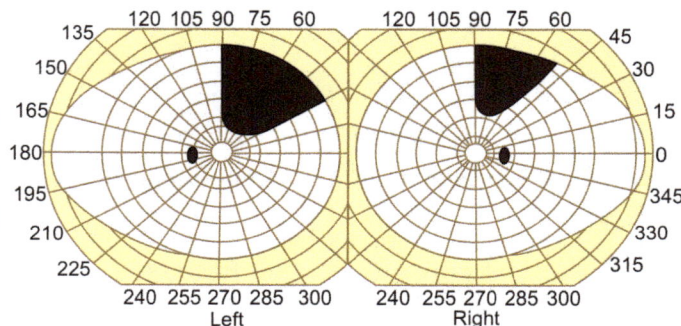

Fig. 3.18: Temporal lobe lesion—superior quadrantanopia.

Inferior Quadrantanopia
- Pie on the floor
- Parietal lobe lesion.

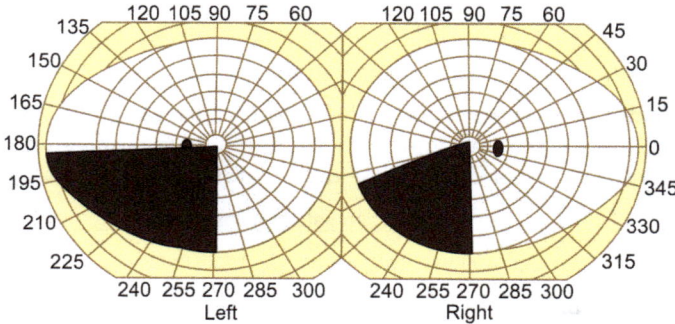

Fig. 3.19: Inferior quadrantanopia.

Occipital Lobe Hemianopia

- Due to infarcts
- Most common
- Congruous paracentral scotoma
- Occipital lobe lesion or injury
- Macular sparing
- Macular splitting in lesion of tip of occipital cortex.

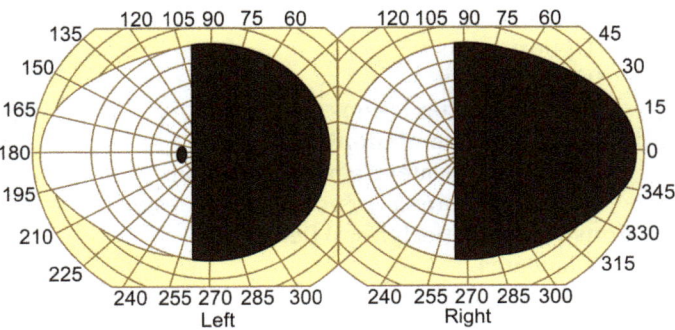

Fig. 3.20: Right homonymous hemianopia with macular splitting.

The temporal crescent of field perceived by nasal crescent of retina is represented in contralateral visual cortex in the most anterior portion of medial surface of occipital lobe along the calcarine fissure.

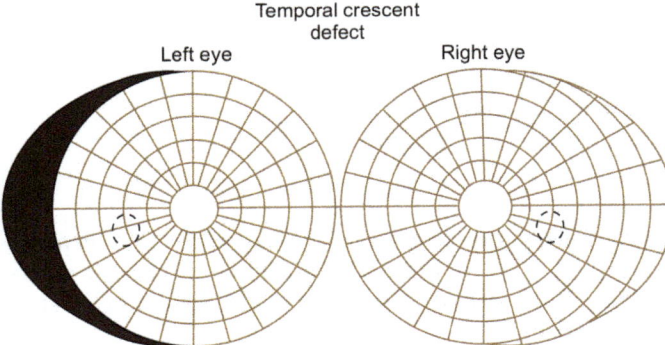

Fig. 3.21: Temporal crescentic scotoma in left eye—anterior calcarine lesion.

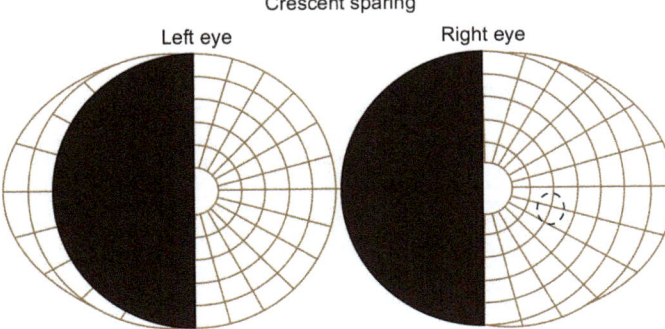

Fig. 3.22: Left homonymous hemianopia with sparing of temporal crescent of the left eye—occipital lobe lesion sparing the anterior calcarine.

Heteronymous Hemianopia
- Binasal
- Bitemporal.

Binasal Hemianopia
- Loss of both nasal fields
- Rare
- Site of lesion—lesions situated on either side of optic chiasma destroying temporal fibers of each retina.

Example: Distention of 3rd ventricle.

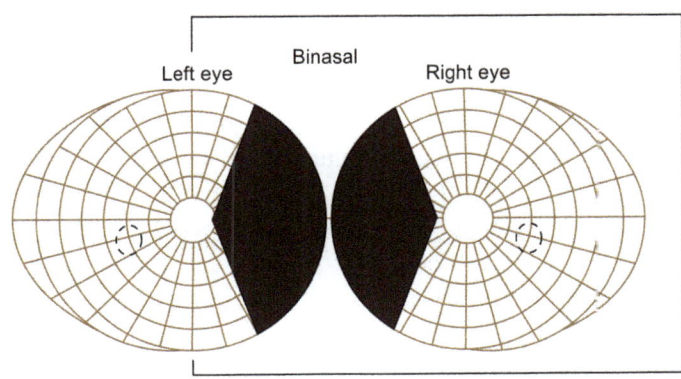

Fig. 3.23: Atheroma of internal carotids or posterior communicating arteries.

Bitemporal Hemianopia
- Loss of both temporal fields—usually starts in superotemporal quadrant then progresses to lower temporal quadrant.
- Site of lesion—lesion of the central part of the chiasma
- **Causes**—pituitary tumors, suprasellar aneurysm or chronic arachnoiditis.

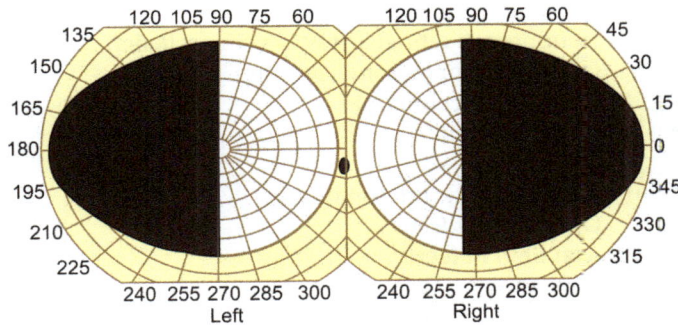

Fig. 3.24: Bitemporal hemianopia.

Bilateral Occipital Infarction
- Cortical blindness
- Anton's sign—denial of blindness
- Riddoch's phenomenon—appreciation of kinetic objects but not static objects.

Altitudinal Hemianopia
Loss of superior or inferior half of field.

Investigations
- Computed tomography (CT) scan
- Magnetic resonance imaging (MRI)
- Positron emission tomography
- Treatment of underlying disease
- Prism glasses expand peripheral field.

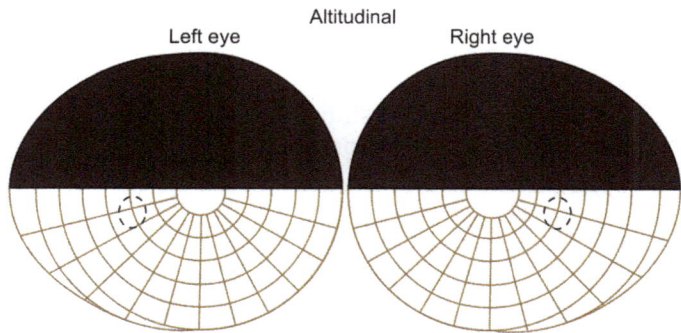

Fig. 3.25: Superior altitudinal hemianopia.

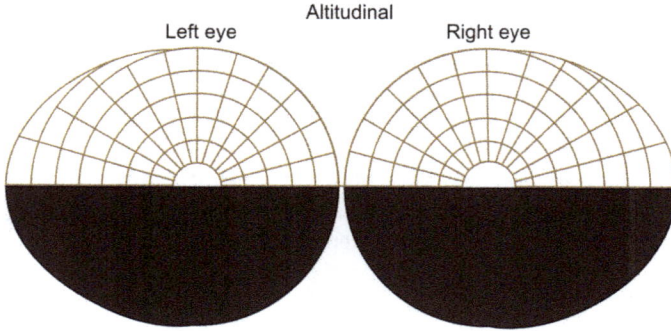

Fig. 3.26: Inferior altitudinal hemianopia.

12. Enumerate the common visual field abnormalities and their causes.

- **Altitudinal field defects:**
  - Ischemic optic neuropathy
  - Hemibranch retinal artery or vein occlusion
  - Optic nerve or chiasmal lesions
  - Optic nerve coloboma.
- **Arcuate scotoma:**
  - Glaucoma
  - Ischemic optic neuropathy
  - Optic disk drusen.
- **Binasal field defect:**
  - Glaucoma
  - Bitemporal retinal disease
  - Bitemporal occipital disease
  - Compressive lesion of both optic nerves or chiasma
  - Functional visual loss.
- **Bitemporal hemianopia:**
  - Chiasmal lesions
  - Tilted optic disks
  - Sectoral (nasal) retinitis pigmentosa.
- **Central scotoma:**
  - Macular lesions
  - Optic neuritis
  - Optic atrophy
  - Occipital cortex lesions.
- **Homonymous hemianopia:**
  - Optic tract or lateral geniculate lesions
  - Temporal, parietal, or occipital lobe lesions.
- **Constriction of peripheral fields:**
  - Glaucoma
  - Retinal disease
  - Bilateral panretinal photocoagulation
  - Central retinal artery occlusion
  - Bilateral occipital lobe lesions with macular sparing.
- **Blind spot enlargement:**
  - Papilledema
  - Optic nerve drusen
  - Optic nerve coloboma
  - Myelinated nerve fibers
  - Myopic disk.
- **Pie in the sky:**
  - Temporal lobe lesion.
- **Pie on the floor:**
  - Parietal lobe lesion.

13. What is visually evoked response?

Visually evoked response (VER) refers to electroencephalography (EEG) recorded at the occipital cortex. It assesses the functional status of the visual system beyond the retinal ganglion cells.

Clinically, VER is used to assess visual acuity in infants and mentally retarded individuals, confirm malingering, and to confirm optic nerve diseases like retrobulbar neuritis.

CHAPTER 4

Ocular Pharmacology

INTRODUCTION

Medications used in ophthalmology are:
- Antimicrobial agents
- Mydriatics and cycloplegics
- Antiglaucoma drugs
- Anti-inflammatory agents
- Corticosteroids and nonsteroidal anti-inflammatory drugs (NSAIDs)
- Viscoelastics
- Local anesthetics
- Diagnostic stains.

1. What are the routes of administration of drugs to the eye?

- Eye drops
- Subconjunctival injections
- Sub-Tenon's injections—anterior and posterior
- Intravitreal injections
- Peribulbar injections
- Retrobulbar injections
- Ocuserts.

2. Name anti-inflammatory agents used in ophthalmology.

- Steroids
- Nonsteroidal anti-inflammatory drugs
- Antihistaminics
- Histamine release blockers
- Antifibrotics
- Immunosuppressive agents.

3. List the steroids used in ophthalmology.

- **Systemic:**
    - Methylprednisolone and prednisolone.
- **Topical:**
    - Prednisolone acetate 1%
    - Dexamethasone phosphate 0.1%
    - Fluorometholone 0.1%
    - Loteprednol etabonate 0.2% and 0.5% suspension.

4. What are the side effects of steroids?

- **Systemic:** Osteoporosis, peptic ulcer, hypertension, diabetes, adrenal insufficiency, muscle weakness, increased infection rate and delayed wound healing.
- **Topical:** Glaucoma, posterior capsular cataract, defective wound healing, corneal and scleral thinning.

5. What nonsteroidal anti-inflammatory drugs are used in ophthalmology and their uses?

It blocks cyclooxygenase pathway preventing conversion of arachidonic acid to prostaglandins.
- **Systemic:**
    - Salicylates—aspirin
    - Indoles—indomethacin
    - Phenylalkanoic derivatives—diclofenac, flurbiprofen, ketorolac, piroxicam, oxyphenbutazone.
    - Side effects—delayed wound healing.
- **Topical:**
    - Diclofenac 0.1%, flurbiprofen 0.03%, ketorolac 0.5%, nepafenac 0.1%, bromfenac 0.09% (0.9 mg in 1 mL).

Uses of NSAIDs

- To inhibit intraoperative miosis, postoperative inflammation and cystoid macular edema
- Steroids can be reduced
- Reduces itching and pain.

6. What antimetabolites (antifibrotic agents) are used in ophthalmology?

- 5-fluorouracil—inhibits cellular proliferation
    - Subconjunctival injection of 5 mg/mL daily given after glaucoma surgery.
- Mitomycin C—inhibits DNA synthesis and fibroblast proliferation
    - Pterygium 0.02% drops qid for 1–2 weeks
    - Recurrent pterygium or after glaucoma surgery
    - 0.2 mg sponge placed for 45–60 seconds
    - 0.4 mg for 39 seconds—irrigated with normal saline.

7. What is the role of antiallergic drugs in ophthalmology?

Mast Cell Stabilizers

- Blocks calcium channel—prevents cell degranulation and stabilizes cell
- Prevents release of histamine and slow reacting substances of anaphylaxis. Prolongs tear breakup time, reduces itching and hyperemia:

- Cromolyn sodium 2–4%
- Lodoxamide 0.1%—more potent
- Olopatadine hydrochloride 0.1%.

Indications

Vernal catarrh and giant papillary conjunctivitis.

8. What is the role of miotics in ophthalmology?

Parasympathomimetic—Cholinergic Agonist

- **Direct-acting:** Activates cholinergic receptors at sphincter pupillae and ciliary muscle—acetylcholine, pilocarpine, carbachol.
- **Indirect-acting:** Inhibits cholinesterase inhibitors
  - Reversible: Neostigmine, physostigmine, edrophonium
  - Irreversible: Echothiophate.

Pilocarpine

- 1–4% eye drops qid.
- It is a direct-acting parasympathetic drug.
- Mechanism of action: In primary open-angle glaucoma, it stimulates longitudinal muscle of ciliary body—pulls scleral spur—widens intertrabecular spaces—increases outflow—decreases intraocular pressure (IOP). In primary angle-closure glaucoma, it reduces IOP by constriction of pupil which moves the iris away from the trabecular meshwork.

Side Effects of Pilocarpine

- **Ocular:** Accommodative spasm, and follicular conjunctivitis.
  - Retinal detachment due to forward displacement of iris lens diaphragm.
- **Systemic:** Headache, perspiration, bronchospasm, bradycardia, abdominal pain and diarrhea.

Carbachol

- 0.75%, 1.5%, 2.25%, 3% eye drops tds.
  - Intrameral (into anterior chamber) 0.01%—0.5 mL irrigation.
- **Ocular toxicity:** Miosis, conjunctival and ciliary congestion, ciliary spasm.

9. Write short notes on phenylephrine.

It is a quick acting mydriatic. It is available in strengths of 2.5%, 5% and 10%.

Action

Synthetic sympathomimetic—acts on alpha-1 receptors.
- Contracts iris dilator and smooth muscle of conjunctival arterioles causing pupillary dilation and conjunctival blanching.
- Acts on Muller muscle—upper lid retraction.
- Reduces IOP.

Uses of Phenylephrine

- Breaks posterior synechiae
- Improves vision in posterior polar cataract due to mydriasis.
- In Horner's syndrome: 1% phenylephrine dilates pupil due to postganglionic sympathetic denervation whereas it is not effective in normal eyes.

Side Effects of Phenylephrine

- **Ocular:** Allergic dermatoconjunctivitis
  - Rebound conjunctival congestion
- **Systemic:** Systolic hypertension
  - Occipital headache
  - Tachycardia.

10. Write short notes on cycloplegics.

- Atropine
- Homatropine
- Cyclopentolate
- Tropicamide.

Action and Uses of Atropine

- 1% ointment or eye drops.
- It is mydriatic and cycloplegic.
- Refraction in children especially with suspected latent hypermetropia or accommodative esotropia.
- Uveitis:
  - Relieves pain by relaxing ciliary spasm.
  - Dilates pupil—prevents posterior synechia.
  - Decreases the excessive permeability of inflamed vessels and thereby reduce leakage of cells and protein into anterior chamber.
  - By reducing pressure on the anterior ciliary artery, it increases blood supply to the anterior uvea thereby more antibodies reach the target tissues and more toxins are absorbed.
- Corneal ulcer—as in uveitis.
- Penalization in amblyopia—alternative to occlusion.
- Myopia—slows progression. Elongation of eyeball is reduced by relaxing accommodation.
  - Homatropine 2%—1/10th potency of atropine
  - Cyclopentolate 0.5%, 1% causes drowsiness
  - Tropicamide—0.5%, 1%.
- 0.01% atropine eye drops—used to delay the progression of myopia in children
- For dilation in premature infants:
  - Retinopathy of prematurity screening
  - 0.5% tropicamide and 2.5% phenylephrine.

Side Effects of Atropine

- Ocular: Allergic contact dermatitis, and risk of angle closure.
- Systemic: Dry mouth, decreased sweating, convulsions, pyrexia
- Hyperactive pupil response in Down's syndrome.

Relative action of cycloplegics.			
Drug	Strength	Maximal action	Recovery
Atropine	1%	40 minutes—mydriasis 1–3 hours—cycloplegics	7–10 days
Homatropine	2%	30–40 minutes	1–3 days
Cyclopentolate	0.5%, 1%	30–60 minutes	1 day
Tropicamide	0.5%, 1%	20–40 minutes	6 hours

11. What are the drugs used for dry eye?

- Artificial tears—water-based polymers
  - Used to enhance viscosity, lubrication, retention time, and stability of tear film.
- Methyl cellulose 0.25–1%.
- Hydroxyethyl or propyl cellulose 0.5%.
- Hydroxypropylmethyl cellulose or carboxymethyl cellulose 1%.
- Polyvinylpyrrolidone or povidone.
- Isotonic or hypotonic.
- NaCl or KCl is added.
- Buffers like phosphate, bicarbonate or borate
  - Are added to make it alkaline.
- Preservatives—sodium perborate.

12. Write short notes on viscoelastics.

Viscoelastics are ocular viscosurgical devices (OVDs) used during cataract surgery.

- **Uses:**
  - To maintain space
  - Helps in pupillary enlargement
  - Capsulorrhexis
  - Maintains anterior chamber
  - Protects corneal endothelium
  - Helps in combating vitreous pressure
- **Types:**
  - Viscoadaptive—high molecular weight.
    Healon 5 (sodium hyaluronate 2.3%)
  - Viscocohesive—high molecular weight
    Healon GV (sodium hyaluronate 1.4%)
    Healon (sodium hyaluronate 1%)
  - Viscodispersive
    Hydroxypropylmethyl cellulose 2%—low molecular weight
  - Viscoat (sodium chondroitin sulfate 4% and sodium hyaluronate 3%)—medium molecular weight.
- **Complications:**
  - IOP rise due to incomplete removal of viscoelastic. More with cohesive than with dispersive type.
  - Postoperative inflammation.

13. What local anesthetics are used in ophthalmology?

Local anesthetics—topical.

Drug	Onset of action	Duration
Cocaine 1–4%	1 minute	20–30 minutes
Proparacaine 0.5%	1 minute	15 minutes
Lidocaine 4%	1 minute	15 minutes

Local anesthetic—regional.

Drug	Onset of action	Duration	Safety limit
Lidocaine 2%	5 minutes	45 minutes	4 mL/kg
Lidocaine + adrenaline	5 minutes	1–2 hours	7 mL/kg
Bupivacaine 0.5%	7–10 minutes	2 hours	2 mL/kg

14. What antibacterials are commonly used in ophthalmology?

- **Polypeptides**—affect cell wall synthesis
  - Bacitracin (gram-positive), polymyxin (gram-negative).
- **Aminoglycosides**—affect protein synthesis
  - Streptomycin, gentamicin, tobramycin, neomycin, amikacin (gram-negative), tetracycline (gram-positive).
- **Cephalosporins**—affect cell wall
  - Cephalexin, cefazolin, ceftazidime, cefixime, ceftriaxone, cefpodoxime (gram-negative).
- **Fluoroquinolones**—affect DNA synthesis
  - Norfloxacin, ciprofloxacin, ofloxacin, gatifloxacin, moxifloxacin (broad spectrum).
- **Macrolides**—affect protein synthesis
  - Erythromycin, ampicillin, amoxicillin, azithromycin, vancomycin (gram-positive).

Drug	Topical	Fortified	Subconjunctival	Intravitreal
Penicillin G	100,000 units/mL	-	-	-
Cipro/Oflox/Gati	0.3%	-	-	-
Genta/Tobra	1–1.4%	20 mg/mL	20–40 mg/mL	0.1–0.2 mg/0.1 mL
Amikacin	2%	20 mg/mL	25–50 mg	0.4 mg in 0.03 mL
Cefazolin/Ceftazidime	5%	50–100 mg/mL	100 mg	2.25 mg in 0.1 mL
Ceftriaxone	10%	100 mg/mL	50 mg	3 mg in 0.1 mL
Vancomycin	2.5–5%		2 mg	1 mg in 0.1 mL

15. What are the fungal organisms affecting the eye?

- **Yeast:** *Candida, Cryptococcus.*
- **Filamentous**
  - Septate
    » *Fusarium, Aspergillus flavus* and *Aspergillus fumigatus*
  - Nonseptate
    » *Mucor.*
- **Dimorphic**
  - Histoplasmosis
  - Causes damage to cell membrane.

16. What antifungals are commonly used in ophthalmology?

- **Polyenes**
  - Eye drops amphotericin B 0.1–0.2%, eye ointment nystatin
  - Eye drops natamycin 5% every 2 hours for 2–3 weeks.
- **Imidazoles:** Clotrimazole, miconazole, fluconazole, itraconazole, voriconazole
  - Ketoconazole 400 mg od orally for 2 weeks.

17. What antivirals are commonly used in ophthalmology?

Drugs affecting DNA of virus
- Idoxuridine (IDU) 0.1% hourly 0.5% ointment h.s.
- Triflurothymidine 1% 4th hourly for 7days
- Acyclovir 3% ointment 5 times for 2–3 weeks
  - Herpes simplex keratitis—acyclovir 400 mg bd orally for 7 days
  - Herpes zoster ophthalmicus—acyclovir 800 mg 5 times a day orally for 7–10 days.
- Vidarabine 3% eye ointment 5 times for 2 weeks.
- Ganciclovir 0.15% ointment for herpes zoster
  - Cytomegalovirus retinitis, posterior ocular retinal necrosis—oral, intravitreal—200–400 µg twice weekly—2 weeks
  - Implant—6 mg, pellet releases 1 µg/hour.

18. Classify and describe antiglaucoma drugs.

- Cholinergic drugs—parasympathomimetic
- Adrenergic drugs—sympathomimetic
  - **Adrenergic stimulators**
    - Nonselective—stimulates alpha- and beta-adrenergic receptors—epinephrine, dipivefrin
    - Selective—alpha-2 agonist—brimonidine
  - **Adrenergic inhibitors**
  - Beta-adrenergic blockers
    - Nonselective—beta-1 and beta-2 antagonist—timolol maleate, levobunolol
    - Selective—beta-1 antagonist—betaxolol.
- Prostaglandin analogs
- Carbonic anhydrase inhibitors
- Hyperosmotics.

Cholinergic Drugs

Parasympathomimetics
- Directly stimulates sphincter pupillae
  - Pilocarpine 2% qid
  - Carbachol 0.75%, 1.5%, 2.25% tid

Anticholinesterases:
Prevents destruction of acetylcholine at neuromuscular junction thereby stimulating parasympathetic system.

Reversible Cholinesterase Inhibitors
- Physostigmine 0.25% od
- Neostigmine 0.25% od
- Demecarium bromide 0.125%, 0.25% bd.

Irreversible Cholinesterase Inhibitors
- Echothiophate 0.03%, 0.06%, 0.12% od
- Diisopropyl pyrophosphate.

Adrenergic Drugs

Sympathomimetics
- Nonselective—stimulates alpha- and beta-adrenergic receptors
- Selective—alpha-2 agonists.

Nonselective Agonists
- Epinephrine 0.25%, 0.5%, 1%, 2% bid
- Dipivefrin 0.1% bid
  Decrease in aqueous production due to initial. Vasoconstrictive effect thus slowing the ultrafiltration and increasing aqueous outflow.

Selective Agonists
- Apraclonidine 1% od—decreases aqueous production
- Brimonidine 0.2%—decreases aqueous production, increases uveoscleral outflow, increases optic nerve blood flow and offers neuroprotection.
- Beta-blockers: Nonselective—beta-1 and beta-2 antagonists
  - Nonselective—beta-1 and beta-2 antagonists
    » Timolol maleate 0.5% bid
    » Carteolol 1%, 2% bid
    » Levobunolol 0.5% od
    » Metipranolol 0.1%, 0.3% bid
    » Reduces aqueous production by 20–30%
  - Selective
    » Betaxolol 0.5% bid
    » Cardioselective beta-1 antagonist
    » Decreases aqueous production
    » No respiratory side effects unlike timolol.

Prostaglandin Analogs
- Latanoprost 0.005%
- Travoprost 0.004%
- Bimatoprost 0.03%—all od in the night
- Unoprostone 0.15%—twice daily
- Tafluprost 0.0015%—Decreases IOP by increase in uveoscleral outflow by relaxation of ciliary muscle.

Latanoprost
- Prodrug, absorbed through cornea, and hydrolyzed into active form.
- Has neuroprotective action by interfering with cyclooxygenase and nitric oxide synthetase activity thereby decreasing apoptosis of retinal ganglion cells.

Carbonic Anhydrase Inhibitors
- **Topical**
  - Dorzolamide 2% tid
  - Brinzolamide 1% tid.
- **Systemic**
  - Acetazolamide 250 mg bd
  - Dichlorphenamide 50 mg bd
  - Methazolamide 50 mg bd.

Hyperosmotics
- **Oral**
  - Glycerol 50%—2 mL/kg body weight
  - Isosorbide 45%—2 mL/kg body weight.
- **Intravenous**
  - Mannitol 20%—5 mL/kg over 30–60 minutes
  - Urea 45%.

CHAPTER 5

Errors of Refraction

INTRODUCTION

Emmetropia is normal optical condition of the eye. When parallel rays come to a focus on the retina with accommodation at rest, the condition is called emmetropia. If they do not come to a focus on the retina with accommodation at rest, it is known as ametropia. There are three types of errors of refraction:
  i. Myopia or short sightedness
  ii. Hypermetropia or long sightedness
  iii. Astigmatism.

1. Discuss the etiology, types, clinical features and treatment of myopia.

Myopia (Short Sightedness)

Dioptric condition of the eye (form of refractive error) in which accommodation at rest, incident parallel rays come to a focus anterior to light sensitive layer of retina.

Etiological Factors

- Pressure of extraocular muscles during excessive convergence in near work causing posterior pole to bulge
- Endocrine deficiencies
- Dietary deficiencies
- Debilitating illness
  - Axial—increased anteroposterior diameter
  - Curvature—increased curvature
    » Cornea—conical cornea
    » Lens—lenticonus
  - Index—increased refractive index of nucleus
    » Senile nuclear cataract
  - Forward displacement lens.

Types

- Congenital (Developmental)
- Simple
- Pathological.

Congenital Myopia
- Present at birth. Usually stationary
- Unilateral or bilateral
- Up to –10 D.

Simple Myopia
- The most common type.
- No degenerative changes in fundus.
- Does not progress after adolescence. Up to –6 D.

Pathological Myopia
- Begins at 5-10 years. Increases steadily up to –15 D to –20 D
- Strongly hereditary. Anterior to equator is normal
- Degenerative changes in posterior part of eyeball.

Symptoms

- Indistinct distant vision
- Floating black spots
- Discomfort after near work
- Disproportion between effects of accommodation and convergence
- Flashes of light
- Defective night vision in high myopia
- Squeezing of eyes (narrowed palpebral fissure enables to see clearly).

Signs

- Prominent eyes
- Deep anterior chamber.

Fundus Changes

- Large optic disk.
- Myopic crescent—gray crescent on temporal side of disk, due to patch of atrophy of choroid.
- Super traction crescent pigment epithelium encroaching over nasal edge of disk.

- Chorioretinal atrophy.
- Tessellated fundus—depigmentation of retinal pigment epithelium.
- Lattice degeneration: Areas of retinal thinning at periphery criss-cross network of fine white lines with retinal tears.
- Cystoid degeneration at ora serrata.

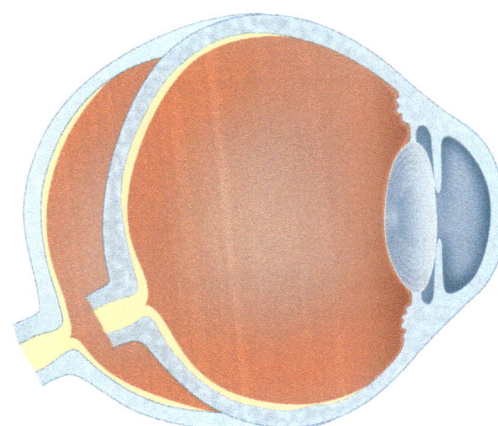

Fig. 5.1: Enlargement of posterior part.

- Posterior staphyloma
- Foster-Fuchs spot—dark pigmented circular areas of intrachoroidal hemorrhage
- Vitreous liquefaction—muscae volitantes
- Lacquer cracks—yellowish white lines due to cracks in Bruch's membrane of choroid.

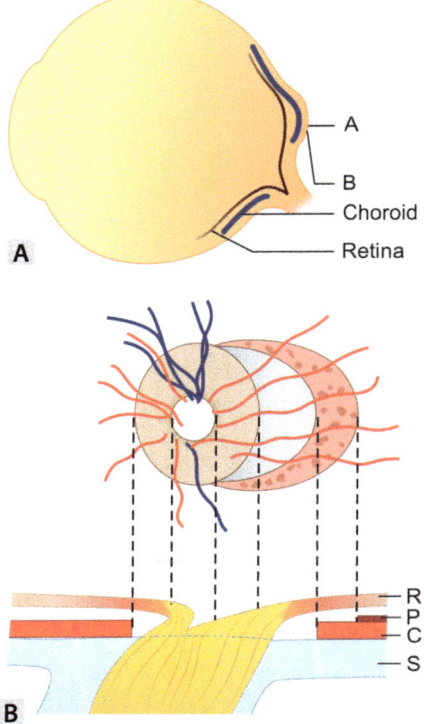

Figs. 5.2A and B: A. Posterior staphyloma; B. Myopic crescent and super traction.

Complications
- Retinal detachment
  - Hole formation in lattice degeneration
  - Fluid vitreous.
- Complicated cataract
- Chronic simple glaucoma
- Divergent squint.

Treatment
- Spherical concave lenses
- Contact lenses
- Operations.

Spherical Concave Lenses
Under correction is preferred—glasses to be worn constantly:
- For proper visual development
- Prevention of amblyopia
- Mental development.

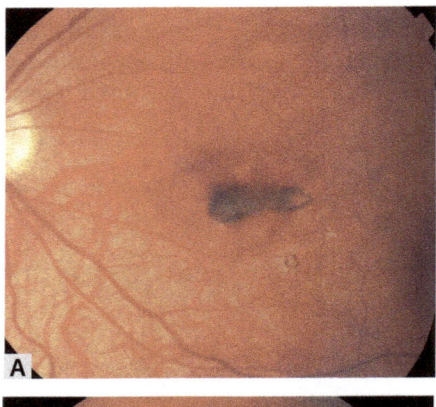
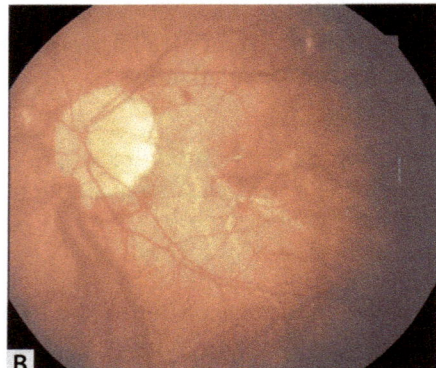

Figs. 5.3A and B: A. Fuchs spot; B. Lacquer cracks.

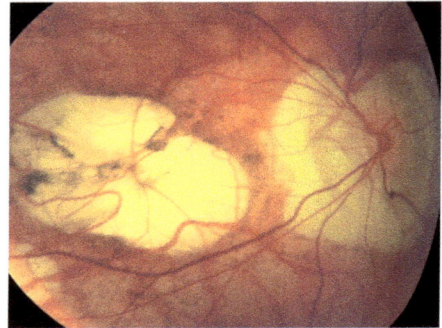

Fig. 5.4: Chorioretinal atrophy.

Errors of Refraction

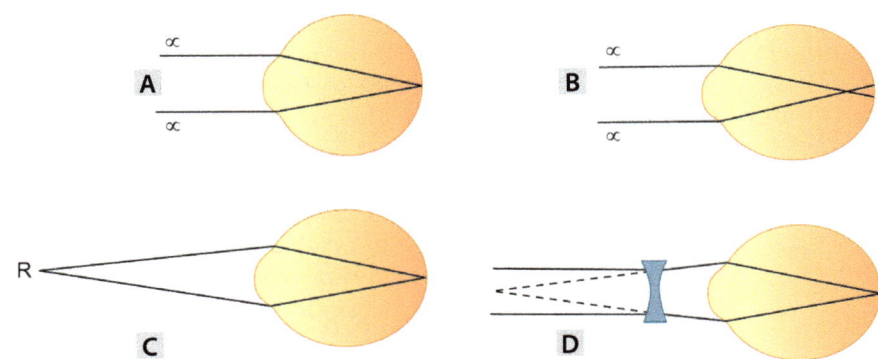

Figs. 5.5A to D: A. Emmetropic eye; B. Parallel rays focusing in front of retina; C. Near objects focusing on retina; D. Parallel rays focusing on the retina with concave lens.

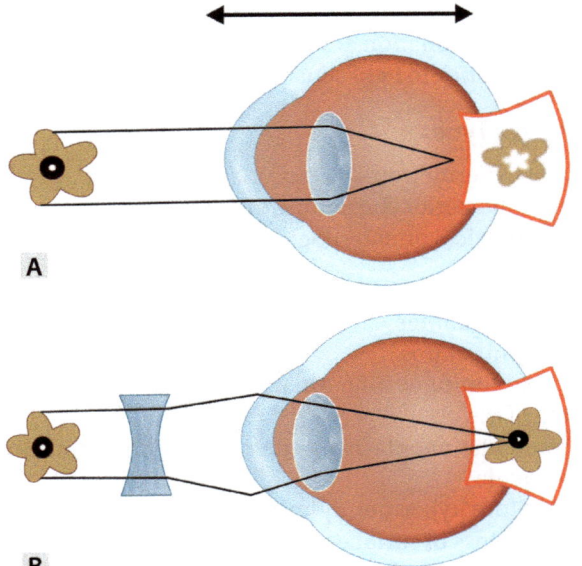

Figs. 5.6A and B: A. Myopic eye—blurred image; B. Clear image after correction.

Contact Lenses
- Normal field of vision
- Aberration of glasses are eliminated
- Cosmetic appearance.

Operations and its possible complications.		
Operation	Power in diopters (D)	Possible complication
Radial keratotomy linear radial incisions 80% depth are made peripherally in the cornea leaving central optic zone making central cornea flatter	1–6 D	Surgically induced astigmatism
Intracorneal rings inserted in paracentral stromal pocket—lead to paracentral bulging and central flattening	1–6 D	Unpredictable results, keratitis
Epikeratophakia: Minus lenticule is used to reshape cornea	Up to 18 D	Glare epithelial defects

Contd...

Contd...		
Operation	Power in diopters (D)	Possible complication
Photorefractive keratectomy (PRK): Excimer laser (193 nm) ablation of cornea after removing epithelium	1–4 D	Delayed visual recovery, corneal haze, glare, loss of contrast sensitivity
Laser-assisted in situ keratomileusis (LASIK): Reshapes cornea by ablating to superficial stroma to predetermined extent after lifting a flap normal cornea with microkeratome. In Intralase, laser is used instead of microkeratome	2–12 D	Infection, diffuse lamellar keratitis, interface debris, epithelial ingrowth flap displacement, thinning and ectasia, regression, glare difficulty in night driving
Laser-assisted subepithelial keratectomy (LASEK): Excimer laser PRK with epithelial flap Methods to reduce overall refractive power of eye	1–6 D	Same as LASIK except there are no microkeratome related complications
Clear lens extraction (Fukala's operation)	>15 D	Endophthalmitis, retinal detachment
Phakic intraocular lens (IOL)	>12 D	Endophthalmitis, cataract

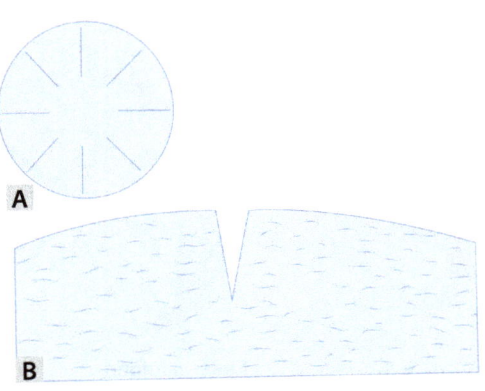

Figs. 5.7A and B: Radial keratotomy.

Photorefractive Keratectomy

Excimer lasers (excited dimer) act by tissue modeling (photoablation).

It is far ultraviolet radiation which allows removal of corneal tissue with the accuracy of a fraction of micron (μm).

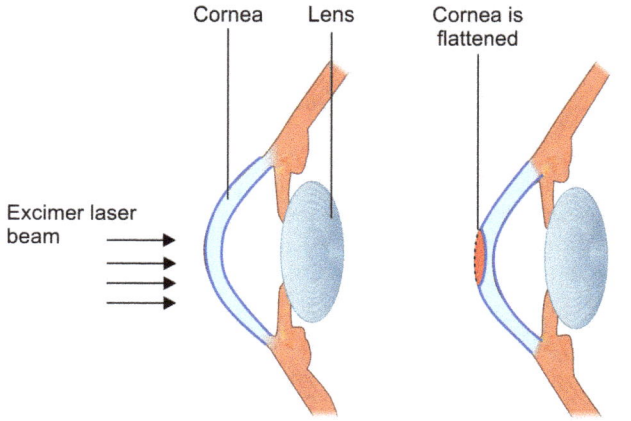

Fig. 5.8: Photorefractive keratectomy (PRK).

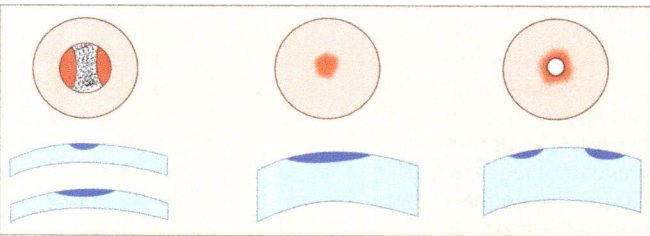

Fig. 5.9: PRK altering central cornea.

The technique of PRK

- Visual axis is marked and corneal epithelium is removed
- Patient fixates on the aiming beam of laser
- Laser is applied to ablate the Bowman's membrane and anterior stroma—takes around 30–60 seconds
- Cornea heals in 48–72 hours.

Laser-assisted in Situ Keratomileusis (LASIK)

Laser-assisted in situ keratomileusis (grinding)—modification of PRK.

160-μm hinged corneal flap is lifted from central 8–9 mm of cornea with microkeratome. The flap is folded to side. Excimer laser used to remove tissue from the exposed surface corneal flap is replaced back.

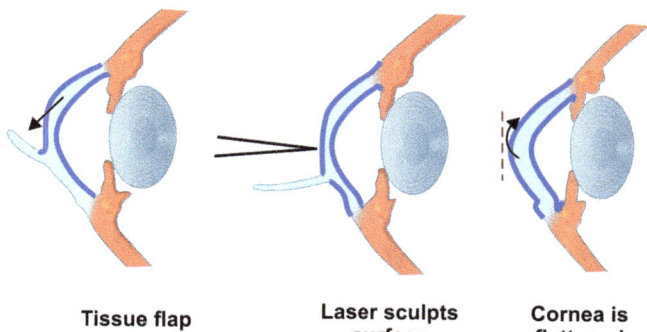

Fig. 5.10: Laser-assisted in situ keratomileusis (LASIK).

Epikeratophakia

- Procedure in which a lenticule of donor tissue used to alter the surface topography of cornea
- The donor lenticule of desired power is sutured with 10-0 nylon suture
- Unilateral myopia up to—18 D can be corrected
- In myopia—minus lenticule used
- In aphakia in children—plus lenticule is used
- In keratoconus—plano lenticule is used
- Complications—glare, epithelial defects.

2. Discuss the etiology, types, clinical features and treatment of hypermetropia.

Definition

Dioptric condition of the eye (form of refraction error) in which accommodation at rest, incident parallel rays come to a focus posterior to light sensitive layer of retina.

Etiological Types

- Axial hypermetropia
- Anteroposterior shortening of the eyeball 1 mm = 3 D
- Physiological or pathological.

Pathological Causes of Axial Hypermetropia

- Microphthalmos
- Nanophthalmos
- Orbital tumor or inflammatory mass indenting posterior pole of the eye
- Intraocular neoplasm or edema displaces retina forward at macula
- Curvature hypermetropia:
  - Flatness of surface of cornea or lens
  - 1 mm flat radius of curvature of cornea = 6 D hypermetropia.
- Index hypermetropia:
  - Decrease in refractive index of lens
  - Hypoglycemia
  - Cortical cataract.
- Posterior dislocation of clear lens—congenital or traumatic
- Aphakia
- Paralysis accommodation:
  - Cycloplegia
  - 3rd nerve palsy
  - Internal ophthalmoplegia.

Components of Hypermetropia

Total hypermetropia
- Latent
- Manifest
  - Facultative
  - Absolute.

Total Hypermetropia

Full amount of hypermetropia revealed only by paralysis of ciliary muscle (by using atropine).

- **Latent hypermetropia:** Part of total hypermetropia overcome physiologically by tone of ciliary muscle.

- **Manifest hypermetropia:** Remaining portion of total hypermetropia which is not corrected by tone of ciliary muscle.
    - Facultative hypermetropia: Which can be overcome by an effort of accommodation
    - Absolute hypermetropia: Which cannot be overcome by accommodation
    - Total hypermetropia = latent + manifest
    - Manifest hypermetropia = absolute + facultative.

Feature	Latent	Facultative	Absolute
Detection	By cycloplegia	Without cycloplegia	Without cycloplegia
Visual acuity	Normal	Normal	Blurred
Vision with convex lenses	Normal	Normal	Improvement
Acceptance of convex lenses	Rejects	Accepts	Readily accepts

Symptoms
- In young subjects—no symptoms
- With low degree of error
- Ocular asthenopia due to excessive accommodation
- Frontal headache increases in evening
- Defective vision for distance and near
- Sensitivity to light.

Signs
- **Eyeball:**
    - Small
    - Decreased axial length
    - Anterior chamber shallow.
- **Fundus:**
    - Disk small
    - Disk margins blurred—pseudopapillitis
    - Watered silk appearance—retina has sheen
    - Vessels tortuous.

Complications
- Uncorrected hypermetropia in children may lead to convergent squint
- Premature presbyopia
- Amblyopia in high hypermetropia particularly in unilateral cases
- Prone for angle-closure glaucoma due to shallow anterior chamber and crowding of iris root at angle of anterior chamber.

Treatment

Correction with convex lens
- When associated with esophoria or esotropia—full correction
- When associated with exophoria or exotropia—under correction
    - For correction, Donders' rule to be applied which is as follows:
        » Manifest hypermetropia +1/4 of latent hypermetropia.
        » Under 16 years
        » < + 3 D—no correction
        » + 3 D—only for near vision.
- Contact lens
- Hyperopic LASIK—midperipheral stroma removed by photoablation
- Conductive keratoplasty—radiofrequency burns are used in corneal periphery
- Laser thermal keratoplasty—Holmium laser burns are used
    - Both types of keratoplasty are used to correct low hypermetropia.

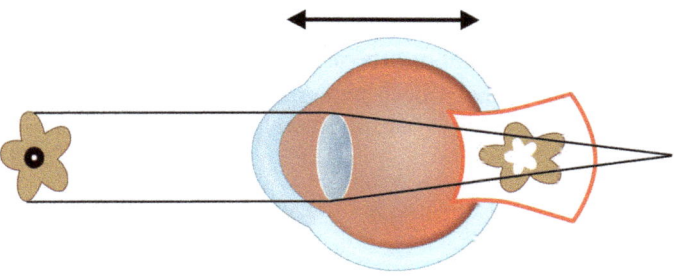

Fig. 5.12: Hypermetropic eye—blurred image.

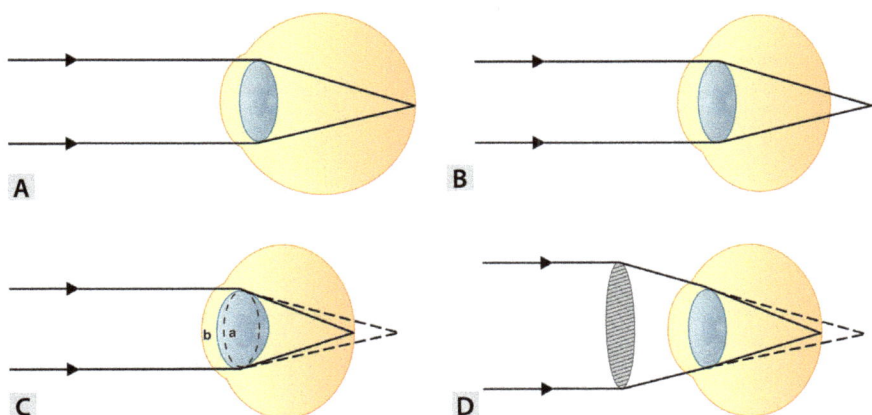

Figs. 5.11A to D: A. Emmetropic eye; B. Parallel rays focusing behind the retina; C. Parallel rays focusing on the retina with accommodation; D. Parallel rays focusing on the retina with convex lens.

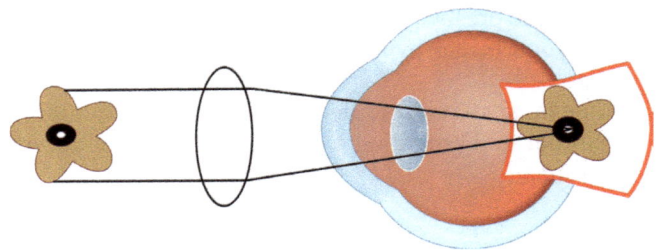

Fig. 5.13: Clear image after correction with convex lens.

3. Discuss the etiology, types, clinical features and treatment of astigmatism.

Definition

It is a dioptric condition of refraction in which a point focus of light cannot be formed upon the retina with accommodation at rest.

Etiology

- **Corneal astigmatism:**
  - Curvature astigmatism—physiological due to constant pressure of upper lid upon the eye. Vertical curvature is > horizontal curvature.
- **Lenticular astigmatism:**
  - Curvature—due to lenticonus
  - Positional—oblique placement of lens or subluxation of lens
  - Index astigmatism—due to small inequalities in refractive index of different sectors of lens.

Types

Depending on focal points on the retina

- Simple hypermetropic astigmatism: One of the foci is on the retina, other is behind the retina.
- Simple myopic astigmatism: One of the foci is on the retina, other is in front of the retina.
- Compound hypermetropic astigmatism: Both the foci are behind the retina at different degrees.
- Compound myopic astigmatism: Both the foci are in front of the retina at different degrees.
- Mixed astigmatism: One of the foci is behind the retina, other is in front of the retina.

Forms of Astigmatism: Related to Principal Meridians of Cornea

- Regular
- Irregular
- Oblique
- Symmetrical
- Asymmetrical
- With the rule
- Against the rule.

Regular Astigmatism

Principal meridians are at right angles to each other. It can be corrected with cylindrical lenses.

Irregular astigmatism

Principal meridians are not at 90° apart due to irregular corneal curvature. It cannot be corrected by cylindrical lenses.

Oblique

Principal meridians are more than 20° from horizontal or vertical meridians.

Symmetrical Astigmatism

Principal meridians of each eye bear a symmetrical position of deviation from the median line. Axes of meridians corrected by cylinders of same sign add to 180°.
Example: Right eye (RE)—Cylinder (cyl) 60° and left eye (LE)—cyl 120°.

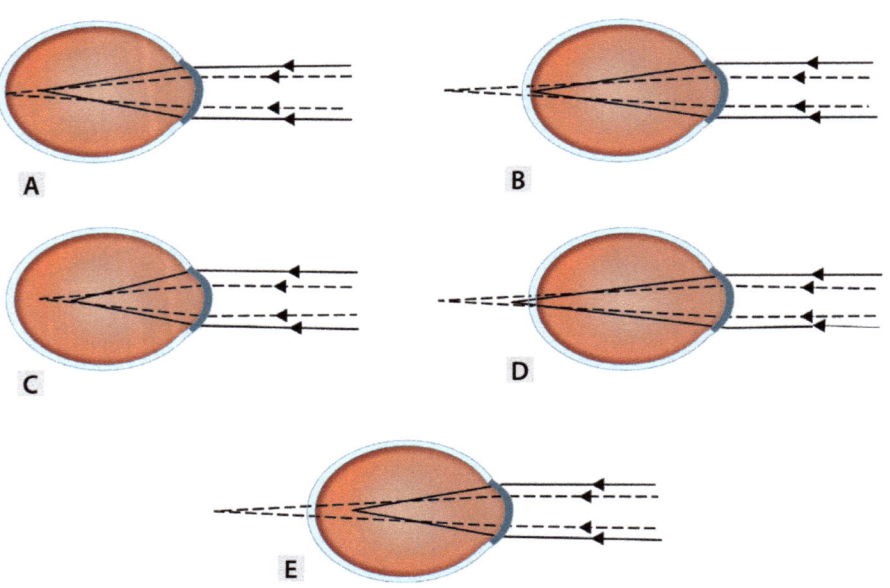

Figs. 5.14A and E: A. Simple myopic astigmatism; B. Simple hypermetropic astigmatism; C. Compound myopic astigmatism; D. Compound hypermetropic astigmatism; E. Mixed astigmatism.

Asymmetrical Astigmatism

No symmetry of principal meridian. They will not add up to 180°.

Example: Corneal scar, keratoconus, lenticonus.

With the Rule

More common, vertical meridian has strong curvature. Corrected by—cyl 180° or +cyl 90°.

Against the Rule

Less common, horizontal meridian has strong curvature. Corrected by—cyl 90° or +cyl 180°.

Symptoms

- **With higher astigmatism:**
  - Blurred vision
  - Tilting of head—high oblique astigmatism
  - Narrowing of eyelids to achieve stenopaeic effect for better vision
  - Holds reading matter close to eye.

	With rule	Against rule
Asthenopia	More	Less
Blurring of vision	Less	More
Full correction acceptance	Poor	Good

Treatment

- Optical
- Surgical

Optical

- **Cylindrical lenses:**
  - No symptoms—no correction
  - Symptoms—initially undercorrect then full correction.
- **Contact lenses:**
  - Rigid gas permeable contact lenses
  - Soft toric lenses.

Surgical

- Usually reserved for iatrogenic astigmatism after cataract or corneal transplant surgery
- Relaxing incisions
- Astigmatic keratotomy—to flatten more curved meridian
- Wedge resection.

4. What is Sturm's conoid?

It is the configuration of rays refracted through the astigmatic surface (toric surface). The distance between the two focal planes is called Sturm's interval. Between the two focal planes, it lies the circle of least diffusion.

Depending upon the position of two focal lines (vertical and horizontal) in relation to retina, the regular astigmatism is classified into three types (simple, compound and mixed) which is shown in Figure 5.16 and described in the following Table.

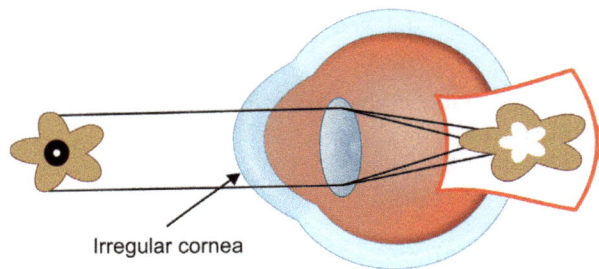

Fig. 5.15: Astigmatism.

- **With low-grade astigmatism:**
  - Asthenopia
  - Transient blurred vision at near relieved by closing or rubbing the eyes
  - Frontal headache on prolonged near-vision task.

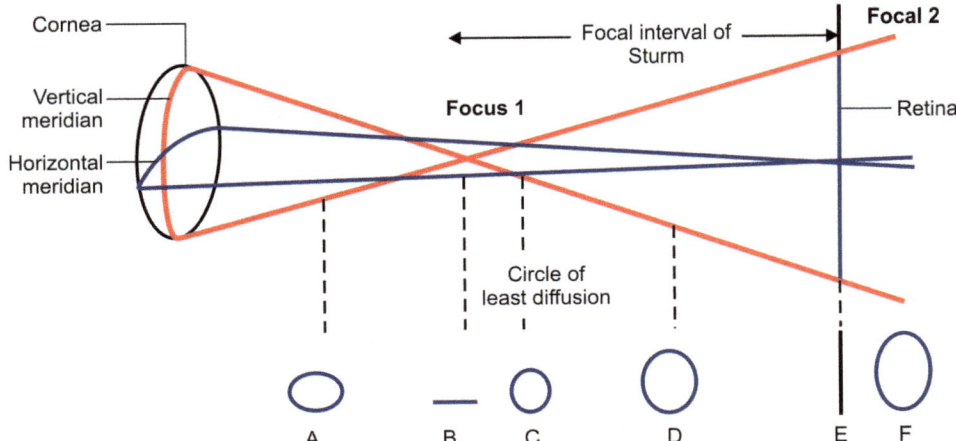

Fig. 5.16: Refraction by an astigmatic lens: Sturm's conoid. VV, the vertical meridian of the refracting body, is more curved than HH, the horizontal meridian. A, B, C, D, E, F and G show different sections of the beam after refraction. At B, the vertical rays are brought to a focus. From B to F is the focal interval of Sturm. D shows the circle of least diffusion.

	Description of rays	Cut section	Type of astigmatism
A	Vertical rays converging more than horizontal rays	Horizontally oval	Compound hypermetropic astigmatism
B	Vertical rays come to focus. Horizontal rays are still converging	Horizontal line (1st focus)	Simple hypermetropic astigmatism
C	Vertical rays are diverging. Horizontal rays still converging	Horizontally oval	Mixed astigmatism
D	Vertical rays diverged as much as horizontal rays have converged	Circle, called circle of least diffusion	Mixed astigmatism
E	Vertical rays diverging more than convergence of horizontal rays	Vertically oval	Mixed astigmatism
F	Vertical rays are diverging. Horizontal rays have come to a focus	Vertical line	Simple myopic astigmatism
G	Both vertical and horizontal rays are diverging	Vertically oval	Compound myopic astigmatism

5. Write short notes on anisometropia.

Optical condition of the eye in which refraction of the two eyes differs in variety and degree.

Types

Congenital
- **Simple anisometropia**
  - One eye is emmetropic, other eye is ametropic.
- **Compound anisometropia**
  - Both eyes ametropic (either myopic or hypermetropic) but differ in degree.
- **Mixed anisometropia**
  - Both eyes are ametropic but differ in variety
  - One eye is hypermetropic
  - Other eye is myopic.

Acquired
- Unilateral cataract extraction
- One eye is hypermetropic
- Other eye is myopic.

Symptoms
- Eye strain due to aniseikonia (difference in size of retinal images)
- Diplopia.

Signs
- 0.25 D of difference causes 0.5% difference in size of retinal images
- Up to 5% difference in size can be tolerated
- > 3 D difference—no binocular single vision
- Uniocular vision one eye—normal, other eye—amblyopic
- Alternating vision:
  - Hypermetropic eye—for distance
  - Myopic eye—for near.

Treatment
- Suitable correcting lenses up to 3 D difference
- Contact lenses
- Secondary intraocular lens in uniocular aphakia
- Lasik correction.

6. Write short notes on presbyopia.

Physiological insufficiency of accommodation due to advancing age.

Etiology
- Hardening of lens with age
- Weakness of ciliary muscle and suspensory ligaments
- Excessive close work
- Prodromal stage of closed-angle glaucoma.

Symptoms
- Blurring of vision for near work
- Vision improves if held further away
- Depends on existing error of refraction
  - In hypermetropia—early onset
  - In myopia—delayed onset.

Treatment

Prescribing suitable convex spherical lenses in diopters:
- 40 years: + 1
- 45 years: + 1.5
- 50 years: + 2
- 55 years: + 2.5
- 60 years and above : + 3

Correction for near work is added to correcting lenses for distant vision. Conductive keratoplasty and multifocal intraocular lens (IOL) are the refractive surgeries done for presbyopia.

7. Write short notes on aphakia.

Aphakia

Absence of lens in pupillary space.

Causes
- Trauma
- Surgical.

Optical Condition
- High hypermetropia: Parallel rays of light reach a focus about 31 mm behind cornea
- Loss of accommodation
- Usually astigmatism against the rule. Surgical scar at the corneoscleral junction in upper part flattens the vertical meridian of cornea.

Symptoms
- Gross dimness of vision because of acquired high hypermetropia.

Signs
- Linear corneoscleral scar mark in upper half of cornea
- Iris—peripheral buttonhole iridectomy near 12 o'clock position
- Anterior chamber—deep
- Iris—iridodonesis (tremulousness of the iris, better appreciated on rapid vertical movement of eye)

- Anterior chamber—deep
- Pupil—jet black
- Purkinje-Sanson image—3rd and 4th absent.

Treatment
- Spectacles
- Contact lens
- Secondary intraocular lens implantation
- Refractive corneal surgery
  - Keratophakia
  - Epikeratophakia
  - LASIK
  - Conductive keratoplasty: Radiofrequency waves are used to create burns in peripheral cornea. It works on the principle of thermokeratoplasty. For emmetropic presbyopes, it is done on the nondominant eye while for a hyperopic presbyope, it is done bilaterally.

Spectacles
Suitable spherical convex lens +10 D spherical and convex cylindrical lens + 1 D to + 3 D cyl at 180°.

Usually prescribed 6 weeks after operation when the scar has healed completely.

Advantages
- Cheap and readily available
- Easy to handle by old person.

Disadvantages
- 25–30% retinal image magnification
- Spherical aberration causes pincushion effect. Greater refraction at periphery than at center
- Image distortion by prismatic effect of spectacle lenses. Distortion at periphery
- Peripheral regions (i.e. corners) are more magnified
- Chromatic aberration
- Peripheral visual fields are reduced
- Difficulty in coordination and orientation
- Cosmetic deficiency
- Jack-in-the-Box Phenomenon due to roving ring scotoma. Ring scotoma at 15° is caused due to prismatic effect at periphery of lens. Scotoma moves in opposite direction to motion of the eye.

When the patient sees an object, he turns his eye toward it. Scotoma moves inward to occlude it. On shifting the eye, scotoma again shifts, the object becomes visible again to pop in and out of view. This is called roving ring scotoma.

Keratophakia
Lenticule prepared from the donor cornea is placed between lamellae of patient's cornea.

Epikeratophakia
Lenticule stitched over the surface of patient's cornea after removing the epithelium.

8. Write short notes on retinoscopy.

Definition
- Also called skiascopy or shadow test.
- Objective method of finding out the error of refraction by the method of neutralization.

Principle
Based on the fact that when light is reflected from a mirror into the eye, the direction in which the light moves across the pupil varies with the refraction of the eye.

Procedure
Patient to sit at a distance of 1 m from the examiner.

Light is thrown from the retinoscope into the patient's eye. Patient fixes a spot of light at the far end of the room to relax accommodation.

Through a hole in the retinoscope, the examiner observes a red reflex in the pupillary area of the patient.

The retinoscope is moved horizontally and vertically and the movement of shadow is observed.

Observation and Inference
- No movement of red reflex—myopia of 1 D.
- Movement of red reflex along the movement of retinoscope—emmetropia or hypermetropia or myopia of < 1 D.
- Against movement of red reflex—myopia of > 1 D.

Greater the ametropia, slower the movement and duller the reflex.

To Assess the Degree of Error
Movement of red reflex is neutralized by the addition of increasing convex lenses when the red reflex moves with the movement of the retinoscope.

Concave lenses are used if the red reflex moves against the movement of the retinoscope.

By altering the lenses, movements both horizontal and vertical meridians are neutralized to assess the degree of error in spherical and cylindrical forms.

End Point in Retinoscope
With plane mirror retinoscope, neutralization of red reflex in all meridians.

With streak retinoscope, streak disappears and pupil appears completely illuminated or completely dark.

Amount of Refractive Error
- Retinoscopy value.
- Deduction for distance (at which retinoscopy is done)
  - 1 D for 1 m
  - 1.5 D for 2/3rd m.
- Deduction for cycloplegics
  - 1 D for atropine
  - 0.5 D for homatropine and tropicamide
  - 0.75 D for cyclopentolate.

If retinoscopy values along the horizontal and vertical meridians are equal, there is no astigmatism. This needs correction only with spherical glasses.

If retinoscopy values along the horizontal and vertical meridians are unequal, it denotes presence of astigmatism which can be corrected by cylindrical lenses or in combination with spherical lenses.

9. Write short notes on contact lens.
Transparent plastic device worn over anterior most part eyeball.

Principle
Alters the vergence power of anterior surface of cornea. It substitutes the anterior surface of cornea.

Types
- Hard
- Semisoft or rigid gas permeable
- Soft.

Hard Lens
- Made of polymethyl methacrylate (PMMA)
- Plastic nontoxic material
- The diameter varies from 8.5 mm to 10 mm.

Advantage: Durable.
Disadvantages: Corneal hypoxia, corneal edema, foreign body sensation.

Semisoft or Rigid Gas Permeable
- Made of hard and soft material
- Silicone, cellulose acetate butyrate (CAB), silicone with PMMA.

Advantage: Minimal corneal hypoxia.
Disadvantage: May break, slight foreign body sensation.

Soft Lens
- Made of hydroxyethyl methacrylate (HEMA) or its polymer
- It is 1–2 mm larger than the corneal diameter.

Advantage: Stable and comfortable.
Disadvantage: Delicate and less durable.

Indications for Contact Lenses
- **Optical**
  - Provides normal field of vision
  - Eliminate aberration of glasses
  - Cosmetically more pleasant when glasses are thick.
- **Therapeutic**
  - Heals epithelial defect in filamentary keratitis and corneal erosion
  - Used as vehicle for drug delivery in glaucoma.
  - Encourages natural healing process in descemetocele and wound leaks.
- **Occupational**
  - In athletics, actors, boxers.
- **Diagnostic**
  - Gonioscopy
  - Fundus photography
  - Corneal thickness measurement.

Complications
If proper precautions like good hygiene are not followed, corneal ulcer and giant papillary conjunctivitis can occur.

Advantages of Contact Lens when Compared to Spectacles
- Produce less magnification
- Better field of vision
- Cosmetically better
- Less aniseikonia and more chances of binocularity in anisometropia
- Rain and fog do not fall on contact lens as in spectacles.

Contraindications
- Active ocular diseases
- Inflammatory diseases of lids, conjunctiva and cornea
- Corneal anesthesia
- Dry eye
- Hot dirty atmosphere.

10. What are the refractive surgeries done for refractive errors?

Refractive error	Cornea	Lens
Myopia	PRK LASIK Radial keratotomy Intrastromal rings	Clear lens extraction Phakic intraocular lens (IOL) Implantable contact lens
Hypermetropia	PRK LASIK Thermokeratoplasty	Phakic IOL
Astigmatism	Arcuate keratotomy	Toric IOL implantation
Presbyopia	Conductive keratoplasty	Multifocal IOL

11. Describe the principles of refractive surgery.

Refractive surgeries aim to reshape the cornea in order to eliminate the refractive errors.
- Radial keratotomy: Radial incisions centered on pupil are performed with diamond knife. These incisions are 80 to 90% of corneal thickness. This produces flattening of cornea thus correcting myopia.
- Laser based photoablation procedures:
  A. Surface ablation procedures
   a. Phtorefractive keratectomy (PRK): Epithelium is removed using laser.
   b. LASEK: Alcohol solution is used to abrade the epithelium
   c. Epi LASIK: Microkeratome is used to scrape off the epithelium.
   In all these excimer laser procedure is performed and a bandage contact lens is placed. Epithelium regenerates in a few days.
  B. Lamellar laser procedures: A microkeratome or Femtosecond laser is used to create a flap. The flap is everted on its hinge and the stroma is exposed for laser ablation. After ablation flap is reflected back in its original position.
- Laser in hyperopia: Central area is steepened by ablation of doughnut shaped area in the midperiphery of cornea.
- Relaxing incisions and astigmatic keratotomy can be done to flatten the more curved meridian in astigmatism.
- Presbyopia: Conductive keratoplasty (radiofrequency burns are applied to corneal periphery) and multifocal lenses are used.

CHAPTER 6

Conjunctiva

INTRODUCTION AND APPLIED ANATOMY

It is the mucous membrane lining the surface of the eye and the inner surface of eyelids. Since it joins the eyeball and the lids, it is called conjunctiva.

It consists of three parts:
i. Palpebral conjunctiva: Inner lining of the lids
ii. Bulbar conjunctiva: Lines the anterior sclera
   - Epithelium ⎤
   - Adenoid layer ⎦ Stroma
iii. Fornices: It joins the bulbar and the palpebral conjunctiva.

Glandular Tissues of Conjunctiva

- **Accessory lacrimal glands**
  - Glands of Krause
    » 42 in upper fornix
    » 8 in lower fornix.
  - Glands of Wolfring
    » Situated along the upper border of superior tarsus and lower border of inferior tarsus.
- **Mucin-secreting glands**
  - Goblet cells—located within the epithelium
  - Crypts of Henle—located along upper third of superior tarsal conjunctiva and lower third of inferior tarsal conjunctiva
  - Glands of Manz—encircles the limbus.

Blood Supply

- Anterior conjunctival artery (branch of anterior ciliary artery)
- Posterior conjunctival artery (branch of lacrimal artery)
- Palpebral branch of nasal arteries.
- The veins drain into venous plexus of the eyelids.

Lymphatics

- From lateral half drain into preauricular nodes
- From medial half drain into submandibular nodes.

Nerve Supply

Ophthalmic division of trigeminal nerve.

Normal Flora of Conjunctiva

- *Staphylococcus epidermidis, Propionibacterium epidermidis*
- *Corynebacterium xerosis* and diphtheroids.

1. Classify conjunctivitis. Discuss the etiology, clinical features and treatment of acute mucopurulent conjunctivitis.

Conjunctivitis

It is the inflammation of the conjunctiva which is characterized by hyperemia and discharge.

Classification of Conjunctivitis

Based on Duration
- Acute: Lasts less than 4 weeks
- Subacute or chronic: More than 4 weeks.

Based on Type of Discharge
- Serous: Viral, allergic or toxic
- Catarrhal: Allergic
- Mucopurulent: Bacterial, chlamydial
- Purulent: Bacterial
- Membranous and pseudomembranous: Bacterial.

Based on Etiology
- Infectious
- Noninfectious.

Infectious

- *Bacterial:* Staphylococcus aureus, Haemophilus aegyptius (Koch-Weeks bacillus), Streptococcus pyogenes, Streptococcus pneumoniae, Neisseria gonorrhoeae, Neisseria meningitidis, Moraxella.
- *Viral:* Herpes simplex, adenovirus, picornavirus, myxovirus (measles), paramyxovirus (mumps), Newcastle virus, molluscum contagiosum.
- *Chlamydial:* Trachoma (A–C), acute inclusion conjunctivitis (D–K).
- *Fungal:* Aspergillus, Candida, Nocardia.
- *Parasitic.*

Noninfectious

Allergic
- Acute or subacute allergic conjunctivitis
- Type 1 hypersensitivity reaction to pollen and other exogenous allergens
- Vernal conjunctivitis
- Giant papillary conjunctivitis
- Phlyctenular conjunctivitis
- *Irritants (physical, foreign body, contact lens use, radiation)*
  - Dry eye
  - Toxic (chemical or drug induced).

Types and causative organisms.

Ocular disease	Caused by
Mucopurulent	*Haemophilus aegyptius*, staphylococci, streptococci
Purulent	Gonococci
Angular conjunctivitis (diplobacillary conjunctivitis)	Morax-Axenfeld
Swimming pool conjunctivitis (adult inclusion conjunctivitis)	Serotypes D to K of *Chlamydia trachomatis*
Trachoma	*Chlamydia trachomatis* (serotypes A to C)
Epidemic keratoconjunctivitis	Adenoviruses type 8 and 19
Pharyngoconjunctival fever	Adenovirus type 3 and 7
Acute hemorrhagic conjunctivitis (Apollo conjunctivitis)	Picornaviruses (enterovirus type 70)

Acute Mucopurulent Conjunctivitis

Etiology
- *Staphylococcus aureus*
- *Haemophilus aegyptius* (Koch-Weeks bacillus)
- Transmission: Contagious
- Transmitted directly by discharge and fomites.

Clinical Features
- **Mild form**
  - Catarrhal inflammation of conjunctiva
  - Hyperemia and mucus discharge
  - Stickiness of lids in the morning.
- **Severe form**
  - Conjunctiva—fiery red
  - Flakes of mucopus
  - Halos may be seen due to mucus passing across the cornea
  - Chemosis.
- **Acute severe form**
  - Purulent conjunctivitis—gonococci infection
  - Lids swelling and copious purulent discharge
  - Presents as:
    » Ophthalmia neonatorum in newborn
    » Acute purulent conjunctivitis in adults.

Complications
Abrasion in cornea may become infected and result in corneal ulcer.

Treatment
- Control of infection
- Often self-limiting
- **Broad-spectrum antibiotic eye drops**—ciprofloxacin, ofloxacin, gatifloxacin, moxifloxacin
  - Six times daily.
  - Eye ointment at bedtime
  - Frequent wash with warm saline to clean crust and discharge.
- **Preventive measure:**
  - The patient must keep his hands clean
  - Towel, handkerchief, pillow or others fomites used by the patient must kept separate.

2. Discuss the etiology, clinical features, complications and treatment of acute purulent conjunctivitis.

It is characterized by profuse purulent discharge. It occurs in two forms:
  i. Purulent conjunctivitis of newborn (ophthalmia neonatorum) (discussed below)
  ii. Purulent conjunctivitis of adult.
  Acute purulent conjunctivitis of adults is usually unilateral and associated with urethritis and arthritis.

Etiology
- More common in men
- Gonococcus is a common causative organism
- Mixed infection can occur with staphylococci and streptococci.

Symptoms
- Swelling of the lids
- Marked sticking of lids
- Purulent discharge.

Signs
- Lids are swollen, red and tender
- Marked conjunctival congestion with chemosis
- Preauricular lymph nodes are tender and enlarged.

Complications
- Cornea becomes hazy and central ulcer may form. Marginal ulcer may also occur.
- Iridocyclitis.

Treatment
- Protect the unaffected eye by prompt control of infection in the affected eye.
- Prophylactic treatment in the normal eye by antibiotic eye drops.
- Treatment of affected eye: Repeated irrigation, intensive therapy with moxifloxacin eye drops 2 hourly and erythromycin or azithromycin eye ointment at bedtime. Atropine is applied if cornea or uvea is involved. Injection ceftriaxone 1 g IM is given as a single dose. In severe cases, the injection is given for 3 days.

3. Describe the etiology, clinical features, differential diagnosis and management of ophthalmia neonatorum.

Bilateral conjunctivitis of newborn is characterized by copious purulent discharge and marked chemosis of conjunctiva and swelling of lids.

Etiology

- Contacted during birth from mother's infected genitourinary tract
- **Established pathogens are:**
  - *Neisseria gonorrhoeae*
  - *Staphylococcus aureus*
  - *Streptococcus pneumoniae*
  - *Staphylococcus haemolyticus*
  - *Escherichia coli*
  - *Chlamydia*
  - Herpes simplex virus.

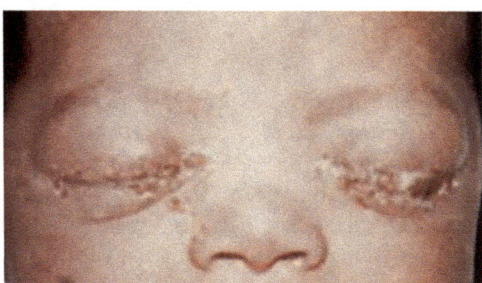

Fig. 6.1: Ophthalmia neonatorum.

Clinical Features

- Manifests in first week after birth
- Watery secretion (Tears are not secreted for first 6 weeks after birth)
- Become mucopurulent and purulent
- Infant is irritable
- Marked chemosis
- Swollen eyelids.

Diagnostic features.			
Causes	Onset	Discharge	Smear and culture
Silver nitrate	Within few hours	Slight watery and mucus	Negative culture
Gonococcus	2–4 days	Copious purulent discharge	Intracellular gram-negative diplococci culture positive on blood agar
Nongonococcal bacteria (S. aureus, S. pneumoniae)	4–5 days	Mucopurulent	Gram-positive or gram-negative organism Positive culture
Herpes simplex	5–7 days	Watery	Multinucleated giant cells, cytoplasmic inclusion bodies and negative culture
Chlamydia	5–14 days	Mucopurulent	Cytoplasmic inclusion bodies and negative culture

Complications

- Corneal ulcer just below the center of pupil prone to perforation
- Leukoma
- Anterior staphyloma
- Phthisis bulbi.

Differential Diagnosis

- Congenital dacryocystitis—only watering and mild discharge
  - No chemosis and edema of lids
- Congenital glaucoma—increased corneal diameter and raised intraocular pressure.

Treatment

Prophylaxis

- Prenatal diagnosis and treatment of birth canal infections
- Aseptic delivery
- Cleaning the lids with sterile gauze
  - Bacitracin and polymyxin B eye drops
  - Povidone-iodine 2.5% drops.

Curative

- Irrigation with warm saline
  - Gonococcus—penicillin or broad-spectrum eye drops
- Penicillin 5,000–10,000 units/mL every minute for 30 minutes
- Every 5 minutes for next 30 minutes till infection is controlled
- Injection ceftriaxone 25–50 mg/kg IV or IM—single dose
  - Nongonococcal bacteria
- Neomycin or bacitracin eye ointment
- Gentamicin, tobramycin or moxifloxacin eye drops
  - Chlamydia
- Topical erythromycin or tetracycline ointment
- Atropine to be used if cornea is involved
- Erythromycin syrup 50 mg/kg/day in four divided doses for 2–3 weeks
  - Herpes simplex
- Acyclovir 3% eye ointment 5 times a day for one week
- Systemic acyclovir for systemic involvement.

4. Write short notes on angular conjunctivitis.

This is chronic bacterial conjunctivitis caused by Moraxella-Axenfeld diplobacillus. It produces proteolytic enzyme which macerates the epithelium of the conjunctiva, lid margin and the skin surrounding angle of eye.

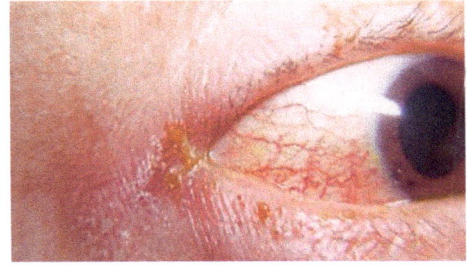

Fig. 6.2: Angular conjunctivitis.

Symptoms
- Redness in the angle of eye.
- Irritation and discomfort with frequent blinking.
- White foamy discharge at the angle of eye.

Signs
- Hyperemia of the conjunctiva limited to intermarginal strip at the inner and outer canthi and neighboring bulbar conjunctiva.
- Excoriation of skin at outer and inner canthi.
- Foamy mucopurulent discharge at the angles.

Complications
Blepharitis and marginal corneal ulcer.

Treatment
- **Prophylaxis:** Treatment of associated nasal infection and good personal hygiene.
- **Curative:**
  - Oxytetracycline 1% eye ointment 2-3 times daily for 10-14 days.
  - Zinc lotion in daytime and zinc oxide ointment at bedtime for the lids. It inhibits proteolytic enzymes and thus helps in reducing the maceration of skin at canthi.

5. Write short notes on follicular conjunctivitis.

Herpes and adenovirus most commonly cause conjunctival reaction by way of follicles particularly in lower conjunctiva.
- **Acute follicular conjunctivitis**
  - Inclusion conjunctivitis by *Chlamydia* serotype D-K (oculogenital)
  - Epidemic keratoconjunctivitis by adenovirus type 8 and 19
  - Pharyngoconjunctival fever by adenovirus type 3 and 7
  - Newcastle conjunctivitis by Newcastle virus
  - Herpetic keratoconjunctivitis by herpes simplex virus.
- **Trachoma—*Chlamydia trachomatis* A-C serotypes.**
- Coronavirus (Covid 19)
- Subacute or chronic follicular conjunctivitis can be caused by drugs such as pilocarpine and local lid lesions by molluscum contagiosa.
- Treatment: As per cause and decongestant and lubricant eye drops.
- Topical antibiotics to prevent superadded bacterial infection.

6. Describe the etiology, clinical features, differential diagnosis and treatment of acute membranous conjunctivitis (and pseudomembranous conjunctivitis).

Acute inflammation of the conjunctiva is associated with formation of a membrane or pseudomembrane on the palpebral conjunctiva.

Etiology
- *Corynebacterium diphtheriae*
- *Streptococcus haemolyticus*
- *Streptococcus pneumoniae*
- *Neisseria gonorrhoeae*
- *Staphylococcus aureus*
- Adenovirus.

Pathology
The membrane may be false or true. It appears as a result of coagulative response to infection or toxic agents. In pseudomembrane, a coagulum consisting of fibrin, mucus and pus is deposited on the surface of epithelium, while in true membrane the epithelial layers undergo coagulative necrosis. The removal of pseudomembrane leaves an intact epithelium, while a raw bleeding surface is left behind following removal of true membrane.

Age group: Common in children 2-8 years.

Clinical Features
- **Mild cases:** Mucopurulent discharge, mild chemosis and lid swelling—pseudomembrane.
- **Severe cases:** Patient toxic and acutely ill, lids—swollen, red and tense.
- **Stages:**
  - Stage of infiltration: Chemosis, membrane, regional lymphadenopathy
  - Stage of suppuration: Cornea may ulcerate, necrosed conjunctiva sloughed out. Lasts for 6-10 days
  - Stage of cicatrization: Symblepharon. Cicatrization of conjunctiva leads to xerosis and entropion.

Differential diagnosis.	
Membranous conjunctivitis	**Pseudomembranous conjunctivitis**
Corynebacterium diphtheriae and Streptococcus haemolyticus	Pneumococcus, streptococcus, adenovirus
Fibrinous exudates over and within conjunctival epithelium	Fibrous exudates over the conjunctival epithelium
Bleeds on peeling	Does not bleed
Rx: Antidiphtheria serum 4–10,000 units in 12 hours	Broad-spectrum antibiotics

Treatment
Preventive
- Immunization
- Isolation of patient.

Curative
- Penicillin eye drops 10,000 units/mL every hour
- Atropine eye ointment if cornea is involved
- Broad-spectrum antibiotic eye ointment at bedtime
- Antidiphtheritic serum (ADS) every 1 hour
- ADS 50,000 units single dose or 10,000 units every 12 hourly
- Crystalline penicillin 500,000 units IM bd.

7. Discuss the etiology, clinical features, differential diagnosis and management of trachoma.

- Trachoma is a chronic keratoconjunctivitis primarily affecting the superficial epithelium of conjunctiva and cornea.

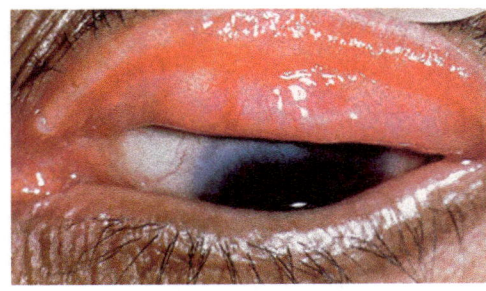

Fig. 6.3: Trachomatous scarring (Arlt's line) in upper lid conjunctiva.

- Also known as Egyptian ophthalmia.
- Endemic in Middle East.
- Common among people living in unhygienic and crowded surroundings.
- Spreads by transfer of conjunctival discharge by fingers, fomites or by flies.
- Incubation period is 7–21 days.

Pathology: Caused by *Chlamydia trachomatis* serotypes A, B and C.

Intracellular parasites are seen as inclusion bodies in epithelial cells. They are called as Halberstaedter-Prowazek bodies.

Clinical Features

- Diffuse congestion of conjunctiva
- Papillary enlargement and follicles
- Upper tarsus is more affected
- Cicatrization of follicles in the lids is seen as Arlt's line or as stellate scars
- Cornea—superficial keratitis—upper part of cornea is involved
- Trachomatous pannus—lymphocytic infiltration with vascularization of upper margin of cornea
- Herbert's pits—follicles at limbus leave pitted scars when they heal.

MacCallan's Classification

- *Incipient stage:* Hyperemia with immature follicles
- *Manifest stage:* Mature follicles, papilla and progressive pannus
- *Healing stage:* Conjunctival scarring, Herbet's pits (scars of healed trachomatous follicles at limbus)
- *Stage of sequela and complications:* Star-shaped conjunctival scarring.

Arlt's line—line of palpebral conjunctival scarring seen—2 mm from upper lid margin.

WHO Classification (FISTO)

- Trachomatous follicular inflammation (TF)
- Trachomatous intense inflammation (TI)
- Trachomatous scarring (TS)
- Trachomatous trichiasis (TT)
- Trachomatous corneal opacity (CO).

Complications

- Lid: Trichiasis, entropion, tylosis, madarosis
- Conjunctiva: Concretions, xerosis, symblepharon
- Cornea: Xerosis, pannus, opacity.

Investigation

- **Laboratory diagnosis:**
  - Study of conjunctival cytology—plasma and Leber cells
  - Inclusion body detection
  - Giemsa stain/immunofluorescent stain
  - Isolation of chlamydia—tissue culture.

Differential Diagnosis

- Follicular conjunctivitis—follicle more on lower palpebral conjunctiva and on fornix
- Spring catarrh (palpebral form)—cobblestone arrangement of papillae.

Treatment

- 1% tetracycline or erythromycin ointment bd × 1 week in each month for 6 months
- Systemic tetracycline 250 mg qid
- Doxycycline 100 mg bd × 4 weeks
- Azithromycin 20 mg/kg—single dose.

Safe Strategy

S—Surgery for trichiasis and entropion.
A—Antibiotics—oral azithromycin—single dose, to be repeated after 6 months.

Blanket treatment in endemic areas recommended by WHO is:
- Topical tetracycline ointment 1% twice daily for 5 days in a month for 6 months.

F—Facial cleanliness (personal hygiene).
E—Environmental hygiene: Supplying piped water, removal of rubbish for fly control, health education in community about spread of trachoma.

8. Write short notes on pannus.

It is a superficial vascularization and infiltration into the cornea between epithelium and Bowman's membrane or replacing Bowman's membrane.

Causes

- *Trachomatous:* Upper lid
  - Progressive—infiltration in front of vascularization
  - Regressive—infiltration recedes vascularization
- *Phlyctenular:* Due to phlycten
- *Lepromatous:* Associated with interstitial keratitis
- *Degenerative:* Bullous keratopathy, Fuchs' dystrophy
- Micropannus:
  - Vernal conjunctivitis
  - Superior limbic conjunctivitis
- Contact lens.

Treatment

- Limbal peritomy and cauterization in progressive cases.
- Treat the cause.

9. Discuss the etiology, clinical features, differential diagnosis and treatment of vernal catarrh.

It is a recurrent bilateral allergic conjunctivitis occurring with the onset of hot weather. It is also known as spring catarrh.

Etiology

- Allergic reaction to exogenous allergen like pollen or dust
- Type I hypersensitivity reaction
- More in summer
- Common in boys (5-10 years)
- 2/3rd—family history
- 3/4th—associated atopy (asthma, eczema).

Clinical Features

- Intense itching—main symptom
- Thick, white, ropy mucus discharge
- Maxwell-Lyon's sign—stringy conjunctival discharge and fibrinous pseudomembrane
- Burning and foreign body sensation
- Photophobia and watering if cornea is involved.

Signs

- **Types:**
  - Palpebral
  - Bulbar
  - Mixed.

Palpebral form

- Conjunctival hyperemia
- Papillary hypertrophy
  - Mostly in upper tarsal region
  - Cobblestone arrangement of papilla
  - Flat-topped polygonal appearance
  - Varying size and shape.
- Epithelium over the nodules which consists of dense fibrous tissue is thickened giving milky hue appearance.
- Fornices are not involved.

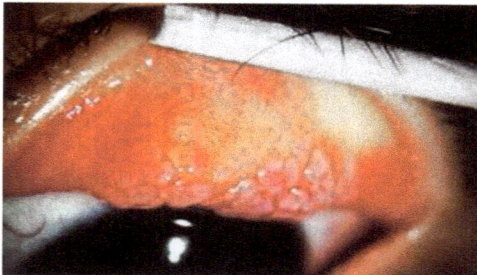

Fig. 6.4: Palpebral form.

Bulbar Form

- Mucoid nodules around limbus.
- Gelatinous thickening of superior limbus—pseudo-gerontoxon or Cupid's bow.
- Dusky red congestion in interpalpebral area.
- **Horner-Trantas spots—seen at limbus**
  - Discrete chalky white superficial spots in cornea composed of degenerated eosinophils and epithelial debris.
- **Keratopathy:**
  - *Punctate epithelial erosion* (micro- and macroerosions)
  - *Plaque formation:* When the base of ulcer gets coated by mucus results in defective wetting—prevents re-epithelialization.

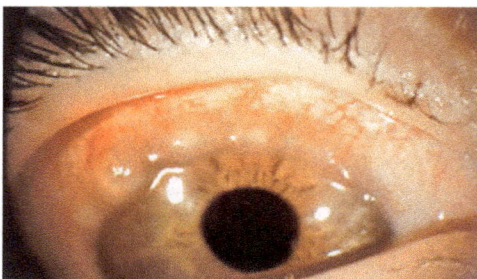

Fig. 6.5: Bulbar form with pseudogerontoxon.

- Pseudogerontoxon—resembles arcus senilis—gelatinous thickening of tissues around limbus—Cupid's bow
  - Shield ulcer: It occurs due to rubbing of hypertrophied papillae in superior cornea as gray-white infiltrates
    » Shallow transverse ulcer in upper part of cornea
    » Ulcer is due to epithelial macroerosions.

Mixed Form

- Both features are seen.

Differential Diagnosis

- **Giant papillary conjunctivitis (GPC):**
  - In spring catarrh, papillae are of varying sizes and shapes resembling cobblestone
  - In GPC, papillae are larger than 3 mm in diameter, similar in shape.
- **Trachoma:**
  - In trachoma, papillae are seen in fornices and scarring is also seen
  - In spring catarrh, milky hue of papilla, sparing of fornices, seasonal nature.

Treatment

- Cold compress and dark glasses provide symptomatic relief.
- **Topical steroids:**
  - 0.1% dexamethasone or betamethasone
  - 3-4 times daily
  - Loteprednol 0.5% or fluorometholone 1%
- Antihistamine eye drops
- **Mast cell stabilizers:**
  - Sodium cromoglycate 2% tds
  - Ketotifen 1%
  - Azelastine HCl 0.05%
  - Olopatadine HCl 0.1% bd
- Acetylcysteine 10 to 20% eye drops, 3-4 times daily for 1 to 2 weeks, for mucolysis of excess mucus.
- Supratarsal injection of betamethasone or triamcinolone in severe cases
- Topical Cyclosporin A eye drops 0.1% twice daily in steroid-resistant cases
- Tacrolimus eye ointment to 0.03% twice daily (immuno-suppressant) in refractory cases
- **Surgical management** is required for severe shield ulcer which is to be scraped to remove superficial plaque before re-epithelialization occurs.
- **Systemic:** Oral antihistamines.

10. Describe the etiology, clinical features, differential diagnosis and treatment of phlyctenular conjunctivitis.

It is nodular lesion of cornea and conjunctiva due to delayed hypersensitivity response (type IV) to endogenous allergen (microbial proteins) TB, staphylococci, parasitic worms infestation.

Phlycten is pinkish white nodule surrounded by hyperemia of bulbar conjunctiva near limbus. It is common in children between 4 years and 14 years. Unhygienic conditions and malnutrition are important predisposing factors.

Symptoms

Reflex lacrimation, irritation and mild discharge. If cornea is involved, pain and photophobia are present.

Pathology: It is composed of compact mass of mononuclear lymphocytes and polymorphs underneath the epithelium.

Types

- Necrotizing: Large nodules with necrosis and ulceration
- Miliary: Several nodules in a ring-like arrangement
- Simple: Single pink nodule near limbus on bulbar conjunctiva.

Corneal Involvement

- Diffuse infiltrative keratitis
- **Fascicular ulcer** with serpiginous character. The fascicular ulcer is followed from periphery by a leash of vessels. Superficial ulcer—does not perforate.

Differential Diagnosis

- Foreign body granuloma
- Acute mucopurulent conjunctivitis
- Episcleritis
- Inflamed pinguecula.

In acute mucopurulent conjunctivitis, congestion is seen on whole conjunctiva, whereas in phlyctenular conjunctivitis congestion is seen only around the phlycten.

	Phlyctenular conjunctivitis	Inflamed pinguecula	Episcleritis
Age	<15 years	>50 years	16–40 years
Site	Usually on limbus	Nasal side of limbus	Away from limbus usually on temporal side
Shape	Small raised round nodule	Flat and triangular	Relatively bigger flat, round nodule
Discharge	Mucopurulent	No discharge	Watery
Regional lymph nodes	Enlarged	Not enlarged	Enlarged

Treatment

- Dexamethasone with antibiotic eye drops or ointment
- Septic foci to be treated.
- Parasitic infection should be treated
- Treatment of tuberculosis if present.

11. Differentiate papillae from follicles.

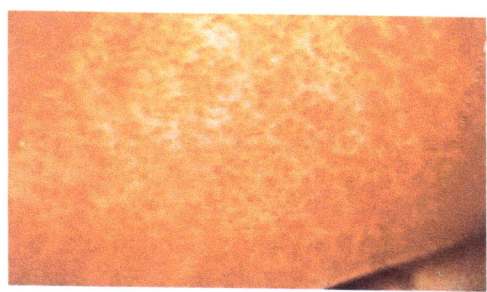

Fig. 6.6: Papillae.

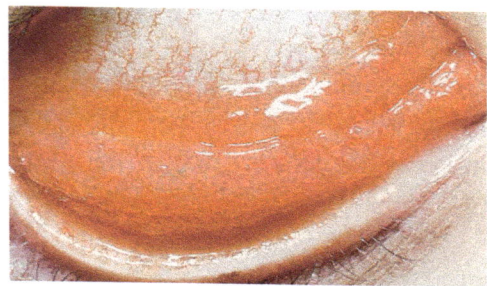

Fig. 6.7: Follicles.

Features	Papillae	Follicles
Appearance	Irregular, flattened conjunctival elevation enclosing vascular core	Opalescent, ovoid elevation similar to rice grains, vessels surrounding the follicles
Structure	Hyperplastic epithelium enclosing vascular tuft, chronic inflammatory infiltration	Foci of hyperplastic lymphoid tissue
Size	<1 mm (except in giant papillary conjunctivitis, GPC)	0.5–5 mm
Site	Common in upper palpebral conjunctiva	Common in lower palpebral conjunctiva
Diseases	Bacterial and allergic conjunctivitis, chronic conjunctivitis	Viral, chlamydial conjunctivitis and toxic reactions Herpes, trachoma, EKC due to drugs—IDU
Pathology	Core of blood vessels surrounded by inflammatory cells. Vascular and epithelial hypertrophy	Hyperplasia of lymphoid tissue followed by secondary vascularization

12. What are the degenerative conditions of conjunctiva?

- Concretions
- Pinguecula
- Pterygium
    - Concretions are yellowish white hard raised spots on the palpebral conjunctiva. These are due to accumulated epithelial cells and inspissated mucus

lodged in depressions called loops of Henle. These are seen in elderly people and in patients with scarring stage of trachoma. If they cause foreign body sensation and scratch the cornea, they can be removed by hypodermic needle under topical anesthesia.
- Pinguecula and pterygium are explained below.

13. Write short notes on pinguecula.

Small yellowish round or triangular spot raised from surface near limbus in the palpebral aperture, the base is toward limbus and apex away from the cornea.

Etiology: Exposure to sunlight, dust, wind, etc.

Pathogenesis: Hyaloid infiltration in substantia propria, elastotic degeneration of collagen of conjunctiva. May get inflamed.

Differential Diagnosis

Malignant epithelioma: Pinguecula and pterygium fluoresce in ultraviolet (UV) light, whereas malignant epithelioma does not.

Pterygium: Pinguecula never invades the cornea. In pinguecula, base is toward limbus, whereas in pterygium, apex is toward limbus.

Treatment

Lubricant eye drops. If yellow spots at edges appear—surgical removal for cosmesis.

14. Describe the etiology, clinical features, differential diagnosis and treatment of pterygium.

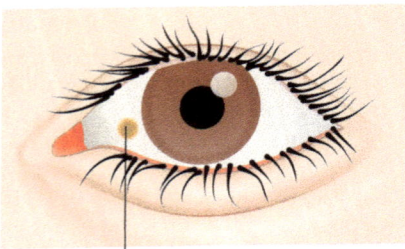
Pinguecula

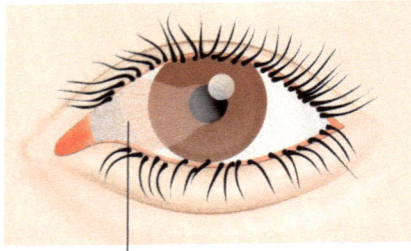
Pterygium

Fig. 6.8: Pinguecula and pterygium.

Definition

Triangular sheet of fibrovascular tissue which invades the cornea.

Etiology

- Damage to limbal stem cells by UV light
- Arises from pre-existing pinguecula
- Nutritional deficiency
- Genetic AD transmission with low penetration
- Exposure to dust, heat, chemicals
- Irritants and allergens
- Tear film deficiency.

Pathogenesis

It is an elastotic degeneration of the collagen fibers of substantia propria of conjunctiva with fibrovascular proliferation of subconjunctival tissue.

Symptoms

- Cosmesis
- Foreign body sensation
- Reduced visual acuity due to induced astigmatism (usually with the rule type due to flattening of horizontal meridian)

Clinical Features

Wing-shaped fold of fibrovascular tissue arising from the interpalpebral conjunctiva and extending onto the cornea. Pterygium is more common on nasal side because of:
- Reflection of light rays from nasal bone
- Irritation by waste products from collection of tears in medial canthus.

Parts of Pterygium

- Cap—infiltration in front of the head
- Head—apical part present on the cornea
- Neck—limbal part
- Body—bulbar part.

Types

Progressive, regressive or atrophic.

Stocker's Line

A curvilinear deposit of iron within the corneal epithelium anterior to the advancing head of pterygium.

Differential Diagnosis

- Pseudopterygium
- Pinguecula
- Conjunctival intraepithelial neoplasia.

Pseudopterygium

Adhesion of fold of conjunctiva to the peripheral corneal ulcer. It is fixed only at its apex to the cornea, whereas pterygium is adherent to the underlying structures throughout.

Conjunctival Intraepithelial Neoplasia

Unilateral papillomatous jelly-like velvety mass—often elevated, vascularized not in wing-shaped configuration, not in typical 3/9 o'clock location of pterygium.

Treatment

Medical

Useful in early stages
- Lubricant and decongestant eye drops
- Ultraviolet protection glasses.

Surgical

Bare sclera technique (D'Ombrains' method)—simple excision. McReynolds' method—diversion of head of pterygium into lower fornix.

- To prevent recurrence—mitomycin C 0.02% drops during and after operation to prevent fibrosis
- Conjunctival limbal autograft or amniotic membrane graft after the excision of pterygium.
- Lamellar corneal graft may be needed for improving vision if pterygium causes corneal scar.

Differences between pterygium and pseudopterygium.		
	Pterygium	*Pseudopterygium*
Etiology	Degenerative process	Inflammatory process
Age	Occurs in elderly	Any age. It occurs due to chemical burns of the eye
Site	Situated in palpebral aperture	Can occur at any site
Stages	Progressive/regressive/stationary	Always stationary
Probe test	Probe cannot be passed underneath	Probe can be passed under its neck

15. Write short notes on nodule at the limbus.

- *Congenital:* Dermoid, dermolipoma, raised nevus
- *Inflammatory:* Episcleritis, nodular form of scleritis
- *Allergic:* Phlycten, vernal catarrh—bulbar type, ophthalmia nodosa
- *Vascular:* Hemangioma
- *Trauma:* Foreign body granuloma, implantation cyst, iris prolapse covered by conjunctiva
- *Degeneration:* Pinguecula, cystic pterygium
- *Nutritional:* Bitot's spots
- *Neoplasm:* Papilloma, epithelioma
- *Miscellaneous:* Intercalary or ciliary staphyloma, filtering bleb, retention cyst
- *Treatment:* Depends on the cause.

16. What is the differential diagnosis of red eye?

Important conditions are:
- Conjunctivitis
  - Infection—viral and bacterial
  - Noninfectious—allergic—episcleritis, scleritis dry eye, toxic/chemical reaction, foreign body.
- Keratitis
  - Infection—bacterial, viral, fungal, protozoal (*Acanthamoeba*)
  - Noninfectious—recurrent epithelial erosion, FB.
- Acute iridocyclitis.
- Acute angle-closure glaucoma.
- Injury—subconjunctival hemorrhage.
- Episcleritis and scleritis.
- Venous congestion.

17. Differentiate conjunctival congestion from ciliary congestion.

	Conjunctival congestion	*Ciliary congestion*
Color	Bright red	Purplish
Level of blood vessels	Superficial	Deep
Site	Intraconjunctival, most marked in fornices	Subconjunctival, marked around limbus
Vessels involved	Posterior and anterior conjunctiva	Ciliary vessels
Movement of conjunctiva	Vessels move with conjunctiva	Does not move
Associated discharge	Mucopurulent	Watery
Causes	Conjunctivitis	Diseases of anterior segment—cornea, sclera, uvea and glaucoma

18. Write short notes on subconjunctival hemorrhage.

Causes
- Local trauma
- Petechial hemorrhages—pneumococcal and apollo conjunctivitis

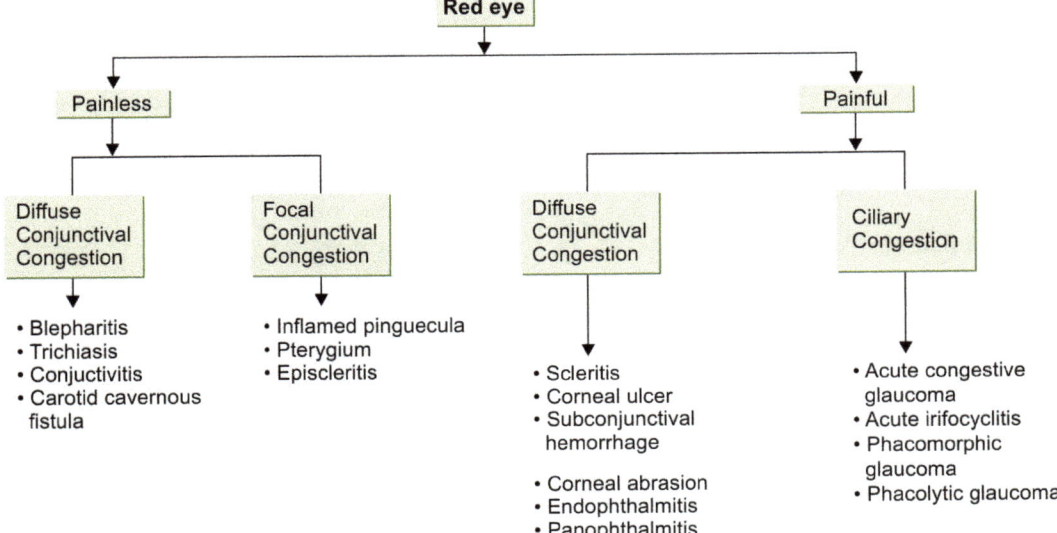

- Children with whooping cough
- Violent bout of vomiting
- Sudden and severe venous congestion of head
- Microvascular diseases—hypertension, diabetes mellitus, arteriosclerosis
- Bleeding disorders
- Injury to orbit and base of skull.

	Local injury	Base of skull
Onset	Immediate	After 12–24 hours
Color	Bright red	Bluish purple
Posterior limit	Seen	Not seen
Spread	Intraconjunctival	Truly subconjunctival
Movement with conjunctiva	Moves	Does not move

Treatment
- Reassurance
- Cold pack to closed eyes
- Vitamin C.

19. Discuss the pathology, ocular manifestations and treatment of vitamin A deficiency (xerophthalmia).

Vitamin A deficiency is one of the major causes of childhood blindness. It usually occurs in children 1–6 years of age. Most common in 1–3 years of age.

Pathology
- Epithelium become epidermoid
- Keratinizing metaplasia
- Vicarious activity of meibomian glands
- Fatty secretion cover instead of watery tears
- Corynebacterium xerosis profuse growth.

Types of Xerophthalmia
- Parenchymatous
- Epithelial.

Parenchymatous
Sequela of local ocular affections:
- Trachoma
- Burns—acids and alkalies
- Ocular pemphigoid
- Diphtheritic conjunctivitis
- Radiation.

Epithelial
- Due to vitamin A deficiency
- Ocular manifestations
  - Conjunctival
  - Corneal.

Conjunctival Manifestations
- Lack of luster
- Unwettability
- Wrinkling
- Pigmentation
- Accumulation of debris.

Xerosis

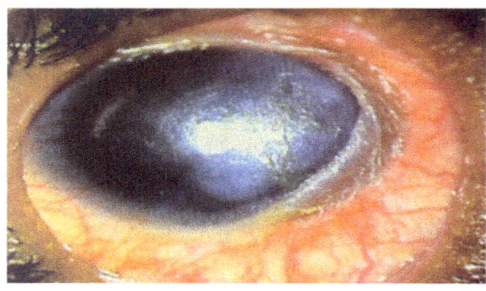

Fig. 6.9: Xerosis.

Bitot's Spots

It is a raised silvery white foamy triangular patch of keratinized epithelium situated on bulbar conjunctiva in the interpalpebral area.
- X1B, as per WHO xerophthalmia classification
- Classical sign
- Cheesy or foamy white material—not wetted by tears
- Seen on temporal conjunctiva
- Foam-like material is due to gas production by *Corynebacterium xerosis*.

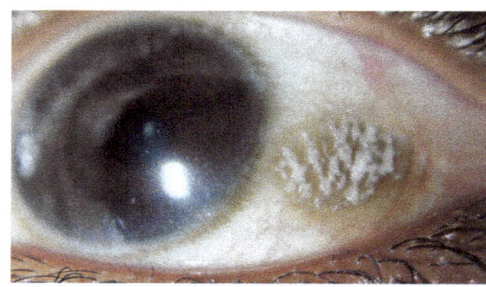

Fig. 6.10: Bitot's spot—foamy type.

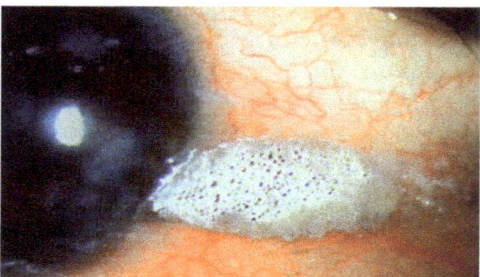

Fig. 6.11: Bitot's spot—cheesy type.

Corneal Manifestations
- Seen in advanced stage
- Lusterless cornea

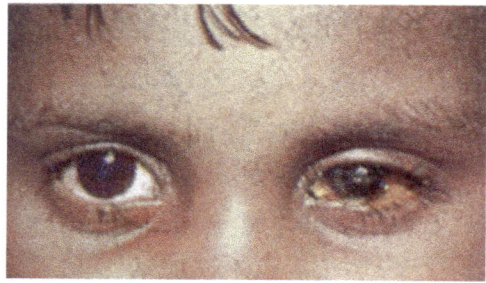

Fig. 6.12: Corneal ulcer with xerosis.

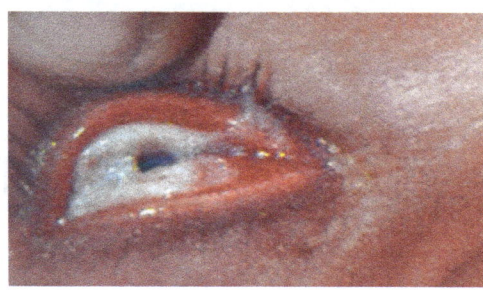

Fig. 6.13: Keratomalacia.

- Hazy cornea
- Exfoliation of epithelium
- Corneal stroma liquefaction
- **Keratomalacia:** It is an advanced stage of xerophthalmia wherein cornea melts and a large ulcer is formed. Perforation of the ulcer or thick corneal scarring results in blindness.

WHO Classification

Conjunctival xerosis	X1A
Bitot's spots	X1B
Corneal xerosis	X2
Corneal ulceration/keratomalacia Involving < 1/3 of cornea	X3A
Corneal ulceration/keratomalacia Involving > 1/3 of cornea	X3B

Secondary Signs

Night blindness	XN
Xerophthalmic fundus	XF (raised whitish lesions scattered in the fundus)
Xerophthalmic scar in cornea	XS

Vitamin A Deficiency

- Primary signs: X1A, X1B, X2, X3A, X3B
- Secondary signs: XN, XF, XS

Primary signs: All together should not exceed 0.01% in below 6 years age group.

Prophylaxis of Vitamin A Deficiency

- Health and nutrition education
- Vitamin A-rich foods
- Greens, spinach, *palak*, amaranth, and drumstick leaves
- Colored vegetables—carrots, beetroots, drumsticks, and cabbages
- Fruits—papayas and mangoes
- Others—milk and fish.

Foods Rich in Vitamin A

- Breastfeeding
- Home gardening
- Environmental sanitation
- Improved water supply
- Child spacing
- Vitamin A fortification
- Measles immunization
- Mega dose of vitamin A.

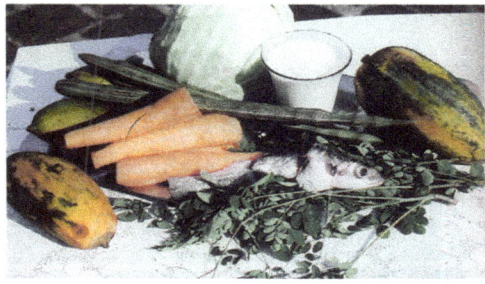

Fig. 6.14: Foods rich in vitamin A.

WHO Prophylaxis against Xerophthalmia

- Infants less than 6 months—50,000 IU orally
- Infants between 6 months and 1 year—100,000 IU orally every 6 months
- Children between 1 year and 6 years—200,000 IU orally every 6 months
- Lactating mothers—20,000 IU orally once at delivery or at next 2 months
- Vitamin A solution is given along with measles vaccination.

Treatment

- Three doses of 200,000 IU of vitamin A on day 0, 1, and 14
- Women of reproductive age with vitamin A deficiency—daily dose of 10,000 IU orally for 2 weeks
- Oral route is preferred
- Half the oral dose for intramuscular injection
- High protein, high calorie diet supplements of Zn, Fe and Cu.

For corneal involvement

- Systemic antibiotics for secondary infection
- Ocular lubricants
- Hydroxypropyl methyl cellulose
- 0.7% eye drops
- 2% ointment.

CHAPTER 7

Cornea

INTRODUCTION

The cornea is the transparent front part of the eye which resembles a *"watch glass"*.

Average diameter:
- Horizontal—12 mm
- Vertical—11 mm.

Thickness:
- Central part—0.5 mm
- Periphery—1 mm.

Structure

Cornea consists of six layers:

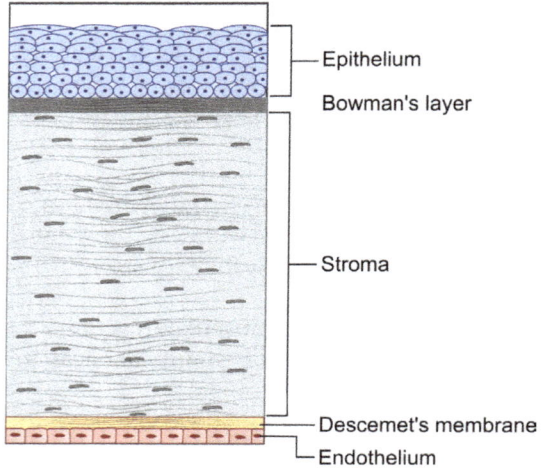

Fig. 7.1: Structure of cornea.

i. **Epithelium**
   - Continuous with the conjunctiva.
ii. **Bowman's membrane**
   - Made up of collagen fibrils
   - Does not regenerate when damaged
   - Leaves opacity on healing.
iii. **Stroma**
   - Consist of keratocytes
   - Corneal lamella arranged in parallel layers continuous with sclera.
iv. **Pre-Descemet's layer of Dua**
   - It is about 15 micrometers thick and strong with collagen fibers.
v. **Descemet's membrane**
   - This is a tough but elastic membrane.
vi. **Endothelium**
   - Single layer of hexagonal cells
   - Cell density 3,000 cells/mm^2
   - Decreases with age
   - Measured by specular microscopy.

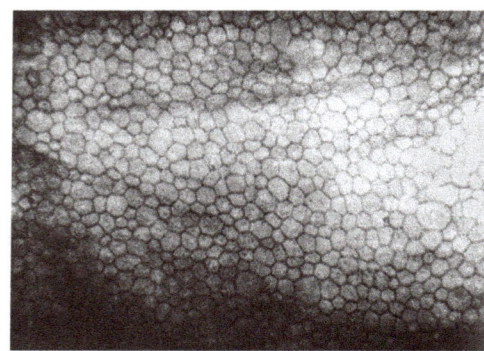

Fig. 7.2: Corneal endothelium.

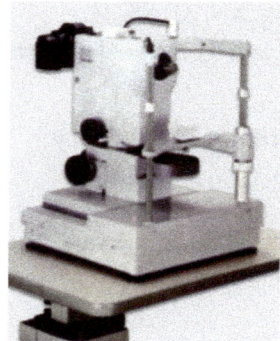

Fig. 7.3: Specular microscope.

Diseases affecting cornea:
- Diseases of conjunctiva affect epithelium
- Diseases of the sclera affect the stroma
- Diseases of the uveal tract affect the endothelium.

Nutrition of the Cornea

- Cornea is avascular
- Derives nutrition from:
  - Perilimbal blood vessels—anterior ciliary vessels
  - Aqueous humor
  - Tear film.

Nerve Supply

Nasociliary branch of ophthalmic division of trigeminal nerve.

Functions

- Two primary functions
  i. Acts as a major refracting medium
  ii. Protects the intraocular contents by maintaining corneal transparency and replacement of the tissues.

Transparency is maintained by:

- Regular arrangement of corneal lamella
- Avascularity
- Relative state of dehydration.

Diseases of the Cornea

- Inflammation
- Degeneration
- Ectasias.

Inflammation of the Cornea

Modes of Infection

- Exogenous—from organisms in the conjunctiva
- Contiguous spread from ocular tissues—owing to anatomical continuity
- Endogenous—due to hypersensitivity reaction.

1. What are the types of keratitis?

Keratitis is inflammation of cornea characterized by corneal edema, cellular infiltration and ciliary congestion. Superficial keratitis which is termed ulcerative keratitis is called corneal ulcer. In corneal ulcer, there is loss of corneal epithelium with inflammation of surrounding cornea.

Classification of Keratitis

Superficial

- Purulent keratitis or corneal ulcer
- Nonpurulent.

Deep

- Interstitial keratitis
- Disciform keratitis
- Sclerosing keratitis.

Superficial Keratitis

- **Purulent keratitis:**
  - Hypopyon corneal ulcer
  - Marginal ulcer
  - Mooren's ulcer.
- **Nonpurulent keratitis**
  - Herpes simplex and zoster
  - Adenovirus.

2. Discuss the etiology, stages, clinical features, and management of uncomplicated corneal ulcer.

Etiology

Two main factors:

i. Damage to corneal epithelium and infection of eroded area.
ii. Pathogens that invade intact epithelium:
   - *Neisseria gonorrhoeae*
   - *Neisseria meningitidis*
   - *Corynebacterium diphtheriae*.

Etiological agents from different corneal ulcers.	
Hypopyon ulcer or ulcus serpens or acute serpiginous ulcer	Pneumococcus
Mycotic corneal ulcer	*Aspergillus fumigatus*
Marginal corneal ulcer	Koch-Weeks bacillus or *Hemophilus aegyptius*
Dendritic ulcer	Herpes simplex
Rapidly progressive sloughing corneal ulcer	*Pseudomonas*
Fascicular ulcer	Phlyctenulosis
Atheromatous ulcer	Degenerative change in old leukoma
Mooren's ulcer or chronic serpiginous ulcer	Antigen-antibody reaction

Staphylococcus aureus, Streptococcus pneumoniae, N. gonorrhoeae, N. meningitidis, and *C. diphtheriae* also cause corneal ulcer.

Predisposing Factors

- **Epithelial damage:** Trauma
- **Virulent organisms:** Pneumococcus, *Pseudomonas*, gonococcus
- Poor resistance
- Xerosis and keratomalacia
- Protein calorie malnutrition
- Corneal edema
- **Neurotrophic keratitis:** 5th nerve palsy, herpes zoster, leprosy
- **Exposure keratitis:** 7th nerve palsy, proptosis.

Stages of Ulcer (Pathology)

- Stage of progressive infiltration
- Stage of active ulceration
- Stage of regression
- Stage of cicatrization.

Stage of Progressive Infiltration

- Infiltration with polymorphonuclear leukocytes and/or lymphocytes into epithelium and superficial stroma associated with necrosis.

Stage of Active Ulceration
Necrosis and sloughing of epithelium, Bowman's membrane and stroma. Ulcer is saucer-shaped with overhanging margins.

Stage of Regression
- Slough is cast off and edema decreases
- Floor and edges of ulcer become smooth
- Epithelium grown over the edges.

Stage of Cicatrization
- Vascularization occurs from limbus near ulcer
- Formation of fibrous tissue which fills the gap.

Clinical Features
Symptoms
Pain, photophobia, decreased vision, and lacrimation.

Signs
- Blepharospasm, corneal opacity
- Ciliary congestion, hypopyon
- Stains with fluorescein
- Slit lamp shows irregular margins of the ulcer.

Management of Corneal Ulcer
Investigations
Microbiological workup to identify invading organisms and drug of choice.

Corneal Scrapings
Under topical anesthesia, edge and base of ulcer are scraped with Kimura platinum spatula or reverse side of no. 15 surgical blade or Took's knife.

Direct Smear
- *Gram stain*—can identify 60–70% of bacterial infections
- *10% KOH mount*—to identify fungal filaments
- *Giemsa stain*—to identify cellular response, inclusion bodies and for cysts and trophozoites of *Acanthamoeba*
- *Gomori's methenamine silver stain*—to identify 90% of fungal infections.

Culture Sensitivity
- Inoculation with blood agar for aerobic organisms
- Thioglycolate broth for anaerobic organisms
- Sabouraud's medium for fungal organisms.

Treatment of Uncomplicated Corneal Ulcer
- Control of infection
- Treatment of pre-existing local conditions
- Rest
- Surgical
- General.

Control of Infection
- Pending smear and culture sensitivity reports, hourly broad-spectrum antibiotics
- 0.3% ciprofloxacin, ofloxacin, gatifloxacin eye drops or 0.5% moxifloxacin eye drops are effective against common pathogens like pneumococcus, *Pseudomonas* and *Staphylococcus*
- Change in antibiotic indicated if there is inadequate clinical response
- Appropriate antibiotics when the test results arrive
- Fortified cefazolin 5% (50 mg/mL)—10 mL of water to 500 mg vial
- Fortified tobramycin 1.3% (13.6 mg/mL)—2 ml of injection (40 mg/mL) to 5 mL of 0.3% eye drops

Differential diagnosis of corneal ulcer.			
S. No.	Features	Ulcer	Abrasion	Opacity
i.	Vision	Markedly affected	Unaffected	Variable, depends on depth and position of opacity
ii.	Pain	Present	Mild	Absent
iii.	Discharge	Present	Absent	Absent
iv.	Watering and photophobia	Present	Present	Absent/mild
v.	Invasion of microorganisms	Yes	No	No
vi.	Corneal epithelial discontinuity	Yes	Yes	Replaced by scar tissue
v.	Surrounding area	Edematous	Normal	Usually normal
vi.	Staining with fluorescein	Present	Present	Absent

Differential diagnosis of types of corneal ulcer.							
S. No.	Features	Bacterial	Fungal	Viral	Protozoal (Acanthamoeba)	Degenerative	Nutritional
i.	Discharge	Mucopurulent	Thick, curdy	Serous	Absent	Absent	Mucopurulent
ii.	Progression	Rapid	Slow	Slow	Slow	Slow	Rapid
iii.	Hypopyon	Present—fluid and mobile	Present—thick and immobile	Absent	Present—fluid and mobile	Absent	Absent
iv.	Corneal sensation	Unaffected	Unaffected	Affected	Unaffected with severe pain	Often impaired	Unaffected
v.	Perforation	Possible	Does not perforate	Does not perforate	Possible	Does not perforate	Possible

- To be administered one hourly during the day, two hourly during night for 48 hours and later 4th hourly till healing
- Fortified vancomycin eye drops 5% for gram-positive organisms
- Fortified ceftazidime eye drops 5% for gram-negative organisms.

Treatment of Fungal Corneal Ulcer

- Topical antifungal eye drops should be used for 6–8 weeks
- Natamycin 5% eye drops for all fungal ulcers
- Amphotericin B 0.2% topical/IV for *Candida*
- Fluconazole 0.2% topical—effective against *Candida*
- Voriconazole 10% eye drops to be used 2 hourly for 6 to 8 weeks. It is effective against *Aspergillus* and *Fusarium*.
- Nystatin 5% eye ointment 5 times a day for *Aspergillus*
- Miconazole 1% ointment for *Aspergillus*
- Ketoconazole 1% for filamentous fungi
- Oral ketoconazole 200 mg or fluconazole 150 mg once daily for 2-3 weeks.

Treatment of Pre-existing Local Conditions

- For chronic dacryocystitis
  - Dacryocystectomy or dacryocystorhinostomy.
- Lagophthalmos or corneal anesthesia
  - Tarsorrhaphy
- Trichiasis, entropion if present to be corrected.

Rest to the Eye

- Cycloplegics
- Pad and bandage.

Cycloplegics

- One percent atropine eye drops twice daily
- **Uses:** Paralyzes the ciliary muscle and provides comfort to the eye by preventing ciliary spasm
- Prevents complication due to iritis
- Dilates limbal vessels and provides nutrition to the cornea.

Pad and Bandage

- If there is no conjunctival discharge, pad and bandage to protect the eye. If there is discharge, green shades or dark glasses to be used
- Analgesics like paracetamol for pain relief.

Surgical

- If ulcer progresses, scrape the floor and edges of ulcer with a spatula to remove slough and organisms
- Cauterize the edges of the ulcer with heat or 5% povidone-iodine.

General

Improvement of general health with nutritious diet—high protein, vitamin A and C.

3. What are the complications of corneal ulcer?

Complications of Corneal Ulcer

- Before perforation
- During perforation
- After perforation.

Before Perforation

- Corneal opacity
- Descemetocele - see Q. no: 17
- Toxic iridocyclitis
- Secondary glaucoma
- Ectatic cicatrix.

During Perforation

- *Small and peripheral*—anterior synechiae.
- *Large*:
  - Prolapse of iris
  - Pseudocornea—consists of two layers viz organized exudates and fibrous tissue covered with epithelium. It may become anterior staphyloma.
  - Intraocular hemorrhage
  - Subluxated and dislocated lens.

After Perforation

- Anterior polar cataract
- Corneal fistula
- Adherent leukoma
- Anterior staphyloma
- Panophthalmitis
- Phthisis bulbi.

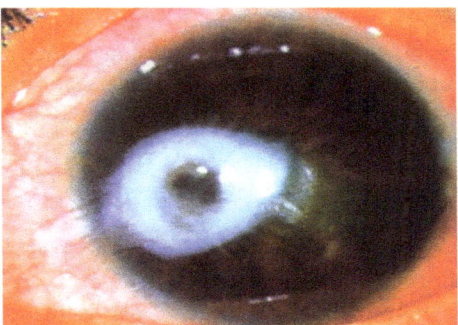

Fig. 7.4: Corneal fistula.

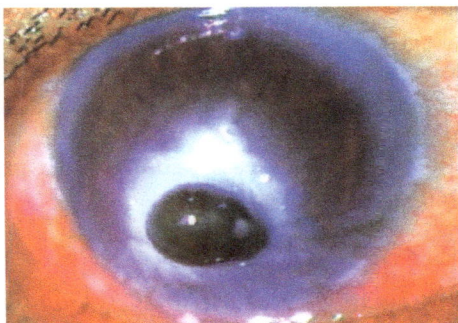

Fig. 7.5: Iris prolapse.

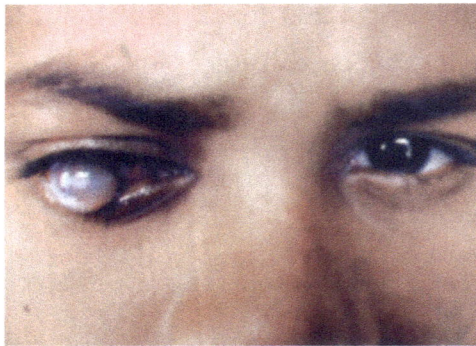

Fig. 7.6: Ectatic cicatrix.

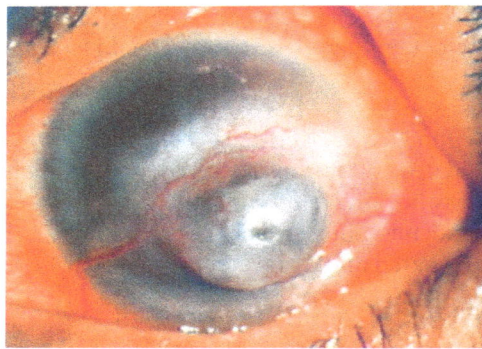

Fig. 7.7: Pseudocornea.

4. Write short notes on hypopyon.

It is accumulation of polymorphonuclear leukocytes and fibrin in anterior chamber (AC) of eye often caused by inflammation.

Nonspecific reaction of diverse etiology usually associated with violent iritis, small pupil and cloudy aqueous.

Toxins liberated by bacteria diffuse through the cornea into anterior chamber.

Mechanism of Hypopyon

- Toxins exert irritative effect upon the vessels of the iris and ciliary body. Hyperemia occurs.
- Leukocytes are poured out by the vessels into the aqueous and gravitate to the bottom of anterior chamber.
- Often it is fluid and fills varying levels of anterior chamber.
- It becomes semisolid due to addition of fibrin.
- Remains sterile as the leukocytosis is due to toxins and the bacteria cannot penetrate intact Descemet's membrane.
- When the ulcerative process is controlled, hypopyon gets absorbed.

Causes

- Ulcerative keratitis—bacterial, fungal, *Acanthamoeba*
- Severe iridocyclitis
- Behcet's disease
- Infective endophthalmitis.

Investigations

- Slit-lamp examination
- B-scan
- Diagnostic paracentesis
- Orbital computed tomography (CT).

Pseudohypopyon

Causes

- Seedling from intraocular tumors—metastasis
- Ghost cell glaucoma
- Lens materials.

Inverse Hypopyon

- Silicone oil in upper part of AC resembles hypopyon
- This occurs due to silicone oil injected into vitreous for sealing superior retinal breaks in retinal detachment surgery.

5. Discuss the clinical features of hypopyon ulcer.

Hypopyon Ulcer

- Corneal ulcer associated with hypopyon
- Hypopyon is accumulation of polymorphonuclear cells and fibrin in the AC of the eye
- It is due to toxins liberated by organisms and not due to actual invasion.

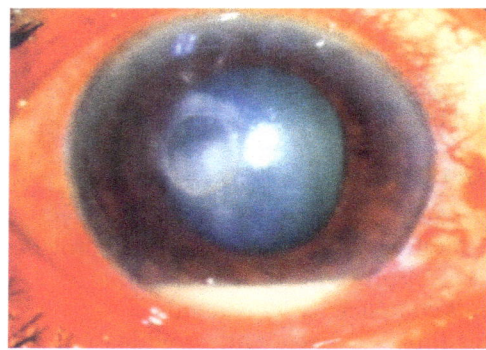

Fig. 7.8: Hypopyon ulcer.

Etiology

Depends on two main factors:
 i. *Virulence of infecting organisms* such as pneumococcus, *Pseudomonas*, staphylococci, gonococci, fungus, etc.
 ii. *Resistance of the host*: Commonly seen in old debilitated, malnourished and immunocompromised patients.
    - It may occur during or after acute infectious diseases such as measles or chickenpox.

Types

Ulcus serpens or bacterial corneal ulcer

Usually caused by pneumococci.

Mycotic hypopyon ulcer

- Caused by filamentous fungi like *Aspergillus fumigatus*, *Fusarium* or nonfilamentous fungi like *Candida albicans*, *Cryptococcus*.

Bacterial versus fungal ulcers.		
	Bacterial ulcer	**Fungal ulcer**
History	Injury with finger nail, iron particle or penetrating injury	Injury with vegetable matter—plant leaves, branch of trees or paddy husk
Onset	Sudden	Insidious, 5–7 days to manifest
Symptoms	Pain and redness are marked	Pain and redness are minimal when compared to signs
Appearance	Ulcer is saucer-shaped with overhanging margins, with surrounding edema and no satellite lesions	Dry looking, grayish white with elevated rolled out margins and delicate feathery finger like extensions into surrounding stroma under intact epithelium. Yellow immune ring is seen when fungal antigen and host antibodies meet Multiple small satellite lesions may be present around the ulcer
Corneal vascularization	Usually present	Usually absent
Contents of hypopyon	Hypopyon usually corresponds to size of ulcer PMN cells and fibrin with absence of bacteria Yellowish white, shifts with posture Hypopyon is mobile and moves to dependent position	Big hypopyon even if the ulcer is small Fungal organisms are present Grayish white stationary Hypopyon is immobile and thick

6. Write short notes on *Acanthamoeba* keratitis.

Etiology
Caused by protozoa found in water and soil.

Risk Factors
- Contact lens wear with poor hygiene
- Swimming pool bathing.

Symptoms
- Severe pain out of proportion to the degree of inflammation.

Signs
- Central or paracentral ring-shaped infiltrates with epithelial defects and associated radial keratoneuritis
- Paracentral ring infiltrates characteristics are as follows:
  - Often unilateral
  - Ring infiltrates
  - Keratoneuritis.

Complications
Descemetocele and perforation are common.

Differential Diagnosis
- Viral keratitis
- Fungal keratitis
- Nonhealing corneal ulcer.

Diagnosis
- KOH and lactophenol cotton blue stain may demonstrate cysts
- Gram or Giemsa stains may also stain cysts and trophozoites of *Acanthamoeba*.

Treatment
- Devastating if not treated early
- Propamidine isethionate 0.1% eye drops and polyhexamethylene biguanide (PHMB) 0.02% eye drops
- Chlorhexidine 0.02% eye drops
- Neomycin 0.175% eye drops
- Miconazole 1% eye drops. To be tapered depending on the response
- Oral ketoconazole or itraconazole 400 mg once a day.

Surgical
- Epithelial debridement
- Penetrating keratoplasty.

7. Write short notes on nonhealing corneal ulcer.

Causes
- Local
- General.

Local Causes
- Raised intraocular pressure (IOP)
- Trichiasis
- Lagophthalmos
- Inadequate therapy
- Chronic dacryocystitis
- Large concretions
- Neuroparalytic ulcer
- Wrong therapy.

General Causes
- Diabetes
- Vitamin A deficiency and dry eye
- Malnutrition
- Immunocompromised patients.

Treatment
- **Medical:** Lubricants, pressure patch, bandage contact lens and anticollagenolytics like tetracycline or doxycycline.
- **Cauterization:**
  - Chemical cautery acts as an antiseptic
  - Povidone-iodine 5%
  - Trichloroacetic acid 10–20%
  - Silver nitrate 1%.
- **Paracentesis:** Improves nutrition of cornea by bringing in fresh aqueous—prevents spontaneous perforation.

- Removal of the cause of nonhealing.
- Conjunctival flap.
- Therapeutic keratoplasty.
- Tarsorrhaphy—for neuroparalytic and neurotrophic keratitis.

8. Write short notes on exposure keratitis.

Exposure keratitis occurs due to incomplete closure of eyelids resulting in dryness of cornea and damage to epithelium.

Etiology

- Paralysis of motor nerve that closes the eyelids due to facial palsy (as in neuroparalytic keratitis)
- Occur in conditions producing lagophthalmos such as:
  - Extreme proptosis
  - Facial nerve palsy (Bell's palsy)
  - Coma
  - Overcorrection of ptosis.

Clinical Features

- Exposure of cornea due to insufficient closure of the eye
- Epithelium becomes desiccated in lower part of the cornea leading to fine punctate epithelial keratitis followed by frank ulceration
- Absence of reflex blinking results in defective closure of the lids during sleep.

Differential Diagnosis

In **neuroparalytic keratitis**, there will be facial palsy but no proptosis. Clinical features and treatment are same as exposure keratitis.

Loss of corneal sensation leads to injury and infection The inferior part of the cornea is most affected.

Treatment

- Keep the cornea covered by eye shade and bandage
- Artificial tear and antibiotic ointment
- Lateral tarsorrhaphy to protect the cornea
- Treat the underlying cause.

9. Write short notes on neurotrophic keratitis.

Neurotrophic keratitis occurs when there is loss of trigeminal innervations to cornea leading to partial or complete corneal anesthesia.

Etiology

- Paralysis of 5th nerve—herpes simplex and zoster
- After radical treatment of trigeminal neuralgia
- Leprosy
- Loss of sensory influence alters the metabolic activity of the epithelium—edema and exfoliation of epithelial cells.

Clinical Features

- Punctate epithelial lesions in the interpalpebral area
- Painless due to corneal anesthesia
- Corneal edema and exfoliation of epithelial cells
- There is desquamation of the epithelium
- Large corneal ulcer due to peeling of the epithelium
- Stroma is cloudy and yellow often associated with hypopyon
- Ciliary congestion.

Treatment

- Protect the eye with eye shield
- Artificial tears and antibiotic eye ointment
- Lateral tarsorrhaphy
- Treat the corneal ulcer in the usual line of treatment
- Closure of lacrimal puncta to conserve moisture.

10. Discuss the etiology, clinical features and treatment of interstitial keratitis.

Interstitial keratitis is nonsuppurative inflammation of corneal stroma without primary involvement of epithelium or endothelium. It is the most common type of deep keratitis.

Etiology

- Occurs between 5 years and 15 years
- Rare after 30 years
- Infective or allergic in origin
- Congenital syphilis—majority
- Acquired syphilis
- Tuberculosis
- Leprosy
- Rarely mumps and malaria
- Cogan's syndrome—interstitial keratitis, vertigo, and deafness
- Manifestation of local antigen-antibody reaction.

Clinical Features

Symptoms

- Photophobia
- Lacrimation
- Pain and diminished vision.

Signs

- Ciliary congestion
- Hazy patches appear in deep layers of cornea near the margin or toward the center
- In 2–4 weeks, whole cornea is hazy with steamy surface ground-glass appearance
- Iris is dimly visible
- Salmon patches—deep vascularization consisting of radial bundles of brush-like vessels covered by hazy cornea—looks dull reddish pink
- Acute stage lasts for 6 weeks and the cornea takes weeks to months to clear
- Iridocyclitis.
- *Hutchinson's triad*: Interstitial keratitis, peg-shaped incisors (Hutchinson's teeth), and vestibular deafness.

Clinical Picture: Three Stages

i. Initial progressive stage
ii. Florid stage
iii. Regressive stage.

Progressive Stage
- Edema of endothelium and deep stroma
- Keratic precipitates
- Diffuse corneal haze resembling ground-glass appearance
- Lasts for 2 weeks.

Florid Stage
- Acutely inflamed
- Salmon patch—deep vascularization of cornea—radial brush-like vessels in deep stroma covered by hazy cornea
- Superficial vascularization near limbus
- Lasts for 2 months.

Stage of Regression
- Clearing of cornea starts from periphery
- Leaves ghost vessels and some opacities
- Lasts for 2 years.

Features in different etiologies.				
	Congenital syphilis	Acquired syphilis	Tuberculosis	Leprosy
Age	5–15 years	>30 years	Any age	Any age
Laterality	Bilateral	Unilateral	Unilateral	Unilateral
Corneal lesions	Starts in upper temporal quadrant later whole cornea is involved	Same as congenital syphilis	Lower 2/3rd of cornea	Upper temporal quadrant
Superficial vascularization	May be present	May be present	Prominent	Prominent

Treatment
- General: Depending on cause
- For syphilis: Injection benzathine penicillin 2.4 million units
- For TB: Isoniazid (INH), streptomycin, pyrazinamide and rifampicin.

Local Treatment

During active inflammation:
- Topical steroids—dexamethasone 0.1% every 2 hours
- One percent atropine eye ointment
- Hot fomentation
- Dark glasses.

After activity has subsided penetrating keratoplasty for corneal opacity.

11. Write short notes on herpes simplex keratitis.

Herpes simplex virus (HSV) is a DNA virus. Ocular infection is more common with HSV-1 and rare with HSV-2 virus.

Type 1 affects above waist and type 2 affects below waist.
- Ocular infection:
  - Primary
  - Recurrent

Primary Infection
- Occurs in children—6 months to 6 years and in teenagers. Usually self-limiting. Virus may travel to trigeminal ganglion and lie dormant. Stroma is not involved.
  - Skin: Vesicles on the lids and lips.
  - Conjunctiva: Acute follicular keratoconjunctivitis with enlarged preauricular lymph nodes.
  - Cornea:
    » Fine and coarse epithelial punctate keratitis
    » Dendritic ulcer.

Recurrent Infection
- Periodic reactivation of the virus lying dormant in the trigeminal ganglion, triggered by:
  - Fever such as malaria or flu
  - Sunlight
  - Use of topical or systemic steroids
  - Immunocompromised patients
  - Mild trauma.

Types of Keratitis

Acute epithelial keratitis
- Punctate epithelial keratitis
- Dendritic ulcer
- Geographical ulcer.

Stromal keratitis
- Disciform keratitis
- Diffuse stromal necrotic keratitis

Punctate Epithelial Keratitis

Superficial punctate keratitis—fine or coarse resembles primary lesion.

Treatment of Epithelial Keratitis
- **Specific**
  - Antiviral:
    » Acyclovir 3% eye ointment 5 times for 7 days
    » Trifluorothymidine 1% 2 hourly till ulcer heals, then 4 times for 5 days.
    » Mechanical debridement of edges and floor with cotton applicator to remove virus-laden cells.
- **Nonspecific**
  - Cycloplegics.
  - Protein and vitamin supplements.

Dendritic Ulcer

Typical lesion is an irregular zigzag linear branching line with knob at the end.
- Double staining—Fluorescein stains the bed of the ulcer and Rose bengal stains the margins of ulcer and virus-laden cells.
- Diminished corneal sensation.

Treatment

Same as epithelial keratitis – Oral Acyclovir 400 mg thrice daily for 7–10 days especially for recurrent and active cases.

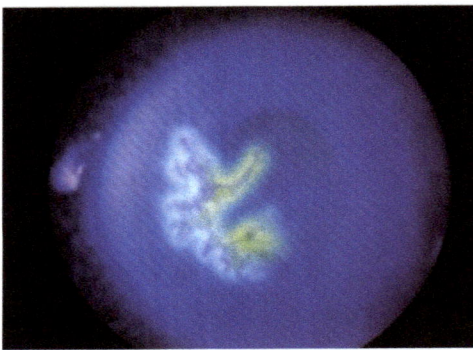

Fig. 7.9: Dendritic ulcer.

Geographical or Amoeboid Ulcer

Branches of dendritic ulcer enlarge and coalesce to form geographical or amoeboidal configuration:
- Use of steroids in dendritic ulcer results in geographical ulcer.

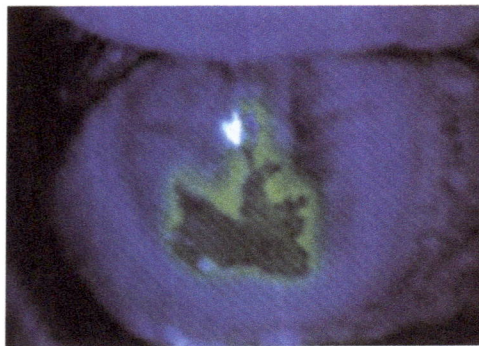

Fig. 7.10: Geographic ulcer.

12. Discuss the etiology, clinical features, and management of herpes zoster ophthalmicus.

Etiology
- Acute infection of dorsal root ganglion of trigeminal nerve by varicella-zoster virus identical to chickenpox virus.
- Both diseases may coexist in an epidemic infection.
- After an infection of chickenpox in childhood, virus lies dormant and may manifest later in elderly people as herpes zoster.

Clinical Features
- Preherpetic stage
- Herpetic stage
- Postherpetic stage

Preherpetic Stage
- Malaise
- Fever
- Severe neuralgic pain on one side of the head and face.

Herpetic Stage
- Unilateral vesicular eruptions along the ophthalmic branch of trigeminal nerves
- Involved branches:
  - Supraorbital
  - Supratrochlear
  - Infratrochlear
  - Nasociliary
- Skin of face becomes red and edematous
- Severe neuralgic pain along the course of the nerve
- Hutchinson's rule: Ocular involvement is usually associated with eruption of vesicles on the skin of tip or side of the nose (nasociliary branch).
- Conjunctivitis
- Corneal lesions:
  - Superficial punctate keratitis
  - Nummular keratitis—coin-shaped
  - Subepithelial punctate keratitis
  - Disciform keratitis
- Sclera—scleritis and episcleritis
- Iridocyclitis
- IOP: Lower in early stage and raised in later stages
- Palsy of 3rd, 6th, 7th nerves may occur
- Exposure keratitis may occur due to 7th nerve involvement
- Optic neuritis.

Postherpetic Stage
- Skin vesicles suppurate and cause pitted scars.
- Postherpetic neuralgia may persist for several months to years.

Differential Diagnosis

Differences between herpes simplex and herpes zoster.			
S. No.	Features	Herpes simplex	Herpes zoster
i.	Type of virus	Dermatotropic virus	Neurotropic virus
ii.	Pain	Less	More
iii.	Dendrites	Linear branching with terminal bulbs with central ulceration	Small dendrites without central ulceration and absence of terminal bulbs
iv.	Skin scarring	Rare	Frequent
v.	Postherpetic neuralgia	Rare	Common
vi.	Iris atrophy	Seen as patches	Sectoral
vii.	Laterality	Can be bilateral	Unilateral
viii.	Other lesions	Vesicles seen on lips and nose commonly	Ocular nerve palsies or optic neuritis can occur. Can be associated with fever and malaise

Treatment

Young patients (<45 years) should be investigated for acquired immunodeficiency syndrome (AIDS).

Preherpetic Stage
- To relieve pain—analgesics 0.5–1 cc IM ergotamine
- Injection of immunoglobulins may protect the eye.

Herpetic Stage
- Skin—calamine lotion
- Eye—keratitis and iridocyclitis
  - One percent atropine, antibiotics and steroids
  - Tablet acyclovir 800 mg 5 times a day for 10 days
- Systemic steroids are indicated in case of optic neuritis and nerve palsies.
- Cimetidine 300 mg 4 times daily—reduces pain and itching due to histamine blockade.
- Antibiotic steroid skin ointment for skin lesion.
- Antiviral therapy to be started within 72 hours of onset of skin lesion to prevent postherpetic neuralgia and uveitis.

Postherpetic Stage
- Tarsorrhaphy—for prevention of exposure keratitis due to corneal anesthesia
- Artificial tears for dry eye
- Skin—cold cream for affected skin
- Pain—analgesics
- Vitamin B_1 and methylcobalamin injection.

Amitriptyline or carbamazepine for severe pain.

13. Write short notes on Mooren's ulcer.

Mooren's ulcer (chronic serpiginous or rodent ulcer) is a severe inflammatory peripheral ulcerative keratitis. It is an autoimmune disease. There is production of antibodies against corneal epithelium.

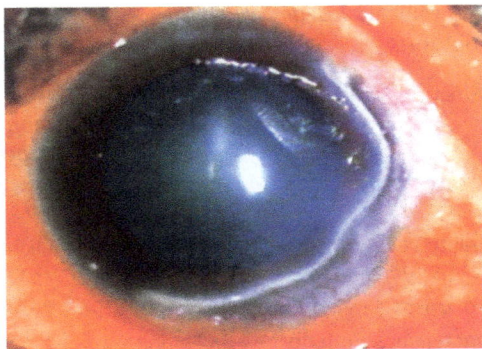

Fig. 7.11: Mooren's ulcer.

Etiology
- Unknown
- Autoimmune disease
- Bilateral form is more painful
- Unilateral form is milder variety.

Symptoms
- Same as corneal ulcer
- Neuralgic pain in head and neck is more severe.

Signs
Shallow furrow with whitish overhanging edges, vascularized base—rarely perforation.

Differential Diagnosis

Differentiation between mooren's ulcer and terrien's marginal degeneration.

S. No.	Features	Mooren's ulcer	Terrien's marginal degeneration
i.	Mode of onset	Aggressive and bilateral in young persons, unilateral in middle aged and elderly	Bilateral, slow in onset and progression
ii.	Symptoms	Severe pain	Mild pain
iii.	Signs	Starts in interpalpebral zone. Leading edge undermines epithelium. Progresses centrally and circumferentially	Starts superiorly and inferiorly. Slope in inner edge of ulcer
iv.	Complications	Increased risk of perforation	Does not perforate

Treatment
- Difficult as ischemia is the underlying cause
- Excision of 4–7 mm strip of adjacent conjunctiva is successful as it eliminates conjunctival source of enzyme collagenase and proteoglycanase
- Cryoapplication of edge of ulcer
- Bandage soft contact lens
- Lamellar keratoplasty
- Intravenous methotrexate in refractory cases.

14. What are the ectatic conditions of the cornea?
- **Inflammations**
  - Ectatic cicatrix
  - Anterior staphyloma.
- **Congenital**
  - Keratoconus
  - Keratoglobus.

15. Write short notes on keratoconus.

Keratoconus is noninflammatory ectasia of cornea resulting in visual impairment owing to high degree of irregular astigmatism.

Etiology
- Congenital weakness of central part of cornea
- Can occur in vernal catarrh or Down's syndrome due to repeated rubbing of the eye.

Incidence
Manifests after puberty and common in girls.

Clinical Features
Impaired vision due to myopic astigmatism.

Signs
- Conical shape of the cornea
- Apex of the cornea is situated below the center of the cornea

- **Placido's disc:** Irregularity in reflection of rings on cornea when seeing through Placido's disc
- **Munson's sign:** Indentation of the lower lid when the patient looks down

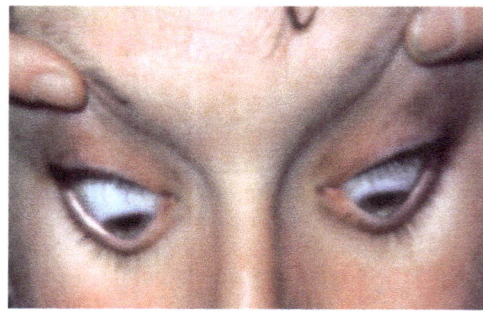

Fig. 7.12: Munson's sign.

- Window reflex—distorted
- Retinoscopy—scissors reflex
- Distant direct ophthalmoscopy—oil droplet reflex
- Keratometry—misalignment of mires
- Corneal topography—early diagnosis of irregular astigmatism.

Slit-lamp Examination
- Vogt's striae—fine parallel lines at apex due to vertical fold of Descemet's membrane
- Fleischer's ring—brownish ring at the base of the cornea due to hemosiderin deposition in epithelium
- Corneal hydrops—in advanced cases, stroma becomes edematous and opaque.

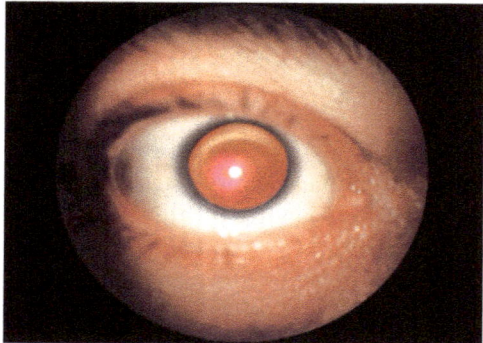

Fig. 7.13: Oil droplet reflex.

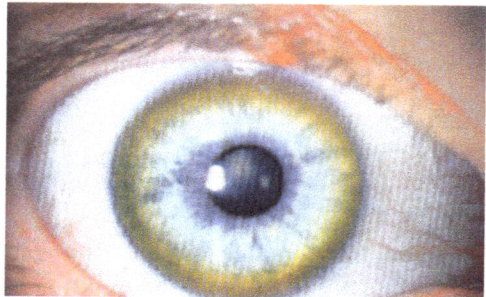

Fig. 7.14: Fleischer's ring.

Ultrasonic Pachymetry
- Corneal thinning
- Ophthalmoscope or plane mirror at 1 m shows ring of shadow in red reflex resembling droplet of oil.

Types of Cones in Keratoconus
- Nipple cone—small size—steep curvature (<5 mm)
- Oval cone—larger and ellipsoidal (5-6 mm)
- Globus cone—very large cone and globe like (>6 mm).

Treatment
- Spectacles
- Gas permeable contact lenses
- Corneal collagen cross-linking to stop progression
- Penetrating keratoplasty
- Deep anterior lamellar keratoplasty (DALK)—risk of rejection is less.
- Intracorneal ring segments (INTACS)—to flatten cornea.

Keratoglobus
- Congenital anomaly and nonprogressive
- Hemispherical protrusion of the whole cornea
- Bilateral, familial and hereditary
- Normal IOP
- Cup-disk ratio is not increased.

Differential Diagnosis
- Buphthalmos: Raised IOP, increased corneal diameter, common at birth to 3 years
- Pellucid marginal degeneration
- Keratoglobus.

S. No.	Features	Keratoconus	Keratoglobus	Pellucid marginal degeneration
i.	Incidence	Most common	Rare	Less common
ii.	Laterality	Usually bilateral	Bilateral	Bilateral
iii.	Age of onset	At puberty	From birth	20–40 years
iv.	Characteristics	Inferior paracentral thinning	Thinning maximal at periphery	1–2 mm band of thinning inferiorly
v.	Area of protrusion	Apex	Generalized	Protrusion superiorly
vi.	Striae	Common	Rare	Rare

16. Discuss the treatment of perforated corneal ulcer.

Incidence of Perforation
More in hypopyon corneal ulcer due to virulence of organisms and if host resistance is less inflammation occurs at three levels:
- Superficial layer
- Deep layers
- Diffusion of exudates between endothelium and Descemet's opposite to the base of the ulcer (posterior corneal abscess).

Treatment for Corneal Abscess
- Evacuation of pus
- Povidone-iodine cautery
- Antibiotics or antifungals.

Perforation
Extension of superficial ulcer and posterior corneal abscess results in perforation:
- Spontaneous
- Increased IOP from blepharospasm or straining. Aqueous escapes and eye becomes soft.

Sequelae of Perforation
- If perforation is small—anterior synechiae and adherent leukoma
- Large perforation—prolapse of iris—sloughing of whole cornea (as in keratomalacia and *Pseudomonas* infection)
- Total prolapse of iris
- Pseudocornea
- Anterior staphyloma.

Treatment of Perforated Ulcer
- Depends on site and size of perforation
- If perforation is small:
  - Rest in bed
  - Atropine and antibiotics ointment
  - Pressure pad and bandage
- Tissue adhesive—cyanoacrylate glue is used to seal the perforation
- Soft contact lenses
- Conjunctival flap covers the perforation and helps in healing
- Large perforation—therapeutic penetrating keratoplasty.

Treatment of Sequela and Complications
- Secondary glaucoma
- Descemetocele
- Perforation
- Corneal fistula
- Corneal opacity
- Anterior staphyloma
- Phthisis bulbi.

Secondary Glaucoma
- Due to hypopyon and iridocyclitis
- The most common cause of failure in treatment of hypopyon corneal ulcer
- Raised IOP results in less nutrition of cornea.

Treatment
- Acetazolamide—250 mg tds.

17. Write short notes on descemetocele.

Descemetocele (Keratocele)
- Descemet's membrane offers great resistance but it may herniate as a transparent vesicle called descemetocele

- It may be surrounded by white cicatricial ring or it may rupture.

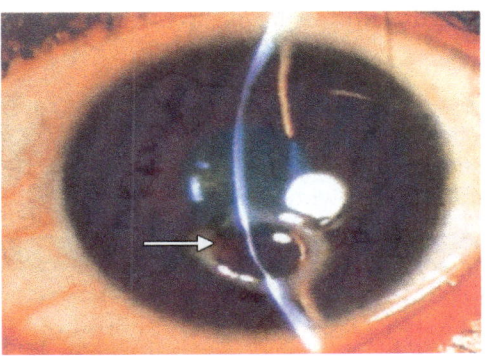

Fig. 7.15: Descemetocele.

Treatment
- Patient is asked not to strain and pressure bandage is applied
- Tablet acetazolamide 250 mg tds
- Therapeutic keratoplasty—lamellar keratoplasty can be done.

18. Write short notes on anterior staphyloma.

Anterior staphyloma is an ectasia of pseudocornea with iris incarcerated in it.

After large corneal perforation, **pseudocornea** forms. Pseudocornea is exudate covering the iris prolapsed which gets organized to form thin layer of connective tissue. Resultant cicatrix formed by the scar tissue is too weak to support the IOP. Cicatrix becomes ectatic. This ectatic cicatrix with iris incarceration results in anterior staphyloma.

Bands of scar tissue on the staphyloma produce lobulated surface blackened with pigment resulting in bunch of grapes.

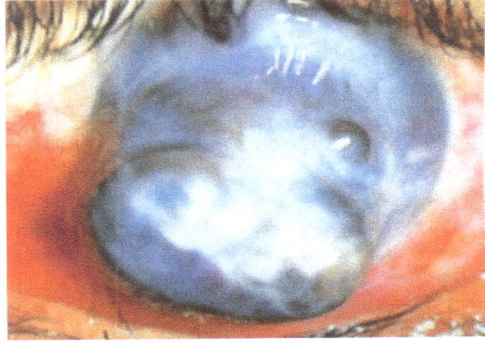

Fig. 7.16: Anterior staphyloma.

19. Write a short note on corneal fistula.

When the exudates filling the perforated ulcer called pseudocornea, is subjected to strain the anterior chamber collapses repeatedly to become permanent corneal fistula.

Perforation opposite to the pupil causes anterior polar cataract, and sudden perforation results in dislocation of lens.

Sudden lowering of IOP also causes expulsive hemorrhage.

Entry of organisms into the eye causes endophthalmitis and panophthalmitis. Final sequela is phthisis bulbi.

20. Write short notes on phthisis bulbi.

Small, shrunken, soft eyeball loses its shape and becomes quadrilateral due to pressure of four recti.

Causes of Phthisis Bulbi
- Perforated corneal ulcer which has lost its contents
- Sequela of panophthalmitis
- Late sequela of chronic iridocyclitis
- Perforated injury with loss of contents.

Differential diagnosis.

Features	Phthisis bulbi	Atrophic bulbi
Size of the eyeball	Shrunken	Normal
Ocular structures	Cannot be identified	Can be identified
IOP	Reduced (marked hypotony)	Reduced
Drooping of eyelid	Present due to lack of support	Absent
Causes	Perforated corneal ulcer or injury	Absolute glaucoma
Cytoarchitecture of the eye	Disorganized	Maintained

Treatment
- Artificial eye or plastic shells can be fitted for cosmetic purposes.
- Enucleation if:
  - Eyeball becomes painful due to intraocular hemorrhage
  - Malignancy such as malignant melanoma is suspected.

21. What are the causes of pigment dispersion on the cornea?

Type of pigment	Disorder	Corneal location
Iron	Keratoconus (Fleischer's ring)	Epithelium
	Pterygium (Stocker's line)	Epithelium
	Filtering bleb (Ferry's line)	Epithelium
Copper	Old opacity (Hudson-Stahli's line)	Epithelium
	Siderosis	Mainly stroma
	Blood staining of the cornea	Mainly stroma
	Wilson's disease; chalcosis Kayser-Fleischer's ring	Descemet's membrane
Melanin	Pigment dispersion syndrome (Krukenberg's spindle—vertical spindle pattern)	Descemet's membrane Endothelium

22. Write short notes on corneal degenerations.

It is seen in:
- Arcus senilis
- Arcus juvenilis
- Pellucid marginal degeneration
- Terrien's marginal degeneration
- Band-shaped keratopathy
- Climatic droplet keratopathy
- Salzmann's nodular degeneration.

Arcus Senilis
Lipoid infiltration in the cornea seen in the elderly persons. It starts as whitish area concentric with upper and lower margin of cornea. They may unite to form a complete ring. It is separated from the limbus by a lucid interval of clear cornea.

Arcus Juvenilis
This is similar to arcus senilis but appears below 40 years of age. It may be associated with abnormal serum lipid profile.

Pellucid Marginal Degeneration
It is characterized by inferior corneal thinning. It has butterfly appearance in corneal topography.

Terrien's Marginal Degeneration
There is progressive thinning of peripheral cornea sparing the limbus. It manifests typically superiorly and more common in men.

Band-shaped Keratopathy
It is seen in chronic uveitis especially in blind shrunken eye and in children with Still's disease. A whitish band appears in the interpalpebral area with round holes in the band.

It is due to hyaline infiltration of superficial stroma followed by deposition of calcareous salts.

It usually starts as fine dust like deposits in Bowman's membrane in interpalpebral fissure. It starts at 3 and 9 o'clock, progresses centrally in ocular surface disease and starts centrally in anterior uveitis. It has peripheral clear zone between the band and limbus.

Treatment:
- Scraping of calcareous material and place bandage contact lens until epithelium heals
- Dissolving it with sodium edetate
- Can also be removed by excimer laser (phototherapeutic keratectomy).

Climatic Droplet Keratopathy
It is also called oil droplet keratopathy. It is characterized by superficial nonvascularized corneal opacity with focal lesion in epithelium resembling droplets of oil. This occurs due to exposure to hot, dry, dusty environment.

Treatment:
- Lamellar keratoplasty
- Phototherapeutic keratectomy.

Salzmann's Nodular Degeneration
It is a slow progressive degeneration due to replacement of basement membrane near superficial stroma by eosinophilic material.

Bluish white avascular nodules appear in superficial stroma in post-traumatic or postviral corneal ulcer.

Treatment:
Lamellar keratoplasty.

23. Write short notes on corneal dystrophies.

Corneal dystrophy is a bilateral, symmetrical, inherited condition that has little or no relationship to environmental or systemic factors.

Classification
- **Anterior**—affecting epithelium and Bowman's membrane:
    - Microcystic corneal dystrophies—dot-like opacities, map-like pattern
    - Reis-Bucklers corneal dystrophies—round and polygonal opacities in the center of the cornea.
    - Meesmann corneal dystrophies—tiny intraepithelial cysts in the interpalpebral area. These are characterized by recurrent corneal erosions.

Treatment: Lamellar keratoplasty.

- **Stromal:**
    - Lattice
    - Macular
    - Granular.

Features	Lattice	Macular	Granular
Inheritance	Autosomal dominant	Autosomal recessive	Autosomal dominant
Deposits	Branching and spider like	Grayish white, cloudy, crust like	Discrete white
Material	Amyloid	Glycosaminoglycan	Hyaline
Periphery	Spared	Involved	Spared
Age of visual loss	25–30 years	10 years	Rare
Recurrence	Common	May occur	Rarely, if visual axis is involved

- **Posterior:**
    - Congenital hereditary endothelial dystrophy: One of the causes of congenital opacity of cornea. It is focal or generalized absence of endothelium causing diffuse bilateral corneal edema.
    - Posterior polymorphous dystrophy: Endothelium displays features of epithelium.
    - Fuchs' endothelial dystrophies: Affects Descemets membrane and endothelium. It typically affects the elderly persons. Corneal endothelial protrusions called cornea guttata begin to appear and lead to corneal edema and bullous keratopathy.

Treatment:
- Hypertonic saline eye drops
- Bandage contact lens
- Penetrating keratoplasty.

24. What are the differences between corneal degeneration and dystrophies?

Features	Degeneration	Dystrophies
Etiology	Acquired	Hereditary
Age of onset	Old age	Presents early (except in Fuchs)
Bilaterality	Unilateral or bilateral	Always bilateral
Progression	Rapid	Slow
Vascularization	Present	Absent
Site	Usually peripheral	Usually central

25. Discuss the etiology, types, clinical features, and management of corneal opacities.

Causes
- Healed corneal ulcer
- Healed keratitis
- Healed injury of cornea—perforating or surgical
- Corneal dystrophy.

Types
- Nebula
- Macula
- Leukoma
- Adherent leukoma.

Nebula
- Faint opacity
- Cloud-like opacity with ill-defined margins
- Involves basement membrane and superficial stroma
- Iris details are clearly visible.

Macula
- It is spot like
- More dense with defined margins
- Involves half of the stroma
- Iris details are seen partially.

Leukoma
- Very dense and white opacity
- Full thickness of stroma is involved
- Margins are well defined
- Iris details not seen through the opacity.

Adherent Leukoma
- It is leukomatous opacity in which iris is incarcerated within the layers of the cornea. It results when healing occurs after perforation of cornea with incarceration of iris.
- It is characterized by:
    - Presence of brown pigment in the leukoma (derived from iris)
    - Varying depth of anterior chamber
    - Pear-shaped pupil drawn toward the opacity.

Sequela of Corneal Opacity
- **Clearing of opacity:** Some degree of clearing in course of time particularly seen in younger patients.
- **Pigmentary changes:** Yellowish brown Hudson-Stahli's line may be seen due to hemosiderin deposition.
- **Degenerative changes:**
  - Calcareous degeneration due to deposition of calcium
  - Atheromatous degeneration due to deposition of yellowish plaques.

Symptoms
Defective vision
- If the opacity is near limbus, there will not be any visual disturbance
- If the opacity is in pupillary area
- Nebula—blurs image by irregularly refracted rays
- Irregular astigmatism—diminishes vision even when the opacity is away from the pupillary area
- Secondary glaucoma—due to peripheral anterior synechia in cases of adherent leukoma
- Amblyopia—when opacity occurs in childhood.

Cosmetic disfigurement
- Obvious when the opacity is large and dense.

Treatment
Diminished vision due to nebular and macular opacities can be improved by contact lenses.
- Optical iridectomy:
  - Indicated for small dense leukoma in central area
  - In lower nasal quadrant to obtain stenopaeic vision
  - In temporal field to improve peripheral field of vision.
- Keratoplasty: May give visual and cosmetic improvement.
- Tattooing: Indicated when opacity is in periphery for cosmetic improvement:
  - One percent gold chloride for brown and
  - One percent platinum chloride for black color. Tinted soft contact lenses for cosmetic improvement.

Treatment for Adherent Leukoma
- Same as for leukoma
- In addition, synechiotomy is done to prevent peripheral anterior synechia, this prevents secondary glaucoma.

26. Write short notes on corneal edema.
Hazy cornea due to accumulation of fluid is called corneal edema.

Causes of Corneal Edema
Ocular trauma, overwear of contact lens, keratitis, corneal dystrophy, bullous keratopathy, acute angle-closure glaucoma, congenital glaucoma and corneal graft rejection.
Treatment is same as for bullous keratopathy (given below).

27. Write short notes on bullous keratopathy.
It is characterized by the presence of corneal edema with epithelial bullae. The main etiological factor is endothelial cell decompensation.

Causes
- Endothelial damage during cataract surgery
- Pseudophakic bullous keratopathy due to anterior chamber IOL touching endothelium or raised IOP following surgery
- Aphakic bullous keratopathy due to vitreous in anterior chamber which touches the endothelium
- Congenital hereditary endothelial dystrophy
- Fuchs endothelial dystrophy
- Posterior polymorphous dystrophy
- Corneal transplant rejection.

Symptoms
Poor vision, halos around light, pain, photophobia and foreign body sensation more pronounced on waking.

Prevention
- Use viscoelastics liberally during cataract surgery to protect endothelium from instrument touch
- Avoid anterior chamber IOL if there is endothelial compromise

Treatment
- Hypertonic saline 5% eye drops or 6% as eye ointment
- A thin high water content bandage contact lens for pain relief
- Remove anterior chamber IOL if it is the cause for bullous keratopathy
- Penetrating keratoplasty.

28. Write short notes on keratoplasty.
Patient's opaque cornea is replaced by donor's clear cornea.

Types
- Full thickness or penetrating: Full thickness of the cornea is replaced
- Partial thickness or lamellar: Superficial layers of the cornea are replaced.

Types of lamellar keratoplasty—three superficial and three deep types

Superficial types:
- Bowman's membrane transplant
- Superficial anterior lamellar keratoplasty (SALK)
- Deep anterior lamellar keratoplasty (DALK)
  - Done for stromal dystrophies and macular corneal opacities

Deep types:
- Descemet's stripping endothelial keratoplasty (DSEK)
- Descemet's membrane endothelial keratoplasty (DMEK)
  - In the above two procedures, mainly endothelium is transplanted. It is done in diseases involving only endothelium as in endothelial dystrophies.
- Pre-Descemet's endothelial keratoplasty (PDEK)

Here Descemet's membrane and endothelium are transplanted.

Indications

Optical
Central corneal opacity is replaced for improvement of vision.

Therapeutic
Bacterial, fungal, viral or *Acanthamoeba* keratitis not responding to treatment is replaced for healing and eradication of infection.

Structural
- To restore the corneal anatomy
- Descemetocele
- Corneal fistula
- After pterygium or dermoid excision
- Keratoconus
- *Cosmetic*—to replace an ugly scar.

Contraindications
- Dry eye
- Marked corneal vascularization
- Absence of corneal sensation.

Method
- Excision of donor eye
- Excision of donor cornea
- Excision of host cornea
- Fixation of donor clear graft.

Excision of Donor Cornea

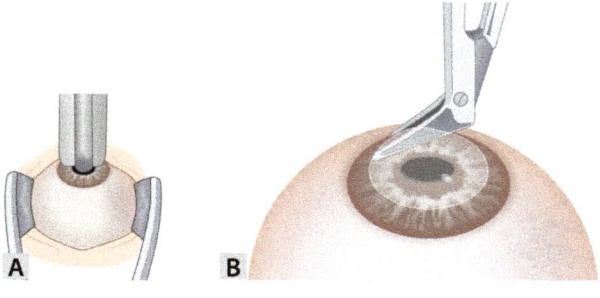

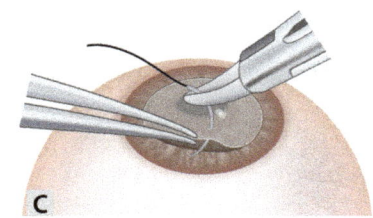

Figs. 7.17A to C: A. Trephining recipient cornea; B. Excision of recipient cornea; C. Suturing the donor cornea.

Complications

Early
- Flat anterior chamber—due to improper suturing and leakage
- Iris prolapse—due to raised IOP
- Infection.

Late
- Graft failure—haziness of cornea
- Secondary glaucoma—due to peripheral anterior synechia
- Astigmatism—due to irregular healing
- Endothelial rejection line with haziness of cornea.

29. Write short notes on eye bank.
- It is the link between donor and recipient/eye surgeon
- Any organization recognized by Government of India to collect and distribute human eyes to those requiring corneal transplantation.

Objectives
- Collection of donor eye
- Preservation of donor cornea
- Distribution of quality donor tissue for corneal transplantation
- Publicity activities
- Promotion of awareness of eye donation.

Procedure for Eye Collection
- Pledges to donate eyes after death
- Eye bank personnel collect eyes (by bilateral enucleation) from dead person after getting consent from close relative of dead person
- Age of person, cause and time of death
- Eyes to be removed within 6 hours.

Contraindications for Eye Collection
- AIDS
- Hepatitis B
- Poisoning
- Severe burns
- Death from unknown cause.

Preservation of Donor Eyes
- **Short-term storage:** Eyeball is kept in moist chamber at 4°C in refrigerator for a maximum of 24 hours.
- **Intermediate-term storage:** Corneoscleral button is excised from donor eye and kept in McCarey-Kaufman (M-K) medium at 4°C can be used up to 4 days.
- **Long-term storage:** Corneal blindness occurs mainly in children and young adults.
  - **Organ culture method:** Calf serum is used for storage. It can be stored at 34°C. It can be preserved for 30–35 days.
  - **Cryopreservation:** Corneoscleral button is excised and frozen to –80°C. It is stored at –160°C. It can be preserved up to 1 year. It can be used for lamellar keratoplasty.
- 40,000 new cases occur in India every year.
- Only 20,000 eyes are collected annually.
- Hospital Cornea Retrieval Programme (HCRP) aimed at motivation of relatives of terminally ill patients, accident victim and other Graves' diseases to donate the eyes by social workers and medical staff.
- Eye Donation Fortnight is organized from 25th August to 8th September every year to promote eye donation/eye banking.

CHAPTER 8

Sclera

INTRODUCTION

Sclera is a strong opaque white fibrous layer which forms the posterior 5/6th of the outer tunic of the eye. It is relatively avascular and is thinnest at the attachments of the muscles.

1. What are the functions of the sclera?

- Gives the correct optical shape
- Supports retina and choroid
- Provides rigid insertion for extraocular muscles.

2. What are the types of inflammation of the sclera?

Two types

i. Episcleritis—superficial
ii. Scleritis—deep.

3. Write short notes on episcleritis.

Episcleritis

It is a common benign self-limiting recurrent disorder of episcleral tissue occurring in young adults. It is seldom associated with a systemic disorder. It never progresses to a true scleritis and is more common in women.

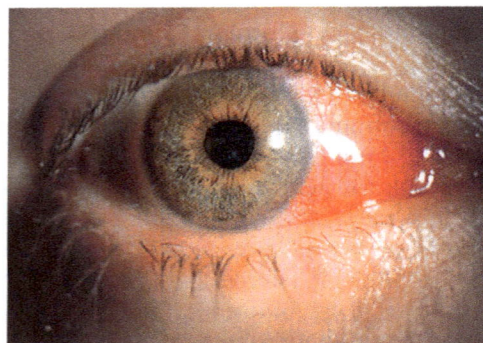

Fig. 8.1: Episcleritis.

Etiology

- Allergic reaction to endogenous protein or toxin
- History of collagen disease or rheumatoid arthritis
- Associated with prior episodes of herpes zoster and gout.

Types

- Simple diffuse episcleritis.
- Nodular episcleritis:
  - *Simple episcleritis*: It is sectorial or diffuse redness seen over the sclera. The conjunctiva looks purple in color. Deep episcleral vessels can be seen over it.
  - *Nodular episcleritis*: Localized nodule of the size of a lentil is seen 2–3 mm away from the limbus. It is hard and immovable and tender. The conjunctiva moves freely over the cornea.

Course

Usually transient lasting for several days or weeks. Recurrence is common. It may become chronic but never ulcerates. Fleeting attacks of episcleritis occur named as episcleritis periodica fugax.

Differential Diagnosis:

- Phlyctenular conjunctivitis
- Inflamed pinguecula
- Scleritis.

Differences between episcleritis and scleritis.		
	Episcleritis	**Scleritis**
Corneal and uveal involvement	Absent	Present
Secondary glaucoma	Absent	Present
Scleral texture	Normal	Thinning uvea seen through
Age group	4th decade	4th–6th decade
Threat to vision	Nil	Serious threat
Pain	Mild	Severe
Thinning of sclera	Absent	Present
Blanching with 2.5% phenylephrine	Present	Absent
Laterality	Usually unilateral	Usually bilateral
Progression	Self-limiting	Runs a long course
Associated diseases	Gout Hypersensitivity to tuberculosis (TB)/ Streptococci/Proteus	Collagen disease, rheumatoid arthritis, systemic lupus erythematosus (SLE), polyarteritis nodosa (PAN), syphilis, TB, leprosy

Complications

- Neuralgia
  - Associated uveitis
  - Rarely scleritis due to deeper infiltration of the inflammation.

Treatment

- Mild cases: No specific therapy. Usually resolves spontaneously within 2–3 weeks especially simple episcleritis
- Nodular type: Topical steroids and oral nonsteroidal anti-inflammatory agents (NSAIDs)
- Recurrent and unresponsive cases: Systemic flurbiprofen 100 mg 3 times daily or systemic indomethacin 50 mg twice daily.

4. Write short notes on scleritis.

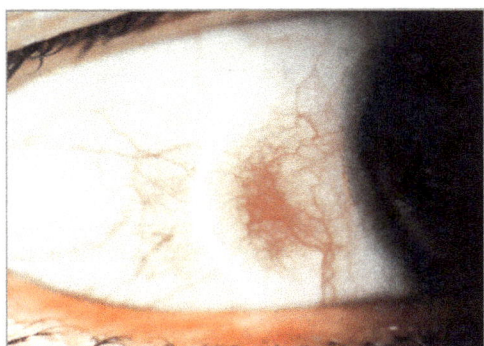

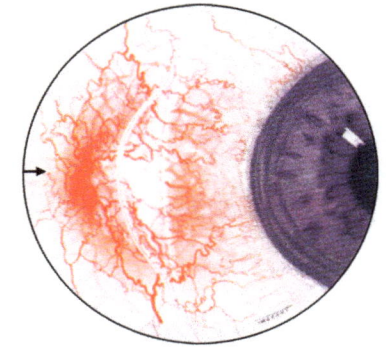

Fig. 8.2: Scleritis.

It is a granulomatous inflammation of the scleral tissue and is less common than episcleritis. It may be a trivial self-limiting episode or progress to sight threatening complications as necrotizing scleritis, uveitis, etc. It is usually bilateral and is more common in women. Age group affected is usually 40–50 years.

Etiology

- Rheumatoid arthritis
- Polyarteritis nodosa
- Systemic lupus erythematosus
- Nonspecific arteritis
- Wegener's granulomatosis
- Dermatomyositis
- Polychondritis
- Herpes zoster
- Ocular surgery.

Classification

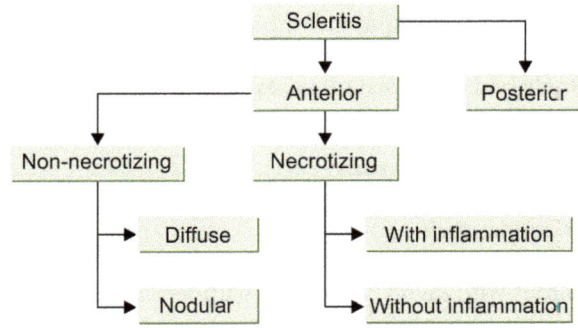

- **Anterior scleritis**
  - Non-necrotizing scleritis
    » Diffuse
    » Nodular.
  - Necrotizing scleritis
    » With inflammation
    » Without inflammation (scleromalacia perforans).
- **Posterior scleritis**
  - In anterior non-necrotizing scleritis (diffuse type), a portion or the entire anterior sclera is inflamed. When entire anterior sclera is inflamed, it is known as brawny scleritis. Distortion of the pattern of the vascular plexus is characteristic. There is loss of radial pattern of the blood vessels. It rarely progresses to nodular type.
  - Nodular scleritis resembles nodular episcleritis. The scleral nodule cannot be moved over the underlying tissue and is less circumscribed than episcleritis. The swelling is dark red or bluish, later it becomes purple and finally porcelain-like sclera results.

Treatment

- Oral NSAIDs—flurbiprofen 100 mg 3 times daily or indomethacin 50 mg twice daily.
- Oral prednisolone 40–80 mg in divided doses when the patient does not respond to NSAIDs.
- Topical steroids—to reduce the associated pain and edema.

Anterior Necrotizing Scleritis with Inflammation

Early cases show distortion and occlusion of the blood vessels in the affected area with avascular patches appearing in the episcleral tissue followed by development of scleral necrosis. The sclera becomes transparent and the uvea is visible. The inflamed areas gradually spread around the globe and join up together. In severe type, it is associated with anterior uveitis.

- Complications—cataract, keratitis, keratolysis and glaucoma.
- 75% of cases are visually impaired.
- 25% of cases die of associated systemic vascular disease within 5 years.

Treatment

Oral prednisolone 60–120 mg daily for 2–3 days. Tapering dose of prednisolone depends upon the clinical features Immunosuppressive drugs such as cyclophosphamide, azathioprine and cyclosporine are given in steroid-resistant cases.

Combined therapy with pulsed intravenous methylprednisolone and cyclophosphamide 500 mg advocated for extremely bad and resistant cases.

Anterior Necrotizing Scleritis without Inflammation (Scleromalacia Perforans)

This is common in women and in long-standing seropositive rheumatoid arthritis.

Starts as a yellow necrotizing scleral patch and spreads to large areas with involvement of the underlying uveal tissue.

Spontaneous perforation is extremely rare even though the sclera is very thin unless intraocular pressure is elevated. There is no effective treatment.

Posterior Scleritis

The inflammation arises posterior to the equator. 20% of the scleritis are posterior. About 30% of the patients have associated autoimmune systemic disease. Diagnosis is confirmed by extreme scleral thinning with ultrasonography.

Clinical Features

Variable and depends upon the site of posterior scleritis and its association with anterior scleritis.

Ophthalmoscopy—optic disk edema, macular edema, exudative retinal detachment, vitritis, choroidal detachment, choroidal folds, subretinal mass, infraretinal white deposits and subretinal infiltrates.

External examination shows lid edema, proptosis, defective ocular motility and defective vision.

Differential Diagnosis

- Optic neuritis
- Retinal detachment
- Choroidal tumor
- Orbital inflammation
- Orbital mass
- Harada's disease.

Treatment

- NSAIDs
- Steroids
- Immunosuppressive drugs.

Investigations for Scleritis

- Total count (TC), differential count (DC), erythrocyte sedimentation rate (ESR)
- Rh factor, antinuclear factor
- Plasma protein and immunoglobulin level
- Uric acid for gout
- Serology for syphilis
- X-ray chest, hand, feet and lumbosacral spine
- Fluorescein angiography for evidence of vasculitis.

5. Write short notes on staphyloma.

Ectasia of outer coat of eyeball with incarceration of uveal tissue.

	Part of ectasia	Part of uvea incarcerated	Causes
Anterior	Cornea, pseudocornea	Iris	Large corneal ulcer, perforation
Intercalary	Limbus and neighboring sclera anterior to anterior ciliary vessels	Root of iris	Glaucoma, scleritis perforating injury
Ciliary	Sclera overlying ciliary body	Ciliary body	Glaucoma, scleritis, ciliary body tumor, sclera perforation due to injury
Equatorial	Equatorial sclera by vortex veins	Choroid	Fungal infections, scleromalacia perforans
Posterior	Posterior pole	Choroid	High myopia, posterior scleritis, posterior perforating injury

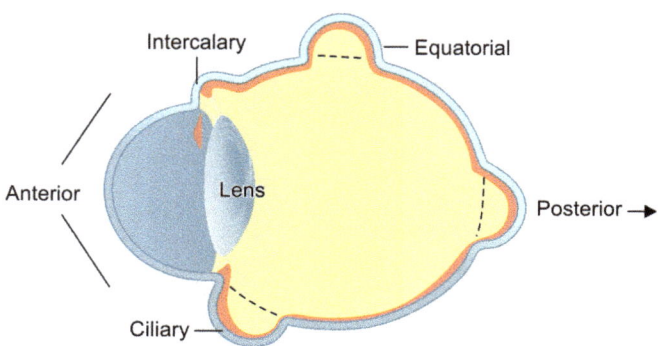

Fig. 8.3: Different types of staphyloma.

Posterior staphyloma is diagnosed by ophthalmoscopy. There is excavation of the area with retinal vessels dipping in it. Its floor is focused with minus power lenses in ophthalmoscope as compared to its margins.

Treatment of Staphyloma

- Localized staphylectomy along with steroids
- Keratoprosthesis may provide some useful vision.

CHAPTER 9

Uvea

1. Describe the anatomy and blood supply of uvea.
- Middle vascular coat
- Parts:
  - Iris
  - Ciliary body
  - Choroid.

Iris

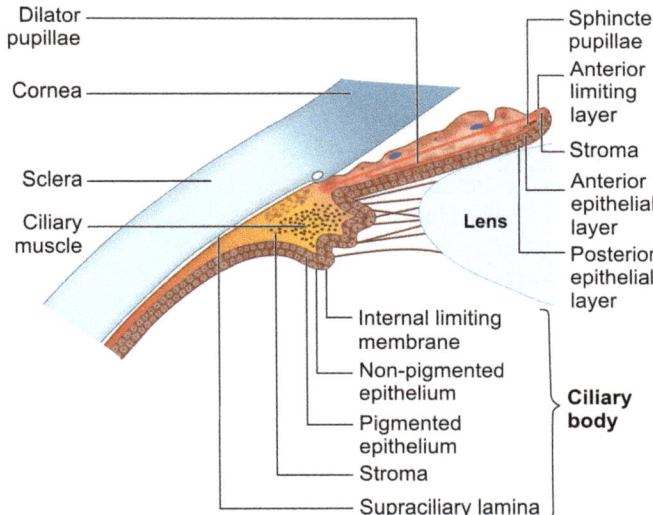

Fig. 9.1: Iris and ciliary body.

- Anteriormost part of uveal tract
- Circular disk—similar to diaphragm of camera
- Central aperture—pupil
- Periphery—attached to middle of anterior surface of ciliary body
- Ciliary zone
- Pupillary zone
- Collarette—zigzag line between ciliary and pupillary zone
  - 1.5 mm from pupillary margin
  - Thickest region of iris.

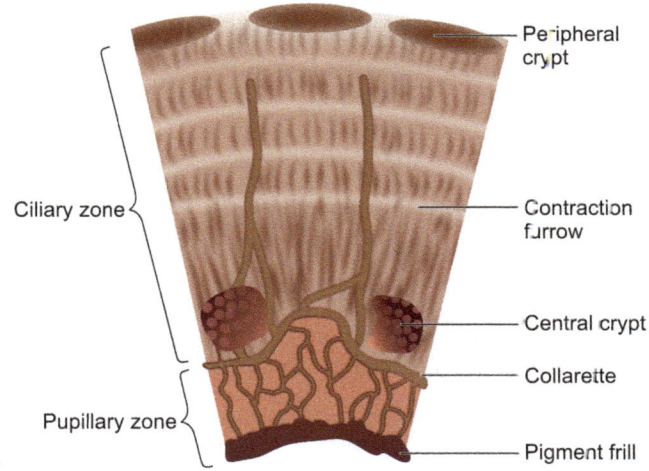

Fig. 9.2: Anterior surface of iris.

Ciliary zone
- Series of radial streaks and crypts
- Crypts: Depressions in which endothelium is missing
- Peripheral crypts: Near iris root, iris thinnest at iris root
- Central crypts: Near collarette.

Pupillary zone
- Smooth and flat
- Lies between collarette and pupillary zone.

Layers of Iris
- Anterior limiting layer
- Stroma
- Epithelial layer (pigmented epithelium—two layers).

Anterior Limiting Layer
- Also called endothelial layer
- Condensed part of stroma
- Consists of melanocytes and fiber.

Iris Stroma
- Loosely arranged connective tissue
- Blood vessels and nerves
- Sphincter pupillae and dilator pupillae.

Sphincter pupillae
- 1 mm circular band at pupillary border
- Supplied by parasympathetic fibers
  - Through 3rd nerve.

Dilator pupillae
- Radial fibers
- Extends from ciliary body to pupillary margin
- Supplied by cervical sympathetic fibers.

Epithelial Layer
- It consists of two layers—anterior and posterior, which are pigmented.

Ciliary Body
- Forward continuation of choroid
- Triangular in cross section:
  - Anterior
  - Outer
  - Inner.

Anterior: Forms part of angle of anterior chamber (AC)

Outer: Lies against sclera

Inner: Two parts:
  i. *Anterior* (2 mm) pars plicata
  ii. *Posterior* (4 mm) pars plana relatively avascular.

Structure of Ciliary Body
From without inward:
- Supraciliary lamina
- Stroma
- Layer of pigmented epithelium
- Layer of nonpigmented epithelium
- Internal limiting membrane.

Stroma of ciliary body
- Consists of collagen and fibroblasts
- Embedded in stroma are ciliary muscle, vessels, nerves, and pigmented cells.

Ciliary muscle
- Longitudinal or meridional fibers help in aqueous outflow.
- Radial or oblique fibers help in aqueous outflow
- Circular fibers help in accommodation
- Pull of these fibers slacken the tension on suspensory ligament—lens becomes spherical.

Ciliary processes
- Finger-like projections from pars plicata
- 70 in number
- 2 mm × 0.5 mm
- White in color.

Functions of Ciliary Body
- Formation of aqueous
- Helps in accommodation.

Choroid
- Dark brown, highly vascular layer
- Extends from optic disk to ora serrata
- Inner surface—smooth, adjacent to pigment epithelium of retina
- Outer surface—rough adjacent to sclera.

Structure of Choroid
- Suprachoroidal lamina
- Stroma
- Basal lamina.

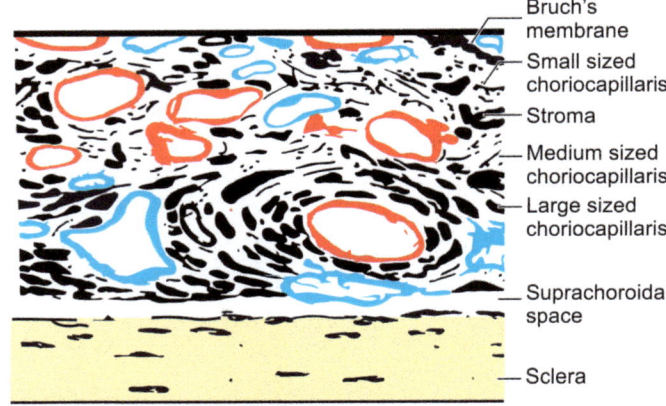

Fig. 9.3: Structure of choroid.

Blood Supply of Choroid
Arterial Supply
- Short posterior ciliary arteries
- Long posterior ciliary arteries
- Anterior ciliary arteries.

All arise from ophthalmic artery.

Venous Drainage
- Three groups
- Short posterior ciliary
- Vortex veins
- Anterior ciliary
- Short posterior ciliary received blood from sclera
- Vortex veins—four in number
- Enters sclera behind equator to open into ophthalmic veins
- Anterior ciliary veins receive blood from outer part of ciliary muscle.

2. Classify uveitis.

Definition
Uveitis is inflammation of uveal tract.
- Endogenous uveitis is a nonpurulent inflammation of uveal tract resulting from organismal invasion or hypersensitive reaction to a variety of infectious and noninfectious agents.
- Exogenous uveitis is caused by either external injury to uvea or invasion of microorganisms or other agents from outside.

Classification
- Anatomical
- Clinical
- Pathological or Morphological
- Etiological.

Anatomical Classification
- *Anterior*: Iritis or iridocyclitis (iris and pars plicata)
- Intermediate or pars planitis—pars plana and ora serrata are involved
- *Posterior*: Choroiditis, chorioretinitis
- Panuveitis—entire uveal tract.

Clinical Classification
- *Acute*: Sudden onset—disease lasts for 6 weeks to 3 months
- *Chronic*: Insidious onset—lasts longer than 3 months.

Pathological Classification
- Suppurative or purulent uveitis.
- Nonsuppurative uveitis:
  - Nongranulomatous
  - Granulomatous.

Etiological Classification
- Infective uveitis
- Allergic uveitis
- Toxic uveitis
- Traumatic uveitis
- Uveitis associated with noninfective systemic disorders
- Idiopathic.

Infective Uveitis
- Exogenous
- Endogenous
- Secondary infection
  - From neighboring structures.
- **Types of infective uveitis:**
  - Bacterial infections
  - Viral infections—herpes and cytomegalovirus (CMV) viruses
  - Fungal—(Rare) aspergillosis, candidiasis, blastomycosis
  - Parasitic—toxoplasmosis, toxocariasis, amebiasis
  - Rickettsial—typhus infections.

Allergic or Hypersensitivity Uveitis

Most Common:
- Microbial allergy: Septic focus elsewhere in the body
- Anaphylactic: Follows systemic anaphylactic reactions
- Atopic: Seasonal iritis due to pollens, dust
- Autoimmune uveitis: Seen in autoimmune disorders—Still's disease, rheumatoid arthritis, systemic lupus erythematosus (SLE), Reiter's disease, etc.
  - Phacoanaphylactic endophthalmitis: Autoantigens are lens proteins
  - Sympathetic ophthalmitis: Uveal pigments human leukocyte antigen (HLA)-associated uveitis:
    » Seen in persons with certain specific HLA phenotypes
    » HLA-B27—associated with ankylosing spondylitis, Reiter's disease
    » HLA-B5—Behcet's disease
    » HLA-DR4 and -Dw15—Vogt-Koyanagi-Harada disease.

Toxic Uveitis
- Endotoxins: Produced inside the body—microbial toxins
- Endocular toxins: Produced from ocular tissues from intraocular hemorrhages and tumors and phacotoxic uveitis
- Exogenous toxins: Irritant substances of chemical, animal or vegetative origin.

Traumatic Uveitis
- Seen in accidental or operative injuries to uveal tissues
- Direct mechanical injuries
- Irritative effects of blood products after intraocular hemorrhage
- Chemical effects of retained intraocular foreign body
- Sympathetic ophthalmitis in the other eye.

Uveitis Associated with Noninfectious Systemic Diseases
- Sarcoidosis
- Collagen diseases
- Metabolic diseases
- Disseminated sclerosis
- Skin diseases.

Idiopathic Uveitis
- **Specific**—pars planitis:
  - Sympathetic ophthalmitis
  - Fuchs heterochromic uveitis.
- **Nonspecific**—where etiology cannot be detected
  - Forms 25% of cases.

3. Discuss the clinical features, complications, differential diagnosis and management of acute iridocyclitis.

Symptoms
- Pain, redness, photophobia, and lacrimation
- Defective vision.

Pain
Dull aching, worse at night, and trigeminal pain

Redness
- Circumcorneal congestion (CCC)
- Hyperemia of anterior ciliary vessels
- Due to the effect of toxins, histamine and axon reflex.

Photophobia
- Associated with blepharospasm
- Sensory fibers of 5th nerve irritated
- Reflex spasm of orbicularis oculi.

Lacrimation
- Lacrimation reflex
- Afferent—5th nerve
- Efferent—secretomotor fibers of 7th nerve.

Defective vision
- Induced myopia due to ciliary spasm
- Corneal haze [due to edema and keratic precipitates (KPs)]
- Aqueous turbidity
- Exudates
- Complicated cataract
- Vitreous haze
- Cyclitic membrane
- Macular edema
- Papillitis
- Secondary glaucoma.

Signs
- Lid edema
- Circumcorneal congestion
- Corneal signs
- Anterior chamber signs
- Iris signs
- Pupillary signs
- Changes in the lens
- Changes in the vitreous.

Lid edema
Usually mild—seen in severe acute attack.

Circumcorneal congestion
- Marked in acute
- Minimal in chronic.

Corneal signs
- Corneal edema
- Due to toxic endotheliitis.

Keratic precipitates
Cellular deposits at back of cornea, composed of epithelioid cells, lymphocytes and polymorphs.

Arlt's triangle
- Deposition of KPs in the form of triangle
  - Apex at center and base inferiorly
- Due to convection currents in aqueous
- Type of KPs:
  - Mutton fat KPs
  - Small and medium
  - Red
  - Old.

Mutton fat KPs
- Occurs in granulomatous iridocyclitis
- Consists of epithelioid cells and macrophages
- Large, thick, fluffy mutton fat like
- Greasy and waxy appearance
- Usually 10–15 in number.

Small and medium KPs
- Occurs in nongranulomatous iridocyclitis
- Consists of lymphocytes
- Small, discrete, dirty white
- Irregular arrangement
- More in number.

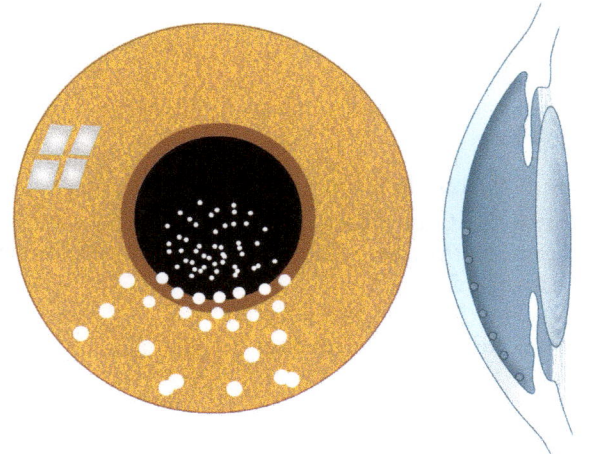

Fig. 9.4: Keratic precipitates. Mutton fat KPs at the bottom, small and medium KPs above.

Red KPs
- Due to hemorrhages
- Consists of RBCs and inflammatory cells
- Seen in herpetic uveitis.

Old KPs
- Sign of healed uveitis
- Pigmented and crenated.

Anterior chamber signs
- Aqueous cells
- Aqueous flare
- Hypopyon
- Hyphema
- Peripheral anterior synechia.

Aqueous cells
- Indicator of activity
- Consists of lymphocytes and plasma cells
- Better seen in slit lamp with 3 mm × 1 mm slit
- Maximum light intensity and magnification.

Grades
- 0: None
- +1: 5–10 cells per field
- +2: 11–20 cells per field
- +3: 21–50 cells per field
- +4: >50 cells per field.

Aqueous flare
- Earliest sign of iridocyclitis
- Due to leakage of protein into anterior chamber from damaged blood vessels
- Breakdown of blood—aqueous barrier
- Better seen with point beam of light in slit lamp
- Protein particles are seen as moving dust particles due to Tyndall phenomenon.

Grades of flare
- 0: None
- +1: Faint—just detectable
- +2: Moderate (iris and lens details clear)

- +3: Marked (iris and lens details hazy)
- +4: Intense (fixated coagulated aqueous).

Hypopyon
- Sterile pus in AC
- Heavy and thick exudates settles down
- Consists of polymorphonuclear leukocytes and fibrin.

Iris signs
- Loss of pattern
- Change in iris color
- Iris nodules
- Posterior synechia
- Neovascularization.

Loss of pattern
- In active phase—due to edema and water logging of iris
- In chronic phase—due to atrophic changes.

Changes in iris color
- In active phase—becomes muddy
- In chronic phase—hyper- and depigmented.

Iris nodules
- Typical of granulomatous uveitis
- Koeppe's nodules:
    - Occurs in pupillary border
    - May initiate posterior synechia.
- Bussaca's nodules:
    - Occurs near collarette
    - Large and less common.

Posterior synechia
- Adhesion between posterior surface of iris and anterior surface of lens or anterior vitreous
- Due to organization of fibrin rich exudate.

Types
a. Segmental
b. Annular or ring synechia
c. Total.

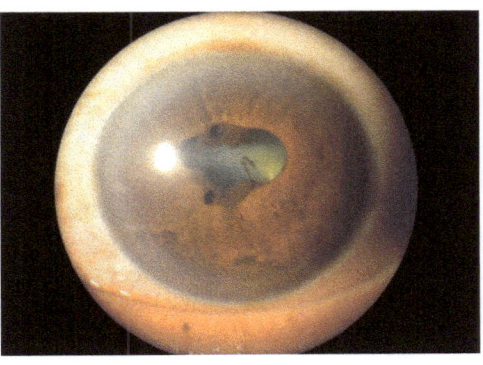

Fig. 9.6: Posterior synechia.

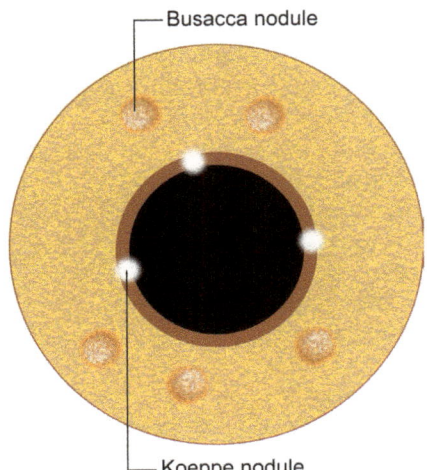

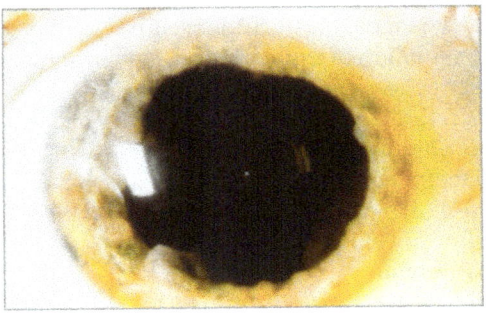

Fig. 9.5: Iris nodules.

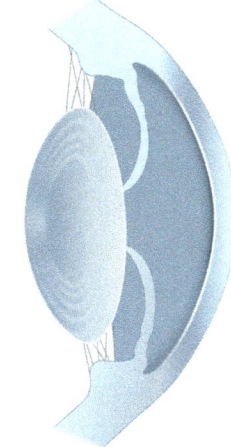

Fig. 9.7: Annular posterior synechia.

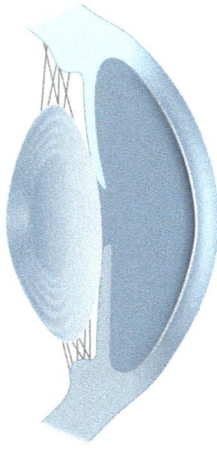

Fig. 9.8: Total posterior synechia.

- Segmental—attached at some points
- Annular—360° of adhesion of pupillary margin posteriorly—results in seclusio pupillae prevents circulation of aqueous from posterior chamber to anterior chamber—lead to iris bombe.
  » Collected aqueous in posterior chamber pushes iris forward.
- Total posterior synechia
  » Due to plastering of entire iris to lens results in deep AC.

Neovascularization of iris
- Also called rubeosis iridis
- Seen in chronic iridocyclitis.

Pupillary signs
- Miosis—seen in acute attack
  - Due to irritation of sphincter by toxins.
- Irregular pupil shape
  - Due to segmental posterior synechia
  - When dilated results in festooned pupil.

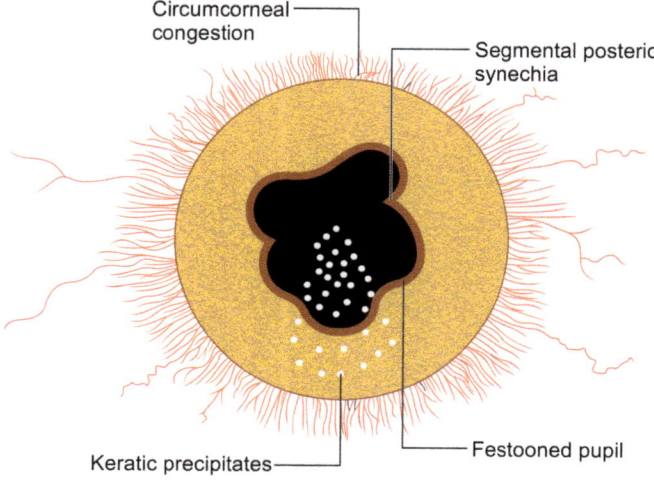

Fig. 9.9: Festooned pupil.

- Ectropion pupillae
  - Eversion of pupillary margin
  - Due to contraction of fibrinous exudate.
- Pupillary reaction
  - Sluggish due to edema and hyperemia which hamper its movements.
- Occlusio pupillae
  - Results when pupil is completely occluded
  - Due to organization of exudates in pupillary area.

Changes in the lens
- Pigment dispersion on the anterior surface of lens.
- Complicated cataract:
  - Polychromatic luster
  - Bread crumb appearance
  - Due to early posterior subcapsular opacities.

Changes in the vitreous
- Vitritis due to exudates and inflammatory cells.

Complications and Sequela

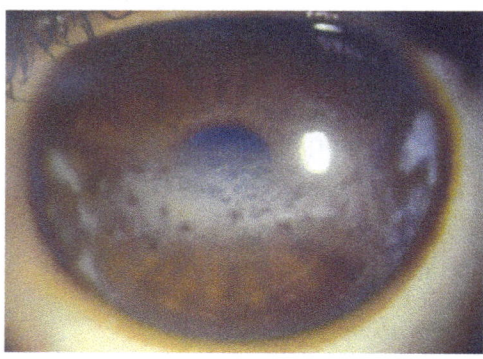

Fig. 9.10: Band keratopathy.

- Sclerosing keratitis
  - Seen in TB, syphilis, rheumatic fever.
- Band-shaped keratopathy
  - Seen in Still's disease due to calcium deposits.
- Keratopathy
  - Seen in long-standing anterior uveitis.
- Posterior synechiae—seclusio pupillae, occlusio pupillae and iris bombe:
  - Seclusio pupillae is annular posterior synechia or ring synechia, which are 360° adhesions of pupillary margin to anterior capsule of lens.
  - Occlusio pupillae results when the pupil is completely occluded due to the exudates across the entire pupillary area.
  - *Iris bombe*: It occurs when there is collection of aqueous behind the iris due to annular posterior synechia which pushes the iris anteriorly leading to iris bombe. This prevents circulation of aqueous from posterior chamber to anterior chamber. This results in rise of intraocular pressure (IOP).
  - Treatment for iris bombe is YAG laser iridotomy.
- Rubeosis iridis:
  - Seen in chronic cases
  - Initially starts at collarette.
- Iris atrophy:
  - Moth-eaten appearance.
- Complicated cataract.
- Secondary glaucoma:
  - Early—trabeculitis
  - Late—peripheral anterior synechia.
- Cyclitic membrane:
  - Fibrosis of plastic exudates behind the lens
  - Seen in acute plastic iridocyclitis
  - Coagulation of exudates on ciliary processes destroys its function.
- Chorioretinitis.
- Retinal complications:
  - Macular edema
  - Exudative retinal detachment.
- Papillitis.
- Phthisis bulbi:
  - End stage of chronic uveitis

- Soft, shrunken, small, and useless eyeball
- Ciliary body is disorganized and aqueous is not secreted.

Differential Diagnosis

- Acute conjunctivitis
- Acute congestive glaucoma.

S. No.	Features	Acute conjunctivitis	Acute iridocyclitis	Acute congestive glaucoma
i.	Onset	Gradual	Usually gradual	Sudden
ii.	Pain	Mid discomfort	Moderate in eye and along the first division of trigeminal nerve	Severe in eye and the entire trigeminal area
iii.	Discharge	Mucopurulent	Watery	Watery
iv.	Colored halos	May be present	Absent	Present
v.	Vision	Good	Slightly impaired	Markedly impaired
vi.	Congestion	Superficial	Deep ciliary	Deep ciliary
vii.	Tenderness	Absent	Marked	Marked
viii.	Pupil	Normal	May be deep	Very shallow
ix.	Media	Clear	Hazy due to KPs, aqueous flare and pupillary exudates	Hazy due to edematous cornea
x.	Anterior chamber	Normal	May be deep	Very shallow
xi.	Iris	Normal	Muddy	Edematous
xii.	Intraocular pressure	Normal	Usually normal	Raised
xiii.	Constitutional symptoms	Absent	Little	Prostration and vomiting

S. No.	Features	Granulomatous uveitis	Nongranulomatous uveitis
i.	Onset	Insidious	Acute
ii.	Pain	Minimal	Marked
iii.	Photophobia	Slight	Marked
iv.	Ciliary congestion	Minimal	Small
v.	Keratic precipitates (KPs)	Mutton fat	Small
vi.	Aqueous flare	Mild	Marked
vii.	Iris nodules	Usually present	Absent
viii.	Posterior synechia	Thick and broad based	Thin and tenuous
ix.	Fundus	Nodular lesions	Diffuse involvement

Investigations

History and clinical examination

Young man with recurrent chronic low back pain
- Usually unilateral anterior uveitis
- Ankylosing spondylitis
  - Unilateral keratouveitis with dendrites—herpes simplex.

Focal sepsis

Total count and differential count

- General information about inflammatory response.

Erythrocyte sedimentation rate (ESR)

- To assess chronic inflammatory condition of body
- Raised in collagen diseases.

Blood sugar: Raised in diabetes mellitus.

Blood uric acid: Raised in gout.

Serum analysis

- Serum viscosity: In rheumatoid arthritis, Eales and Behcet's disease
- Serum calcium: In sarcoidosis
- Serum protein: In collagen diseases.

Serum antibodies

- Syphilis:
  - VDRL
  - FTA ABS
  - TPI.
- Rheumatoid factor
- Toxoplasma antibodies:
  - Dye test
  - Indirect fluorescent antibody test
  - Enzyme-linked immunosorbent assay (ELISA) test.

CMV complement fixation test

HLA typing

- Skin test
- Indication of specific delayed hypersensitivity
- Tuberculin test
- Toxoplasmin test
- Behcet's skin test
- Kveim reaction—for sarcoidosis.

X-ray

- Chest
- Paranasal sinuses
- Sacroiliac joints
- Lumbar spine.

Paracentesis and study of aqueous

Tissue biopsy

Fluorescein angiography, ultrasonography

Vitreous aspiration—for posterior uveitis.

Treatment

Aim of Treatment

- To prevent vision-threatening complications

- To relieve patient discomfort and pain
- To treat underlying cause of uveitis.

Specific Treatment

Directed at the cause of disease.

Nonspecific Treatment
- Aim at reducing the inflammatory response
- Physical measures:
  - Dark glasses—give comfort
  - Hot fomentation:
    » ↑circulation
    » ↓venous stasis
- Mydriatics and cycloplegics
- Nonsteroidal anti-inflammatory drugs (NSAIDs)
- Steroids
- Immunosuppressive agents.

Mydriatics and Cycloplegics
- Relieves spasm of ciliary muscles
- ↓ vascular permeability:
  - Thus exudation is curbed.
- Dilates pupil:
  - Prevents posterior synechia
  - Breaks down recently formed synechia.

Drugs used
- Atropine 1%—long-acting and powerful
- Homatropine 2%—duration of action 24 hours
- Cyclopentolate 1%—duration of action 24 hours
- Phenylephrine 10%—duration of action 3 hours
- Tropicamide 1%—duration of action 6 hours.

Nonsteroidal Anti-inflammatory Drugs
- Antiprostaglandin effect
- Drugs:
  - Aspirin
  - Phenylbutazone
  - Oxyphenbutazone
  - Diclofenac
  - Aceclofenac.
- More useful in rheumatoid diseases.

Steroids
- Mainstay of treatment
- Nonspecific anti-inflammatory action
- Phagocytosis is decreased
- Fibrosis is curbed
- Inhibition of neovascularization
  Routes of administration:
  - Topical—eye drops/ointment
  - Periocular injection
  - Systemic.
- **Topical steroids**:
  - Only for anterior uveitis
  - Dexamethasone
  - Betamethasone
  - Prednisolone acetate
  - Fluorometholone or loteprednol—weak steroid
  - Frequency of administration varies with severity of inflammation.

One drop every 15 minutes for a few hours gradually tapered to 4 times daily, further reduced by 1 drop per week for about 6 weeks.

Periocular injection
- Long-acting effect:
  - Triamcinolone acetonide
  - Methylprednisolone acetate.
- Anterior or posterior sub-Tenon's injection.

Indications
- Severe acute anterior uveitis
- Resistant cases
- Intermediate uveitis
- Poor patient compliance with topical/systemic medication at the time of surgery in eyes with uveitis.

Systemic therapy
- Indication:
  - Severe anterior uveitis resistant to topical therapy
  - Intermediate uveitis unresponsive to posterior sub-Tenon's injection or panuveitis.

Dosage
- High dose of steroids
- 60–100 mg daily for 2 weeks
- Decreased at weekly intervals and tapered in 8 weeks.

Immunosuppressive agents
- Sight-threatening uveitis
  - Bilateral cases
  - *For example*: Vogt-Koyanagi-Harada syndrome, Behcet's disease and sympathetic ophthalmitis.
- Steroid-sparing therapy: Intolerable side effects from steroid therapy
  Preparations used:
  - Antimetabolites
    » Azathioprine
    » Methotrexate.
  - T-cell inhibitors
    » Cyclosporine
    » Tacrolimus.

Specific Treatment

Treat the etiological factor

- Syphilis
- Leprosy
- Toxocariasis
- Tuberculosis
- Sarcoidosis
- Toxoplasmosis.

Nonspecific treatment has to be started before any etiological diagnosis is made.

4. What is intermediate uveitis (also called pars planitis)?

Intermediate Uveitis

It is the inflammation of ciliary body, peripheral retina and anterior vitreous. It may be infectious or noninfectious.

Symptoms: Blurred vision and floaters.

Signs
Fine white KPs on the back of cornea. Mild aqueous flare, posterior subcapsular opacities, cells in anterior vitreous, snow banking on the pars plana of ciliary body.

Treatment
Periocular steroids if unilateral and systemic steroids if bilateral. In refractory cases, immunosuppressives are given.

5. Write short notes on choroiditis (posterior uveitis).
Choroiditis refers to inflammation of choroid.
Etiology: Same as anterior uveitis.

Clinical Types
- Suppurative choroiditis: It is almost a part of endophthalmitis.
- Nonsuppurative choroiditis: It may be granulomatous or nongranulomatous. It is usually bilateral.

Classification
Depending on the number and site of lesion, it is classified as follows:
- Diffuse choroiditis—involves most of choroid
- Disseminated choroiditis—multiple small areas of inflammation spreading all over the choroid
- Circumscribed choroiditis (localized/focal).

Depending on the location, it is as follows:
- Central choroiditis—involves macula
- Juxtacecal choroiditis—involves area adjoining optic disk
- Anterior/periphreral choroiditis—involves peripheral part of choroid anterior to equator
- Equatorial choroiditis—involves equator.

Symptoms
- Defective vision
- Photopsia
- Seeing black spots floating in front of eye
- Metamorphopsia
- Micropsia
- Macropsia.

Signs
- Anterior segment is usually normal
- Vitreous opacities—fine, coarse, stringy or snowball

Fundus

S. No.	Active choroiditis	Healed choroiditis
	Differences between active and healed choroiditis.	
i.	Vitreous haze is present	Vitreous is clear
ii.	Ill-defined yellow patch with feathery margins	Well-defined white patch
iii.	Lesion is deeper to retinal vessels. Overlying retina is often cloudy and edematous	Large choroidal vessels may be exposed. Borders are pigmented

Complications
Iridocyclitis, complicated cataract, vitreous degeneration, macular edema, secondary periphlebitis and retinal detachment.

Treatment
- Nonspecific: Posterior sub-Tenon's injection of triamcinolone and systemic steroids. Rarely, immunosuppressive drugs.
- Specific: Treatment of cause such as tuberculosis, toxoplasmosis, toxocariasis and syphilis.

6. Discuss the etiology, clinical features, and management of sympathetic ophthalmitis.

Definition
- Severe inflammation of the sound eye after injury to the other eye
- Serious bilateral granulomatous panuveitis which follows penetrating ocular trauma particularly to the ciliary body
- The injured eye is the exciting eye and the fellow eye is the sympathizing eye.

Etiology
Unknown
- Considered to be autoimmune
  - T-cell mediated disease
  - Allergen—uveal pigment
  - Viral infection—may be initiating factor
  - Modifies the uveal protein to become antigenic or damages cells to uncover previously sequestrated antigen
  - Usually starts 4–8 weeks after injury to the first eye—earliest—9 days
  - May be delayed for months or years
  - Children—more susceptible
  - 65% after penetrating trauma
  - 25% after surgery
  - 10% after perforated corneal ulcer.

Pathology
- Same in both eyes
- Granulomatous uveitis
- Nodular aggregation of lymphocytes, plasma cells, epithelioid cells, and giant cells scattered throughout the uveal tract.

Dalen-Fuchs Nodule
Seen in granulomatous uveitis as small, and yellowish white spots in the choroid. They are nodular aggregation of lymphocytes and epithelioid cells with proliferation of retinal pigment epithelial cells.

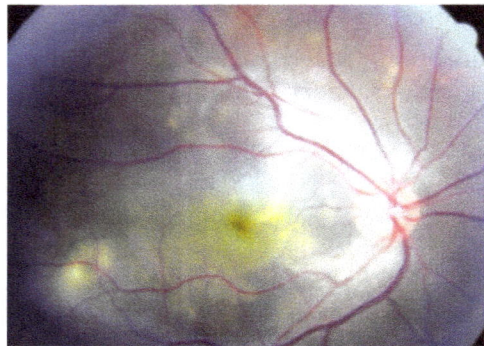

Fig. 9.11: Dalen-Fuchs nodules.

Symptoms
- Photophobia and lacrimation
- Impaired near vision due to irritation of ciliary body.

Signs
- Mild to moderate ciliary congestion
- Tender eyeball
- Keratic precipitates
- Vitreous floaters
- Retrolental floaters—earliest sign
- Optic disk edema may occur
- May present as acute plastic iridocyclitis.

Prophylactic Treatment
- Early use of corticosteroids and broad-spectrum antibiotics
- Meticulous repair of wound
- Taking care that uveal tissue is not incarcerated in the wound
- Evisceration of injured eye is done if there is no chance of saving useful vision
- Rarely occurs after excision of injured eye unless it has commenced before excision.

Curative Treatment
- Corticosteroid by all routes (systemic, periocular and topical)
- Intravenous methylprednisolone 1 g, followed by 100 mg of prednisolone orally, tapered slowly. 15–20 mg of prednisolone to be continued for many months
- Severe cases—immunosuppressive drops, cyclosporine A
- Topical atropine thrice daily
- Severe cases—immunosuppressive drops, cyclosporine A
- Oral cyclosporine 3–5 mg/kg/day
- Azathioprine 1–2 mg/kg/day
- Both can be given with steroids
- Topical atropine thrice daily.

7. Write short notes on rubeosis iridis.

Definition
- Neovascularization of iris particularly near its root and angle of anterior chamber
- Causes neovascular glaucoma.

Etiology

Ischemic
- Central retinal vein occlusion
- Proliferative diabetic retinopathy
- Eales disease
- Central retinal artery occlusion
- Carotid artery disease.

Inflammation
Chronic uveitis.

Neoplastic
- Retinoblastoma
- Malignant melanoma
- Metastasis.

Symptoms
- Pain and defective vision.

Signs
- Hyperemia of conjunctival and episcleral vessels
- Increased IOP
- Corneal edema
- Dilated capillary tufts in iris.

Stage 1
New vessels between pupil margin and iris.

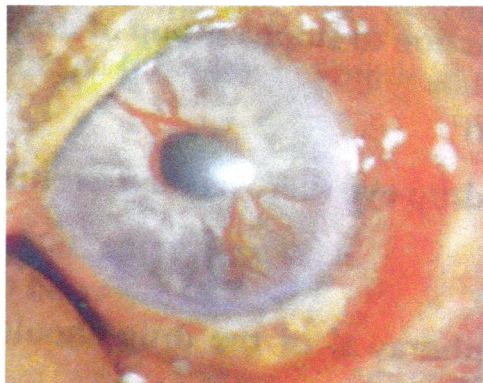

Fig. 9.12: New vessels on the iris.

Stage 2
- New vessels extending across the whole iris with involvement of angle which remains open.
- New vessels arborize and form a fibrovascular membrane which blocks the trabeculum and gives rise to secondary open-angle glaucoma.

Stage 3
- Stage 2 + Peripheral anterior synechia and angle-closure contraction of fibrovascular tissue in the angle with pulling of peripheral iris over trabeculum. The angle closes circumferentially in a zipper-like fashion.

Uvea

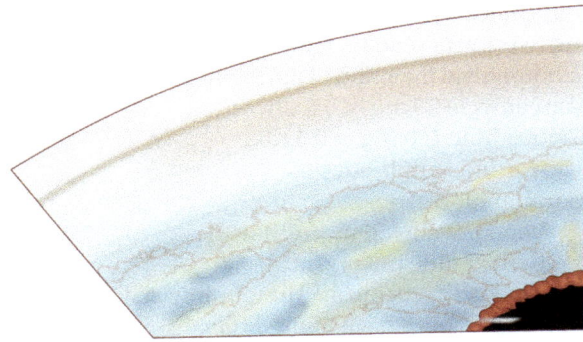

Fig. 9.13: Early angle neovascularization.

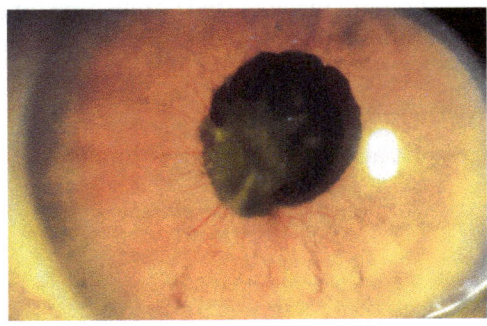

Fig. 9.14: Severe rubeosis iridis.

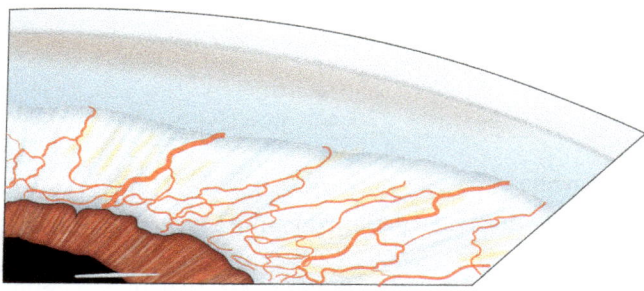

Fig. 9.15: Total angle closure.

Treatment

- Atropine eye drops twice daily
- Steroids eye drops 6 times daily
- 0.5% timolol maleate twice daily
- Panretinal photocoagulation
- Uncontrolled IOP:
  - Trabeculectomy with mitomycin C
  - Valvular shunts.

8. Discuss the etiology, clinical features, and management of endophthalmitis.

Definition

Inflammation of internal structure of the eye viz choroid, retina, and vitreous.

Etiology and Types

- Infective
- Noninfective (sterile).

Infective Endophthalmitis

Mode of Infection

- Exogenous:
  - Following perforating injuries
  - Perforation of infected corneal ulcer
  - Postoperative infections.
- Endogenous or metastatic:
  - Through blood spread from septic foci.
- Secondary infection from surrounding structures:
  - Eyelids, conjunctiva and lacrimal passage.

Causative Organisms

- **Bacterial endophthalmitis**
  - Gram-positive bacteria (90%):
    » *Staphylococcus epidermidis*
    » *Staphylococcus aureus*
    » Streptococci
    » Pneumococcus
    » *Propionibacterium*.
  - Gram-negative bacteria (7%):
    » *Pseudomonas*
    » *Proteus*
    » *Haemophilus influenzae*
    » *Escherichia coli*.
- **Fungal endophthalmitis:**
  - Aspergillosis
  - *Fusarium*
  - *Candida*.

Noninfective Endophthalmitis

Caused by toxins or toxic substances

- Postoperative
  - Toxic reaction to chemicals adherent to IOL or instruments.
- Post-traumatic
  - Toxic reactions to retained intraocular foreign body, e.g. pure copper.
- Intraocular tumor necrosis
  - Presenting as Masquerade syndrome.
- Phacoanaphylactic
  - Induced by lens proteins in Morgagnian cataract.

Clinical Features

- Acute bacterial endophthalmitis:
  - Occurs within 7 days of operation
  - Severe ocular pain, redness, and lacrimation
  - Photophobia and loss of vision
  - Lids—red and swollen
  - Conjunctiva—chemosis and circumcorneal congestion
  - Cornea—cloudy
  - Anterior chamber—hypopyon
  - Iris—edematous and muddy
  - Pupil—yellow reflex due to purulent exudation in vitreous. Absence of red fundus reflex—inability to visualize fundus even with indirect ophthalmoscope

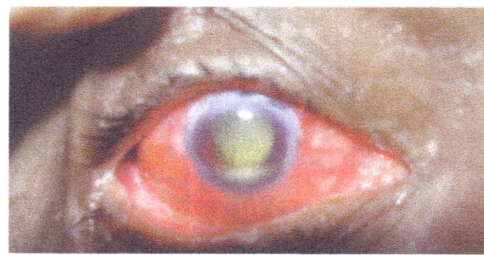

Fig. 9.16: Postoperative posterior endophthalmitis.

- Vitreous—filled with exudates and pus
- Intraocular pressure—raised in early stages. Low in severe cases due to destruction of ciliary processes.
- Fungal endophthalmitis:
  - Longer incubation period of several weeks mild pain and redness with hypopyon.
    Vitreous may be filled with granulomatous mass.

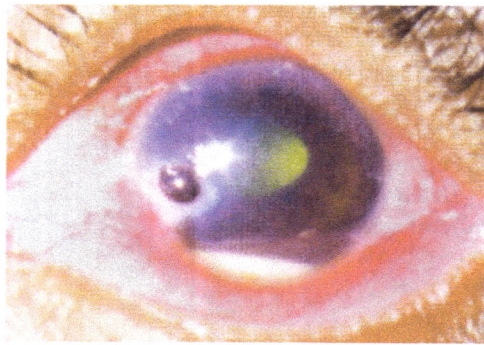

Fig. 9.17: Endophthalmitis following penetrating injury.

Differential Diagnosis
Panophthalmitis
- Associated inflammation of extraocular tissue
- Painful limitation of movements of eyeball.

Complications
- Panophthalmitis
- Papillitis
- Phthisis bulbi.

Investigations
Identification and culture and sensitivity of causative organism from aqueous and vitreous taps.

Treatment
- Antibiotics
- Steroids
- Supportive therapy
- Vitrectomy.

Early diagnosis and vigorous therapy is essential:
- Intravitreal antibiotic at the earliest, combination of two antibiotics—one for gram-positive, another for gram-negative organisms.
- First choice—vancomycin 1 mg in 0.1 mL and ceftazidime 2.25 mg in 0.1 mL.

- Second choice—vancomycin 1 mg in 0.1 mL and amikacin 0.4 mg in 0.1 mL—can be repeated after 48 hours.
- Subconjunctival injection of antibiotics daily for 5–7 days
  - Vancomycin 25 mg in 0.5 mL
  - Ceftazidime 100 mg in 0.5 mL.
- Topical fortified antibiotics
  - Combination of:
    » Vancomycin (50 mg/mL) with
    » Ceftazidime (50 mg/mL)
    » Amikacin (20 mg/mL) or tobramycin (15 mg/mL).
- Systemic antibiotics have limited role.

Steroid therapy
- Limits the tissue damage caused by inflammatory process:
  - Intravitreous injection of dexamethasone 0.4 mg in 0.1 mL in bacterial endophthalmitis.

Supportive therapy
Cycloplegia—1% atropine or 2% homatropine tds.

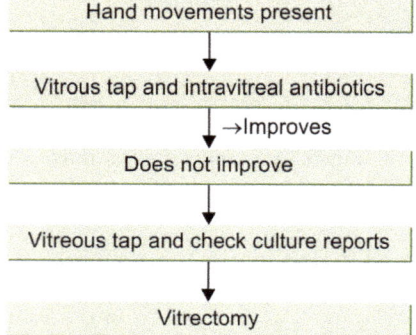

Vitrectomy:
- To be performed if patient does not improve within 48–72 hours
- Severe infection with vision reduced to light perception
- Helps in removal of infecting organism present in infected vitreous mass.

Endophthalmitis vitrectomy study (EVS):
- Vision–only perception to light
  - Early vitrectomy with intravitreal antibiotics.

9. Write short notes on panophthalmitis.
Definition
- Intense purulent inflammation of whole eyeball including the Tenon's capsule.

Etiology
- Exogenous
  - Usually due to infected wound which may be due to trauma, operation or after perforation of corneal ulcer
- Common pathogens
  - *Pneumococcus, Staphylococcus, Streptococcus, E. coli*
  - *Pseudomonas, Bacillus subtilis, Clostridium welchii*, etc.
- Endogenous etiology
  - Due to metastasis of infected embolus in the retinal artery and choroidal vessels.

Uvea

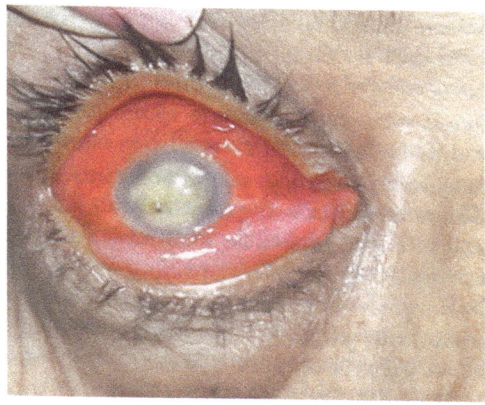

Fig. 9.18: Panophthalmitis.

Clinical Features
- Severe pain and headache
- Complete loss of vision
- Purulent discharge
- Marked redness and swelling of eyes
- Constitutional symptoms—malaise, fever.

Signs
- Lids—marked edema and hyperemia
- Eyeball—slightly proptosed
- Movements—limited and painful
- Conjunctiva—marked chemosis. Conjunctiva and ciliary congestion
- Cornea—cloudy and edematous
- Anterior chamber—full of pus
- Vision—no perception of light
- IOP—raised
- Globe perforation may occur at limbus. When pus comes out, IOP falls.

Complications
- Orbital cellulitis
- Cavernous sinus thrombosis
- Meningitis and encephalitis
- Phthisis bulbi.

Treatment
- Visual prognosis is poor
- Anti-inflammatory and analgesics to relieve pain
- Broad-spectrum antibiotics to prevent further spread of infection in the surrounding structures
- Evisceration.

10. Write short notes on evisceration.
- Removal of contents of eyeball leaving behind the sclera
- Frill evisceration—3 mm frill of sclera is left around the optic nerve.

Indication
- Panophthalmitis with no perception of light.
  - To prevent extension of infection to brain.
- Bleeding anterior staphyloma
  - To control excessive bleeding from the uveal tract.

Surgical Steps
- Conjunctiva and Tenon's capsule are separated all over the limbus posteriorly
- Cornea is excised with corneal scissors after incising it by 11 blade
- Uveal tissue is separated from sclera with the help of evisceration spatula. Contents are scooped out using evisceration curette
- Extraocular muscles separated as in enucleation
- Sclera excision by curved scissors leaving 3 mm frill of sclera around optic nerve
- Tenon's capsule and conjunctiva closed.

11. Write short notes on enucleation.
Eyeball is excised as a whole by cutting the optic nerve.

Indications
- Malignant tumors in eyeball:
  - Retinoblastoma
  - Malignant melanoma, to prevent spread of malignant cells to brain.
- Severely injured eye with no perception of light, to prevent sympathetic ophthalmitis in good eye.
- Painful, blind eye
  - Absolute glaucoma to prevent severe pain.
- In eye donation
  - Done within 6 hours after death.

Contraindication
- Panophthalmitis—because infection may spread to brain through meningeal sheaths leading to meningitis or encephalitis.

Technique

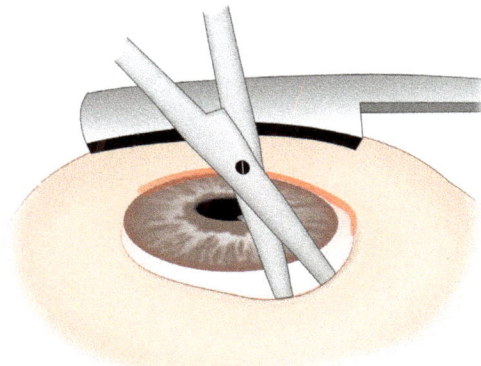

Fig. 9.19: Cutting the conjunctiva around the limbus.

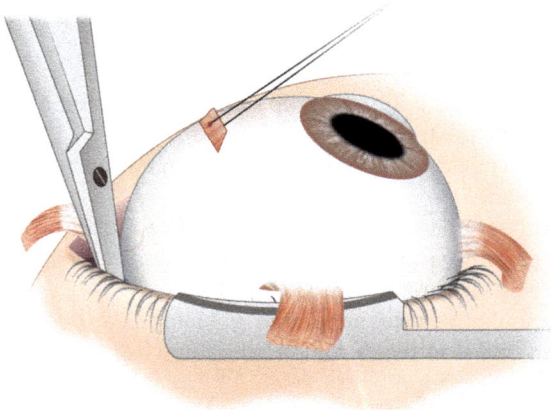

Fig. 9.20: Cutting the extraocular muscles.

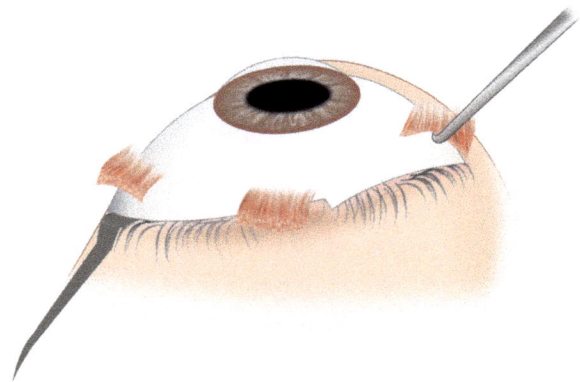

Fig. 9.21: Cutting the optic nerve and removal of eyeball.

- Conjunctiva cut all around cornea just outside the limbus
- Rectus muscles hooked with muscle hook and divided close to globe one by one
- Optic nerve is cut as far back as possible by enucleation scissors from medial side
- Eyeball is freely drawn forward and removed
- Conjunctiva sutured.

CHAPTER 10

Lens

1. Describe the anatomy of lens.

The lens is a transparent bi-convex avascular structure. It is suspended between iris and the vitreous by the zonules, which connect it with the ciliary body. The lens continues to grow throughout life and its thickness increases with age.

The lens consists of 3 parts:
 i. Lens capsule
 ii. Lens epithelium
 iii. Lens fibers.

The lens capsule is a highly elastic envelope. It is thicker in front than behind. It is secreted by the epithelium. The lens epithelium is a single layer of cuboidal cells that forms the anterior subcapsular epithelium. The posterior epithelial cells elongate to form the lens fibers and they are composed of proteins called crystallins. The fibers formed earlier lie in a deeper plane, the newer ones occupy the more superficial plane. The deeper part forms the embryonic nucleus surrounded by fetal, infantile and adult nucleus. The peripheral part of the lens consists of cortex surrounded by a lens capsule.

Dimensions
- Diameter of lens—9 mm
- Lens thickness—4 mm
- Weight at birth—65 mg; at 80 years—250 mg
- Curvature of lens—anterior surface—10 mm, posterior surface—6 mm.

2. Describe the types, stages, clinical features, investigations and treatment of senile cataract.

A cataract is an opacity of the lens or its capsule.

Types of Senile Cataract
- Cortical:
  - Cuneiform: 70%—starts at the equator and extends axially as radial spokes—vision affected lately
  - Cupuliform: 5%—posterior subcapsular cataract,
  - In South India, it is about 50%.
  - It starts as saucer-shaped opacity in the posterior cortex and extends outwards
  - vision affected early
- Nuclear—25%:
  - Increased sclerosis of the nucleus starts centrally and spreads peripherally
  - Color is due to an accumulation of urochrome pigments which is due to oxidation of aromatic amino acids or lipids in the lens.

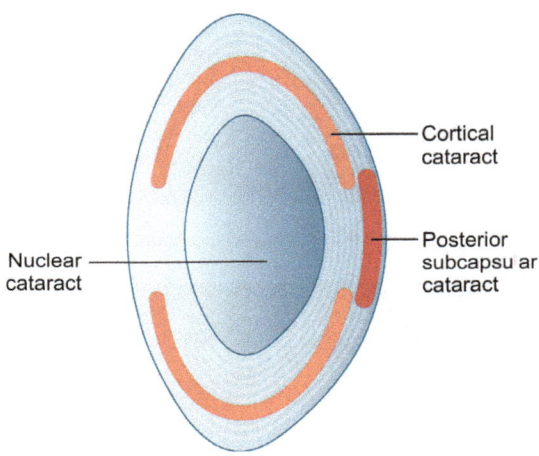

Fig. 10.1: Types of senile cataract.

Etiological Factors
- Aging—altered autoxidation system of lens
- UV radiation (from sunlight)
- Deficiency of amino acids (glutathione) and riboflavin
- Genetic predisposition
- Exposure to smoke (firewood smoke or from smoking)
- Dehydration.

Biochemical Changes
- Hydration followed by dehydration
- Acidification
- Increase in insoluble proteins
- Reduced metabolism and oxidative changes.

Stages of Cortical Cataract

Lamellar Separation

Cortical fibers are separated by fluid. Seen better by slit lamp examination. These changes are reversible.

Incipient Cataract
- In cuneiform cataract, wedge-shaped opacities in cortex extend from equator to center. Starts in lower nasal quadrant. On distant direct ophthalmoscopy, the opacities

are seen as dark opacities against red fundal glow. Visual disturbance occurs at comparatively late stage as the opacities start in periphery
- In cupuliform cataract (also called posterior subcapsular cataract), saucer-shaped opacities start in posterior cortex. Since the opacities are in visual axis, it causes early diminution of vision.

Immature Cataract

Diffuse and irregular opacification. When light is thrown on the eye from the side, iris throws shadow upon the grayish white opacity until clear lens substance exists between the iris (pupillary margin) and the opacity.

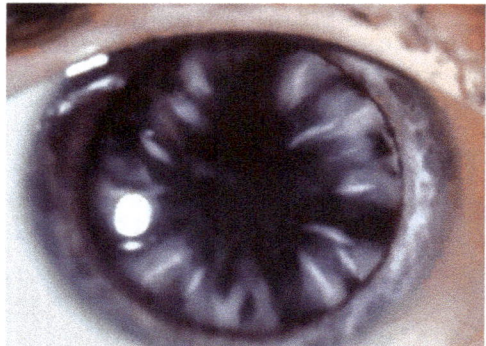

Fig. 10.2: Cuneiform cataract.

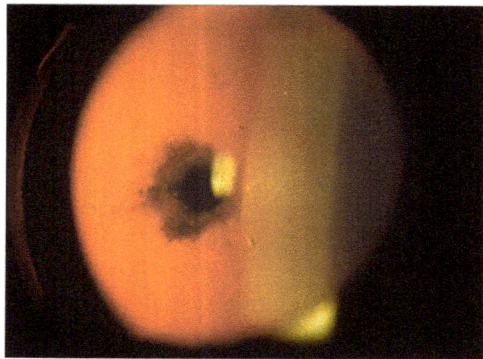

Fig. 10.3: Cupuliform cataract.

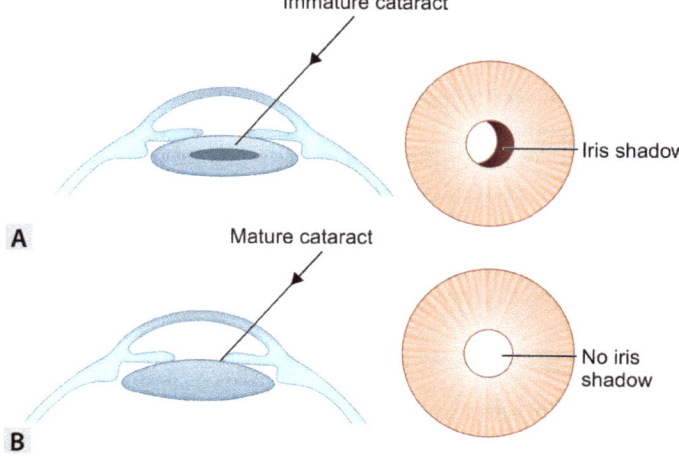

Figs. 10.4A and B: Iris shadow. (A) Present in immature cataract; and (B) Absent in mature cataract.

Differential diagnosis of immature cataract.				
Features	Cortical immature cataract	Nuclear sclerosis	Nuclear cataract	Mature cataract
Color	Grayish white	Gray	Amber brown or black	Milky white
Iris shadow	Present	Absent	Absent	Absent
Improvement with pinhole or glasses	May be possible	Possible as it is an aging process in which lens nucleus becomes inelastic and hard	Not possible	Not possible
Distant direct ophthalmoscopy	Multiple dark shadows against red fundal glow	No black spots seen	Central dark shadow against red background	No fundal glow

Mature Cataract

Opacification of the lens becomes complete and partly white. Iris cannot throw its shadow on the complete opacity.

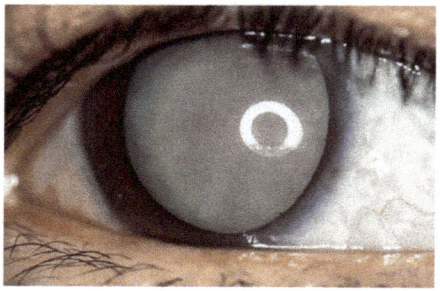

Fig. 10.5: Mature cataract.

Hypermature Cataract

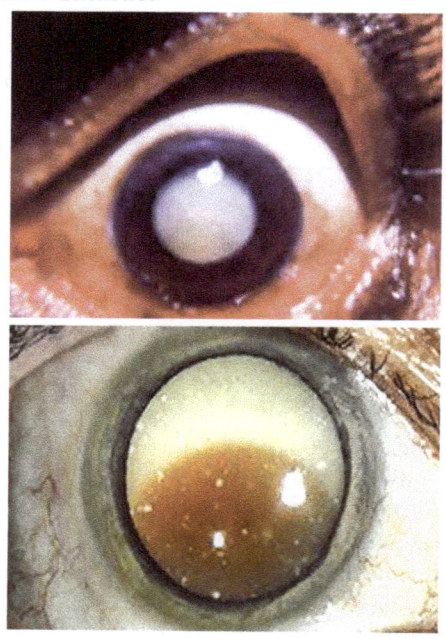

Fig. 10.6: Hypermature cataract.

Two forms:

i. *Morgagnian cataract:* Whole cortex liquefies. The capsule is filled with milky fluid and the nucleus sinks to the bottom. It may cause phacolytic glaucoma.

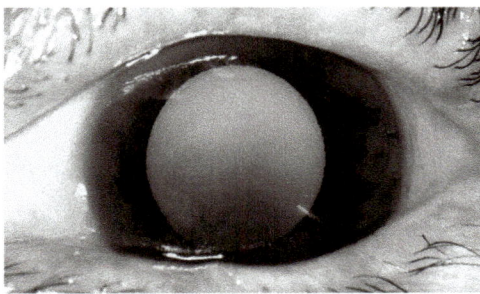

Fig. 10.7: Morgagnian cataract.

ii. *Dry and shrunken (sclerotic type):* The lens becomes shrunken due to the leakage of water. The anterior chamber becomes deep and tremulousness of the iris occurs. Intumescence can occur in immature and mature stages. It may cause phacomorphic glaucoma.

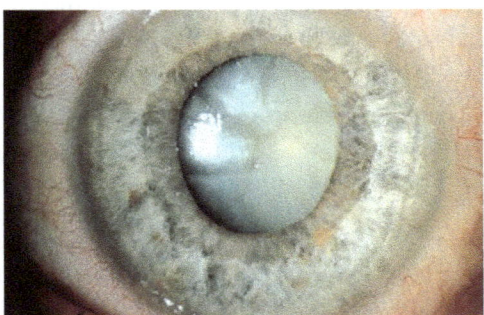

Fig. 10.8: Intumescent cataract.

In nuclear cataract, lens becomes diffusely cloudy and it is inelastic and hard. It may be tinted amber, brown or black.

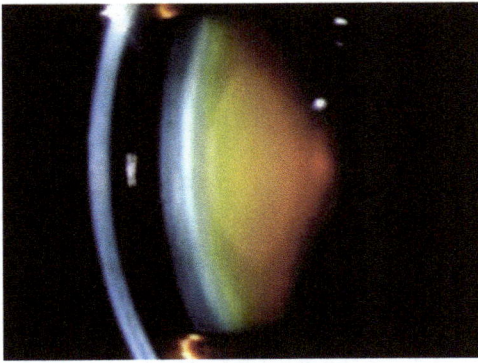

Fig. 10.9: Nuclear cataract.

Features	Nuclear	Cortical
Vision	Poor in day time, better in dim illumination, improves with concave lenses	Poor at night time, better with bright light, improves with convex lenses
Age of onset	Usually starts in forties	Starts in fifties
Lens opacity	Central	Peripheral
Color	Brown/black	Grayish white/white
Maturity	Takes long time	Matures early
Hypermaturity	Usually does not occur	Reaches hypermaturity

Symptoms

All types of cataract will have diminished vision. Symptoms which are peculiar to certain types are as follows:
- Posterior subcapsular cataract:
  - Glare to bright sunlight or headlights from vehicles
  - Near vision is affected > distant vision
- Cuneiform cataract:
  - Wedge-shaped opacities with clear lens in between
  - Uniocular polyopia
  - Frequent change of glasses due to sectorial alteration in the refractive index of lens
  - Bright illumination—improves vision
- Nuclear cataract:
  - Change in color values. Pigment in lens absorbs blue light
  - Red and yellow light are perceived better
  - Second sight: Increased refractive index of nucleus induces myopia, which facilitates reading without presbyopic glasses.

Investigations

- Examination of an eye:
  - Pupillary reaction
  - Vision and projection of rays
  - Intraocular pressure
  - Patency of nasolacrimal duct
  - Conjunctival smear
- Systemic examination:
  - Check blood sugar levels – diabetes
  - Check blood pressure – hypertension
  - Look for chronic obstructive pulmonary disease/myocardial ischemia
  - Focal sepsis—ENT/dental/genitourinary/joints/skin/lungs.
- Fundus examination—to view disc, macula and retina
- When fundus cannot be visualized:
  - Macular function tests
  - B scan.

Macular Function Tests

- 2-point discrimination—2 pinholes, 2 cm apart 2 feet from the eye to appreciate 2 lights. If patient cannot appreciate 2 lights, macula is defective
- Maddox rod test—light from pen torch will show unbroken, illuminated, straight line when seen through Maddox rod. If discontinuity in the line is seen, the macula is defective.

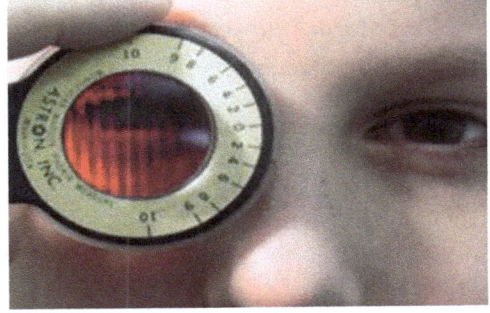

Fig. 10.10: Maddox rod test.

- Photostress test—bright light is shown for 10 seconds. Restoration of vision prior to viewing the bright light (visual recovery time) is 60 seconds. Delayed visual recovery indicates defective macula
- Entopic phenomenon—Blue field entoptoscopy—in the strong blue light of the instrument, leucocytes in parafoveal capillaries are seen moving if the macula is normal
- Foveal electroretinogram
- Laser interferometry—Most accurate.

B Scan Ultrasonography

To detect retinal detachment, tumors or vitreous pathology.

To Calculate Intraocular Lenses (IOL) Power

- Keratometry—to measure corneal power in diopters (Figs. 10.5A and B).
- A-scan—to find axial length of eyeball (Fig. 10.6).

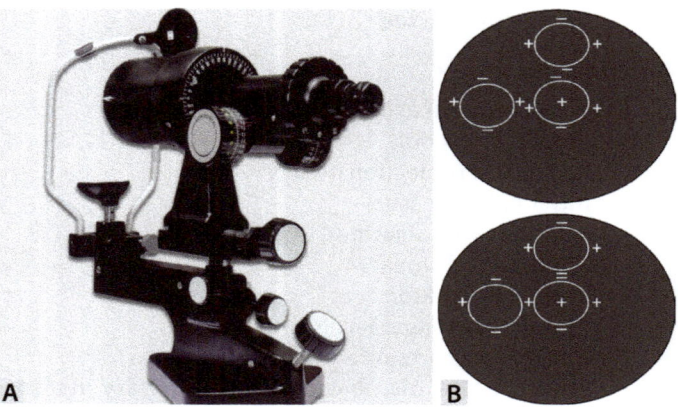

Figs. 10.11A and B: Keratometry—to measure corneal power in diopters.

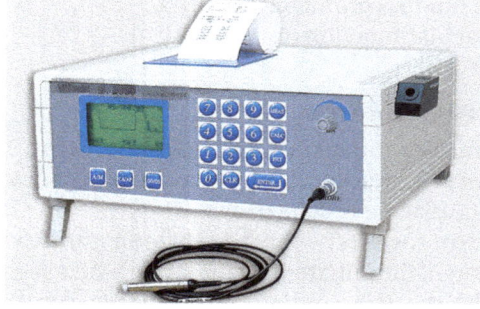

Fig. 10.12: A-scan—to find axial length of eyeball.

Indications for Cataract Surgery

- Usually visual improvement < 6/18
- Mainly depends on individuals visual requirement and type of work
- Medical causes:
    - Phacomorphic glaucoma
    - Phacolytic glaucoma
    - Retinal diseases like retinal detachment, diabetic retinopathy, etc.

Grades of Nuclear Hardness

- Grade 1: soft—white
- Grade 2: soft—yellow
- Grade 3: soft to hard—amber
- Grade 4: hard—brown to black.

Treatment

Medical

In incipient and immature stages. Vision can be improved by correction of refractive error.

Patients with small axial cataract may be benefited by pupillary dilation (5% phenylephrine or 1% tropicamide).

Surgical Management

- Intracapsular cataract extraction—removing the entire lens along with its capsule
    - Forceps—mechanical pulling at equator of lens by forceps
    - Cryo—pulling the lens by cryo probe which freezes at tip
    - Erysiphake—pulling the lens by vacuum suction
- Extracapsular cataract extraction—removal of lens leaving behind posterior capsule (for IOL support)

Conventional Extracapsular Cataract Extraction (ECCE)

Incision is made at superior limbus from 10 o'clock to 2 o'clock. Anterior capsulotomy is done through 2 mm entry into anterior chamber after injecting viscoelastic substance. Hydrodissection is done to separate cortical fibers from its capsule. Nucleus delivered with lens expressor and spatula. Cortical lens matter is removed with Simcoe's irrigation aspiration cannula. Intraocular lens inserted into posterior chamber. Viscoelastic substance is removed from anterior chamber. Limbal wound closed with 5 interrupted sutures (8-0 or 10-0 nylon suture).

Small Incision Cataract Surgery (SICS)

Self-sealing scleral tunnel incision is made 2 mm from superior limbus. Anterior chamber entered with keratome and viscoelastic is injected. Anterior capsulotomy is done with cystitome. Incision is extended to 6 mm tunnel incision. Hydrodissection is done to separate cortex from capsule. Nucleus is rotated and brought into anterior chamber by Sinski's hook. Viscoelastic is injected in front and back of lens. Nucleus is delivered by irrigating vectis or by wire vectis and lens hook. Cortical matter is aspirated with Simcoe's irrigation aspiration cannula. Posterior chamber intraocular lens is inserted into the capsular bag. Viscoelastic is removed. Conjunctiva reposited over the scleral incision.

Phacoemulsification

- **Principles of Phacoemulsification**:
    - Fragmentation of lens by ultrasonic vibration
    - Irrigation and emulsification
    - Aspiration
- **Advantages of Phacoemulsification**:
    - Early visual rehabilitation
    - Minimal astigmatism

- **Disadvantages:**
  - High cost of equipment and maintenance
  - Learning curve
  - Difficult in black cataract.

3. Describe the complications of cataract surgery.

- Anesthesia related
- Intraoperative
- Early postoperative
- Late postoperative
- IOL related.

Anesthesia Related

- Xylocaine allergy
- Retrobulbar hemorrhage
- Oculocardiac reflex particularly in general anesthesia.

Intraoperative

- Hyphema
- Detachment of Descemet's membrane
- Vitreous loss
- Rupture of posterior capsule
- Suprachoroidal hemorrhage
- Lens subluxation or dislocation.

Early Postoperative

- Striate keratitis
- Prolapse of iris
- Anterior uveitis
- Shallow anterior chamber
- Updrawn pupil
- Acute bacterial endophthalmitis.

Late Postoperative

- Posterior capsular opacification and after cataract
- Secondary glaucoma
- Cystoid macular edema
- Chronic endophthalmitis—fungal
- Retinal detachment.

IOL Related

- Anterior chamber IOL related:
  - Pupillary tuck
  - Pupillary block
  - Uveitis glaucoma hyphema (UGH) syndrome
  - Bullous keratopathy
- Posterior chamber intraocular lens (PCIOL) related:
  - Pupillary capture
  - Decentration of IOL
    » Sunset syndrome(inferior subluxation of IOL)
    » Sunrise syndrome (superior subluxation of IOL)
  - Toxic IOL syndrome due to uveal inflammation.

4. Write short notes on after cataract.

It is an opacity which persists or follows after extracapsular cataract extraction.

Types

- Thin membrane
- Ring of Soemmering—new lens fibers are formed by proliferation of anterior capsular cells
- Elschnig's pearls—the subcapsular cells proliferate to form large balloon-like cells
- Fibrous membrane—usually formed when there is associated iritis.

Treatment

- YAG laser capsulotomy
- Surgical incision.

5. Write short notes on aphakia.

Absence of lens in pupillary space.

Signs

- Limbal scar
- Deep AC
- Iridodonesis
- Jet black pupil—due to total internal reflection
- Purkinje images—3 and 4 absent
- Fundus—small disc
- Retinoscopy—high hypermetropia.

Correction of Aphakia

- Spectacles
- Contact lens
- Intraocular lens implantation (secondary).

Disadvantages of Aphakic Glasses

- Image magnification 25–30%
- Limited field of vision
- Spherical aberrations—Pin cushion distortion
- Roving ring scotoma—Jack in the box phenomenon
- Chromatic aberrations
- Loss of accommodation
- Thick glasses.

6. Write short notes on traumatic cataract.

It is usually caused by the blunt or perforating injury. A blunt injury to the eye may occur by a fist or a tennis or cricket ball injury and may produce Vossius ring, traumatic cataract and subluxation or dislocation of the lens.

- Vossius ring: Imprint of pigment from the papillary margin on the anterior lens surface in a ring form.
- Rosette-shaped cataract: Axial in a location involving posterior lens capsule. It can be early or late. Early rosette has star shaped cortical suture with radiating feathery lines of opacities from the suture. Late rosette develops after 1–2 years as feathery lines seen in posterior cortex. Its suture extensions are shorter and more compact than the early rosette cataract. Early rosettes are more commonly seen in concussion cataract.
- The sudden expansion of the globe in an equatorial plane may occur due to rupture of zonular fibers may result in subluxation or dislocation of the lens.

Penetrating injury may occur due to needle, thorn, arrow or a flying foreign body. Small perforating injury may heal and only a small opacity is formed. Sometimes entire lens may become cataractous.

Treatment depends on vision. If the vision is < 6/18, it is better to remove the lens by phacoemulsification and implant intraocular lens.

7. Write short notes on metabolic cataract.

A metabolic cataract is caused by endocrine disorders and biochemical abnormalities. Some are associated with inborn errors of metabolism such as galactosemia.

- **Diabetic** (blood sugar > 200 mg/mL):
  - Snowflake opacities in cortex causing the milky white appearance
  - Due to sorbitol in lens fibers
  - Causes osmotic imbalance
- **Galactosemia:**
  - Oil droplet cataract
  - Due to dulcitol accumulation
  - Inability to metabolize galactose
- **Wilson's disease:**
  - Sunflower cataract in the anterior capsular region
  - Defective copper metabolism
- **Lowe's syndrome:**
  - Oculocerebrorenal involvement
  - Defective amino acid metabolism.

8. Mention types of cataract in systemic diseases.

- **Diabetic cataract**: Snow flake cataract—white punctate opacities appear in the anterior or posterior cortex
- **Galactosemic cataract:** Oil droplet cataract—opacities are initially lamellar but eventually becomes total
- **Hypoparathyroidism:** Small discrete opacities in the cortex coalesce to form large shining crystal like flakes
- **Myotonia dystrophy:** Christmas tree appearance in superficial cortex, can occur in anterior and posterior sub capsular areas
- **Lowe's syndrome**: Lens opacities are nuclear, lamellar or total. Congenital cataract, congenital glaucoma and blue sclera may also be present.
- **Down's syndrome:** Punctate subcapsular cataract along with mental retardation.

9. Write short notes on complicated cataract.

Occurs as a result of any disease or pathology in the eye. The main factor is disturbance in lens metabolism.

Etiology

- Inflammatory diseases:
  - Iridocyclitis
  - Choroiditis
- Degenerative diseases:
  - High myopia
  - Retinitis pigmentosa
  - Retinal detachment.

Symptoms

Marked impairment of vision due to opacity near nodal point in posterior cortex.

Signs

- Inflammation of anterior segment causes opacification of cortex.
- Progresses and matures rapidly
- Posterior segment disease causes posterior cortical cataract.

Slit Lamp Examination

- Bread crumb appearance
- Polychromatic luster
- Rainbow colors.

10. Write short notes on ectopia lentis.

Ectopia lentis is defined as displacement of crystalline lens from its normal anatomical position in the patellar fossa. The characteristic clinical feature is phacodonesis which is tremulousness of the lens which is better seen on rapid movement of the eye.

- Subluxation—Partial displacement
- Dislocation—Lens not in Buerger/patellar space.

Causes

- Congenital:
  - Ectopia lentis—Bilateral, symmetrical and usually upwards.
  - Associated with systemic anomalies:
    » Marfan's syndrome—Subluxated up and out
    » Homocystinuria—Subluxated down and in
    » Weill-Marchesani syndrome—Subluxated down
    » Spherophakia and subluxation
    » Ehler-Danlos syndrome—blue sclera, keratoconus and angiod streaks with subluxation
    » Hyperlysinemia
    » Sulphitoxidase deficiency
- Traumatic displacement.
- Consecutive or spontaneous displacement
  - Hypermature cataract
  - Buphthalmos
  - High myopia
  - Intraocular tumors.

Complications

- Optical distortion due to lenticular myopia
- Astigmatism
- Lens edge effect
- Glaucoma
- Lens induced uveitis.

In Marfan's syndrome: Lens subluxation is usually upwards, zonules are intact and stretched—some accommodation is retained

In homocystinuria: Lens subluxates downwards due to acquired zonular degeneration; there is loss of accommodation

In Marchessani syndrome: Inferior subluxation, disorder of connective tissue, micro- spherophakia.

11. Describe the etiology, types, and management of congenital cataract.

Etiology

- Maternal malnutrition—vitamin A, C, D and B2 deficiency
- Infection in mother—Rubella, toxoplasmosis, CMV, varicella
- Hereditary predisposition
- Placental hemorrhage—due to anoxia:
  - 5th–8th week—critical period in lens development
  - 33%—idiopathic
  - 33%—inherited
  - 33%—with systemic diseases.

Other ocular anomalies are present in 50% of cases.

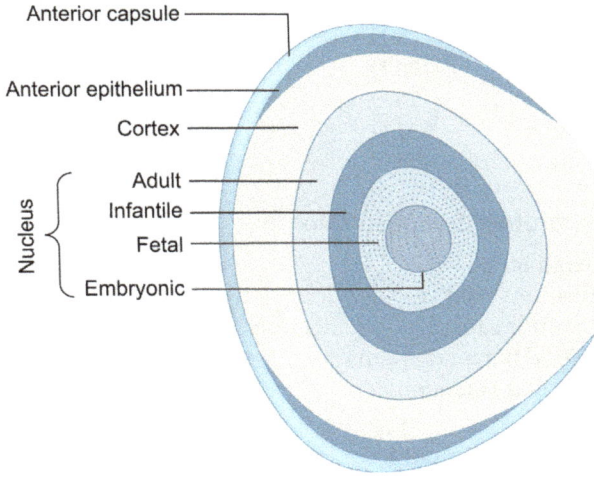

Fig. 10.13: Types of nuclei in crystalline lens.

Types

- Involving embryonal nucleus
  - Central nuclear cataract—rubella in mother
- Involving the fetal nucleus
  - A lamellar or zonular cataract forms 50%. It is the most common type which causes visual impairment
- Involving infantile and cortical nucleus

  Occurs in 10–20 years:
  - Congenital punctate cataract (blue dot)
    » Most common type but it does not cause visual impairment
  - Coronary cataract:
    » Club shaped opacities in the cortex

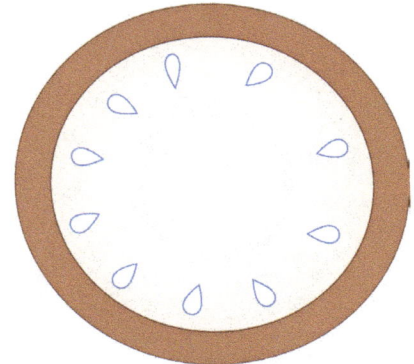

Coronary cataract

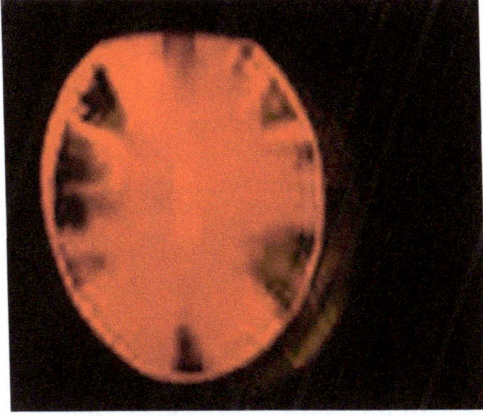

Fig. 10.14: Coronary cataract.
» Radial distribution
» Occurs at deep layers of the cortex
- Coralliform cataract:
  » Spindle-shaped cataract occurs in an axial region resembling coral

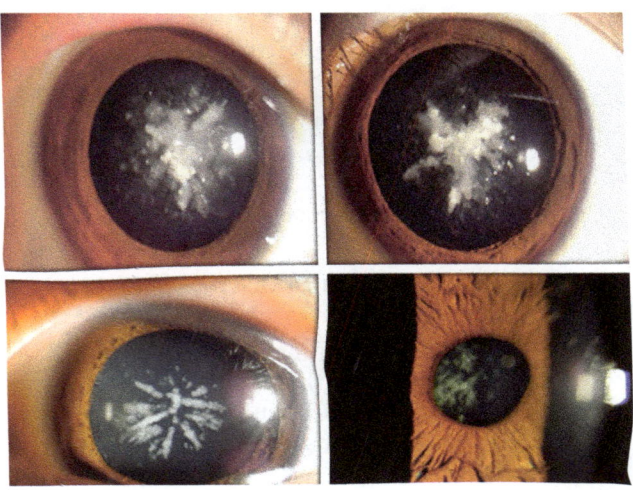

Fig. 10.15: Coralliform cataract.

- Sutural cataract:
  - Punctate opacities around a suture

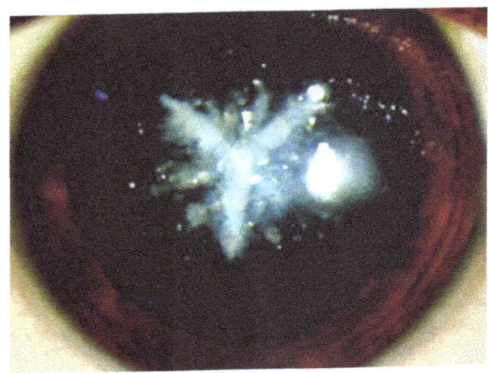

Fig. 10.16: Sutural cataract.

- Involving an anterior pole
  Anterior polar cataract:
  - Remnants of anterior vascular sheath
    » Perforated corneal ulcer
- Involving posterior pole
  - Associated with remnants of the hyaloid artery
  - Posterior polar cataract.

Investigations

- Blood tests:
  - Blood glucose, calcium and phosphorus
  - RBC transferase and galacto kinase levels
  - Antibody titers for TORCH and hepatitis B virus

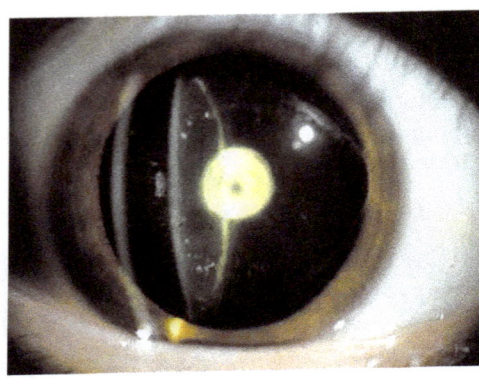

Fig. 10.17: Posterior polar cataract.

- Urine tests:
  - Urine assay for reducing substance after milk feeding (for galactosemia)
  - Screening for an amino acid in the urine (if Lowe's syndrome is suspected)
- B scan, if fundus cannot be seen:
  - To assess the posterior segment
  - Retinal detachment
  - Retinoblastoma
- A scan to compare the axial length of both eyes.

Treatment

- Not required if vision is not impaired
- Central cataract: Pupil can be dilated to improve vision through clear cortex around it
- Watch the progression of cataract till puberty.

Indications for Surgery

- Visually significant cataract:
  - > 3 mm in the visual axis
- **Unilateral cataract** - Squint, nystagmus:
  - Early surgery (6-8 weeks) to prevent amblyopia
  - Before 2 years ECCE by aspiration, soft contact lens, amblyopia therapy, after 2 years PCIOL

Lens aspiration can be performed either by manual SICS or by phacoemulsification. Lens aspiration is to be combined with primary posterior capsulotomy in children below 6 years of age and should be combined with anterior vitrectomy in children below 2 years of age.

IOL Power for Children
- Emmetropic power > 8 years
- 90% of IOL power 2-8 years of age
- 80% of IOL power < 2 years
- IOL power varies with an axial length of the eyeball.

Axial Length	IOL Power
21 mm	22 D
20 mm	24 D
19 mm	26 D
18 mm	27 D
17 mm	28 D

Postoperative Complications

- Astigmatism
- Fibrinous uveitis
- Posterior capsular opacification
- Cystoid macular edema
- Secondary glaucoma.

12. Write short notes on intraocular lenses (IOL).

It is a plastic device used to replace the original cataractous crystalline lens to restore normal vision.
- Types
- Parts and dimensions
- Indications
- Contraindications
- Power
- Sterilization
- Complications.

The Types of Intraocular Lenses are Classified:

- Based on the method of fixation
- Based on the material of the lens
- Based on refractive status.

Based on the method of fixation

- Anterior chamber IOL
- Iris fixation

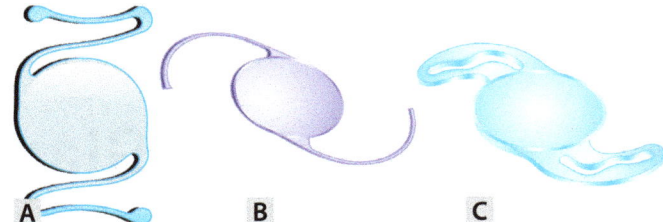 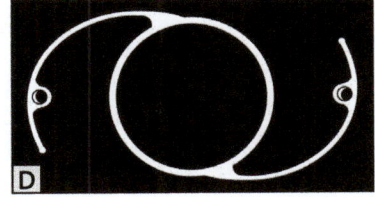

Figs. 10.18A to D: Types of intraocular lenses: (A) Anterior chamber lens; (B) Rigid posterior chamber lens; (C) Foldable posterior chamber lens; (D) Scleral fixation lens.

- Posterior chamber IOL
- Scleral fixation
- Glued IOL
- Phakic IOL

Based on material of lens
- Rigid lens—polymethyl methacrylate (PMMA)
- Foldable lens:
  - Hydrophobic acrylic—water content <1%
  - Hydrophilic acrylic—water content 18–35%
  - Silicon
- Rollable acrylic.

Based on Refractive Status
- Unifocal
- Multifocal:
  - Refractive—good distant and intermediate
  - Diffractive—good near reading
  - Trifocal lens—corrects distance, intermediate and near vision
  - Accommodative
- Toric lens—to correct astigmatism.

Parts of Intraocular Lenses and Dimensions
- **Optics:** 5–6.5 mm in diameter. It is made up of PMMA, silicon or acrylic.
- **Haptic or Loop:** It is made up of PMMA, polyamide, polypropylene, polyethylene or acrylic:
  - Overall diameter of IOL is 13–14 mm
  - Diameter of the optic is 5–6.5 mm
  - Thickness of IOL is 1.5–2 mm
  - Weight of IOL is 15 mg in air and 5 mg in aqueous.

Indication for IOL
Cataract with vision usually < 6/18.

Contraindications
- Proliferative diabetic retinopathy
- Uncontrolled recurrent iridocyclitis
- Rubeosis iridis.

Power of IOL
It is calculated by Sanders-Retzlaff-Kraff (SRK) -I formula as follows:
- Power of lens = $A - 2.5L - 0.9K$
  - A: Constant for the IOL given by the manufacturer. It is usually 118 for posterior chamber IOL and 116 for anterior chamber IOL
  - L: Axial length of the eyeball. It is usually 24 mm
  - K: Corneal power in diopters. It is usually 43D to 45D

In SRK-II formula correction is given for axial length:
- 22–24.5 mm—no correction
- 21–22 mm—add 1
- 20–21 mm—add 2
- Below 20 mm—add 3
- Above 24.5 mm—subtract 0.5.

Sterilization

Sterilization of IOL is done by ethylene oxide gas.

Complications
- Anterior chamber IOL related:
  - Pupillary tuck
  - Pupillary block
  - Uveitis-glaucoma-hyphema (UGH) syndrome
  - Bullous keratopathy

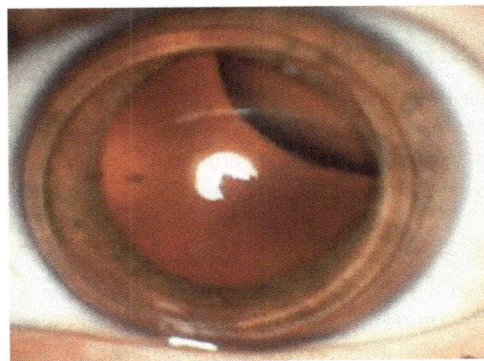

Fig. 10.19: Superior subluxation of lens (sunrise syndrome).

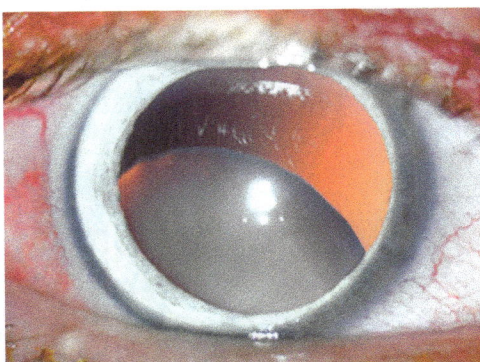

Fig. 10.20: Inferior subluxation of lens (sunset syndrome).

- Posterior chamber IOL related:
  - Pupillary capture
  - Decentration of IOL—sunset syndrome, sunrise syndrome
  - Toxic IOL syndrome due to uveal inflammation.

11. Glaucoma

INTRODUCTION

- It is a chronic progressive optic neuropathy characterized by loss of retinal ganglion cells and their axons—retinal nerve fiber layer (RNFL).
- Intraocular pressure (IOP) measurement is indirect evidence of glaucoma.
- RNFL assessment helps in early detection and monitoring progression of glaucoma.

Visual field changes occur only after 40% of nerve fiber layer damage has occurred.

Normal range of IOP is 10–20 mm Hg.

CLASSIFICATION OF GLAUCOMA

- Congenital glaucoma
- Primary open angle glaucoma (POAG)
- Primary angle closure glaucoma (PACG)
- Secondary glaucoma.

1. Define glaucoma.

Primary open angle glaucoma is a chronic progressive optic neuropathy characterized by morphological changes at the optic nerve head and nerve fiber layer in the absence of other ocular diseases/congenital anomalies with or without raised IOP.

2. How is aqueous produced and circulated?

Aqueous is produced by
- Diffusion
- Ultrafiltration
- Active secretion

Aqueous outflow
- Trabecular: 80%
- Uveoscleral: 15–20%
    - Rate of production—2.3 µL/min.

3. List investigations in glaucoma.

- Tonometry
- Gonioscopy
- Optic nerve head analysis:
    - Direct ophthalmoscopy
    - Scanning laser polarimetry—GDX
    - Scanning laser ophthalmoscopy—HRT
    - Optical coherence tomography—OCT
- Perimetry.

4. What is Van Herick's sign?

Depth of anterior chamber is compared with corneal thickness by slit lamp beam at 1 mm inside the limbus.

Van Herick's slit lamp grading.		
Grade 4	PAC > 1 CT	Wide open
Grade 3	PAC = ¼–½ CT	Mild narrow
Grade 2	PAC = ¼ CT	Moderately narrow
Grade 1	PAC < ¼ CT	Extremely narrow

(CT: corneal thickness; PAC: peripheral anterior chamber)

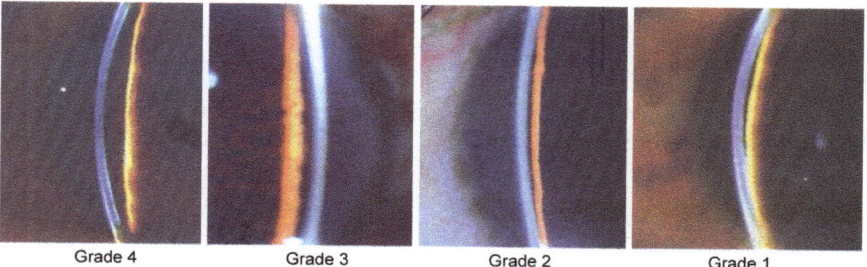

Fig. 11.1: Van Herick's slit lamp grading comparing peripheral anterior chamber with corneal thickness.

5. What are the types of tonometry?

Measurement of IOP by tonometer is called tonometry.

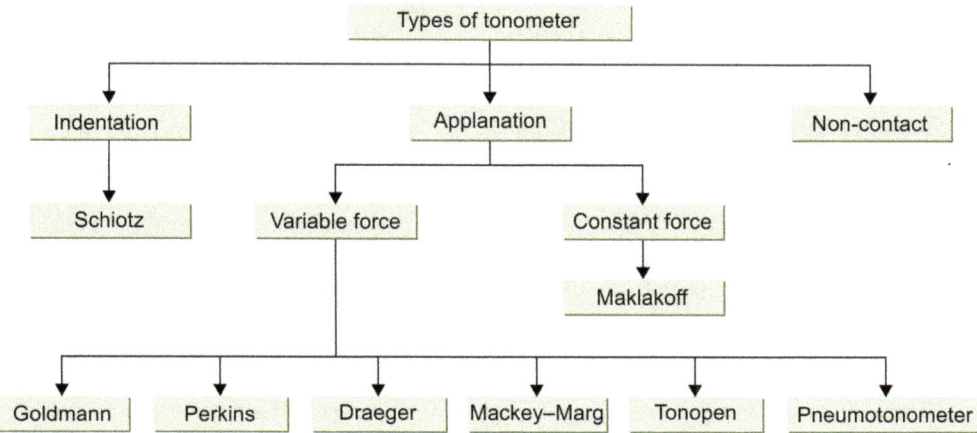

Schiotz

It is easy to use. It uses a plunger with a preset weight to indent the cornea. The amount of indentation is converted into millimeters of mercury by the use of a table.

Disadvantages
- Error due to ocular rigidity
- Repeated measurements reduce IOP
- Steeper or thickness of cornea give false high pressure measurements.

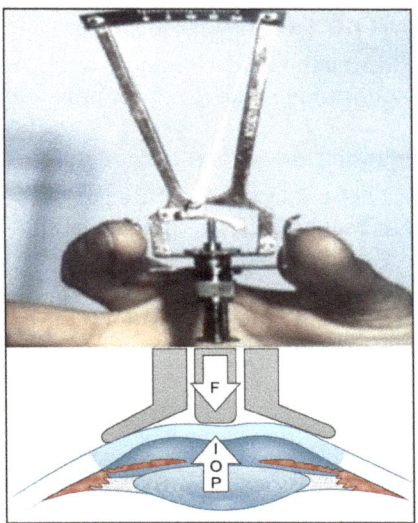

Fig. 11.2: Schiotz indentation tonometer.

Applanation Tonometry

It is based on Imbert Fick law which states that pressure inside a sphere (P) is equal to the force (F) required to flatten the surface divided by the area of flattening (A).

Hence, $P = F/A$

It is attached to the slit lamp. The tear film is stained with fluorescein dye and by adjusting the two mires the IOP is measured. The measurement is determined by how much pressure is applied to make the cornea flat.

Goldmann accuracy is optimal with 520 µ corneal thickness. 14 µ thickness equals 1 mm difference. For thicker cornea subtract and thinner cornea add. Applanation area—3.06 mm.

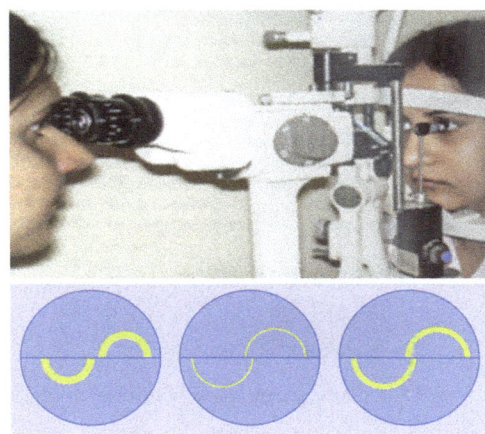

Fig. 11.3: Mires in Goldmann applanation tonometer.

Mackay-Marg—Plunger size 1.5 mm diameter:
Combined applanation and indentation tonometer. The plunger is electronically controlled. It overestimates IOP. It is useful in eyes with corneal edema and corneal scar.

Perkins—same principle as Goldmann
- Can be performed in any posture
- Useful for infants and children
- Portable.

Draeger—similar to Perkins
- Operates with motor adjusting the force.

Disadvantages
- Large size
- Needs training to use.

Tonopen
- Similar to Mackay-Marg
- Portable.

Pneumotonometer—similar to Mackay-Marg

Maklakoff—measures diameter of cornea flattened by a fixed weight, popular in Russia and China.

Non-contact Tonometer
- Deforms corneal apex by jet of air
- Accurate if IOP is near normal
- Accuracy is decreased in high pressure, abnormal cornea, poor fixation
- Useful in postoperative patients
- Time required for air jet to flatten cornea is proportional to IOP.

6. Write short notes on gonioscopy.

Visualizing angle of the anterior chamber by the gonioscopic lens is called gonioscopy. Angle structures seen from anterior to posterior are:
- Schwalbe's line
- Trabecular meshwork and Schlemm's canal
- Scleral spur
- Ciliary band (anteromedial surface of ciliary body)
- Root of iris.

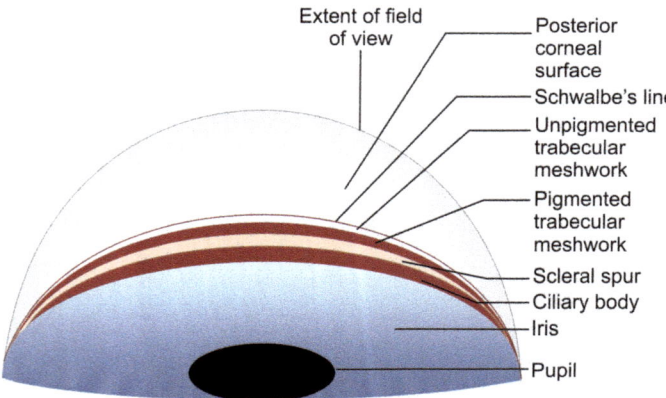

Fig. 11.4: Gonioscopic view of normal angle.

Types of Gonioscopic Lenses

Direct
- Koeppe lens
- Barkan's
- Swan Jacob.

Indirect
- Goldmann
- Zeiss four mirror
- Posner
- Sussman.

Shaffer's grading of angle of anterior chamber.

Grade 0	0°	Angle closed	None of angle structures visible
Grade 1	10°	Very narrow angle	Schwalbe's line seen
Grade 2	20°	Moderately narrow	Trabecular meshwork seen
Grade 3	25–35°	Open angle	Up to scleral spur seen
Grade 4	35–45°	Wide open angle	Ciliary body band seen

Spaeth's Grading-Reverse of Shaffer

Use of indirect lens—can perform indentation gonioscopy to determine whether angle closure is appositional or synechial.

7. Briefly describe the methods of optic nerve head analysis.

- Direct ophthalmoscope–Red free light
  - Slit lamp examination with + 78D or + 90D lens
  - Nerve fiber layer (NFL) visibility is enhanced with short-wavelength light
- Fundus camera with red free filter
  - Stereo photograph
- Scanning laser ophthalmoscope (HRT)
  - 3-Dimensional construction of retinal surface
  - Measures retinal height particularly optic nerve head.
  - Height is related to nerve fiber layer thickness
- Optical coherence tomography
  - Uses reflected and backscattered light to create images of various retinal layers analogous to the use of sound waves in B-scan
  - Can differentiate layers within the retina including nerve fiber layer with 10µ resolution
  - Correlates with known histology
- Scanning laser polarimetry—GDX
  - Uses a confocal scanning laser with an integrated polarimetry to detect changes in light polarization from axons to measure NFL thickness—quantitative analysis
  - NFL thickness detects early glaucomatous damage
- Optic nerve blood flow measured by color Doppler imaging and flowmetry.

8. Write short notes on perimetry.

Perimetry is testing the field of vision. There are types:
 i. **Kinetic** – stimulus is moved from non-seeing to seeing area
 ii. **Static** – stimulus does not move but its intensity varies

A stimulus is a light or target presented to the patient.
- Bjerrum's screen and Lister's perimeter are of kinetic type
- Humphrey's or Octopus belongs to static type
- Goldmann bowel perimetry is both kinetic and static

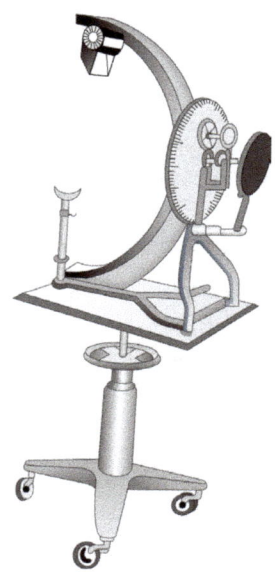

Fig. 11.5: Lister's perimeter.

Glaucoma

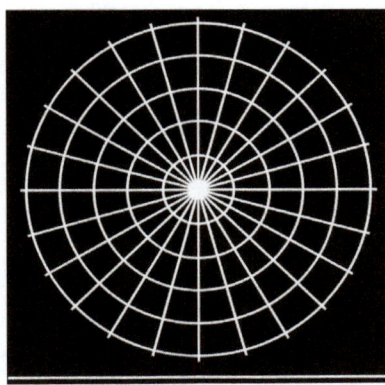

Fig. 11.6: Bjerrum's screen for central 30° field.

Bjerrum's Screen
- Tangent screen: Maps central 30° of field
- 7.5 FC (foot candle) 1 meter distance – 2 × 2 meter screen
- 2 meter distance – 4 × 4 meter screen
- Light behind patient's head.

Goldmann Bowl Perimetry
It measures retinal receptors ability to perceive light—kinetic and static:
- **Kinetic:**
  - Tested on a flat screen with test objects that move back and front between non-seeing areas and zones in which they are detected
- **Static:**
  - One attempts to find in the visual field sensitivity of eye at a preselected location.

Automated Perimetry
It is of static type. It is reliable and repeatable. It measures retinal sensitivity on the threshold at different locations by varying the brightness of the test target.

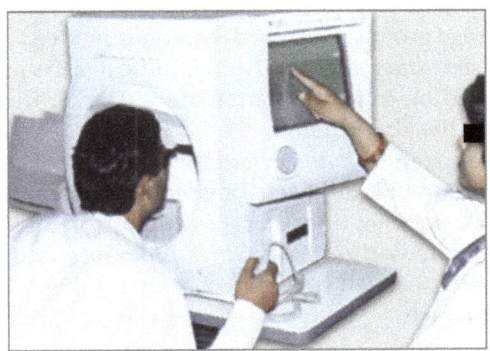

Fig. 11.7: Automated perimeter.

Humphrey
Static type:
- Test distance 0.33 m
- Stimulus duration 0.2 sec
- Programs—central 30°, 24°, 10°
- *Reliability indices:*
  - Fixation loss: Patient responds when a target is projected in a blind spot. If it is 20%, field is unreliable
  - False positive: Patient responds when there is no stimulus
  - False negative: Patient fails to respond to a super threshold stimulus—loss of attention
  - If false positive and false negative are 20% the field is unreliable

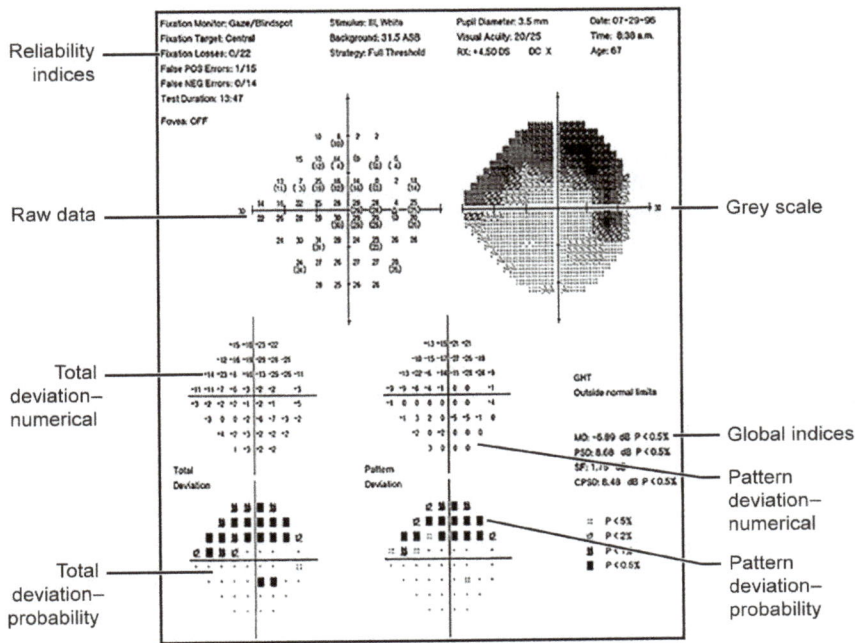

Fig. 11.8: Bjerrum's superior arcuate scotoma.

- *Grey scale:* Helps in identifying general pattern of field loss and highlighting abnormal areas
- *Raw data:* Gives measurement of exact retinal sensitivity of the patient
- *Total deviation numerical plot:* Raw data compared with same age groups. Decibel deviation is plotted
- *Total deviation probability plot:* Indicates the probability of deviation in general population. Darker the symbol, greater the abnormality
- *Pattern deviation numerical plot:* Represents true focal depression. It is adjusted for generalized depression due to lens opacities, miosis or refractive error
- *Pattern deviation probability plot:* It is important to identify localized field loss. Lower P value has greater significance
- *Global indices:*
  - Mean deviation (MD)—average departure of each test point from age adjusted normal values. A measure of overall field loss
  - Pattern standard deviation (PSD)—standard deviation of differences between threshold and expected values for each test point. A measure of focal field loss
  - Short-term fluctuation (SF)—variability in responses when the same point is retested - measure of consistency
  - Corrected pattern standard deviation (CPSD)—adjustment of PSD by subtracting out the component due to SF. A measure of variability within field after correction for short-term fluctuation.
    $$CPSD = PSD - SF$$

9. Discuss the etiology, clinical features and treatment of congenital glaucoma.

Glaucoma appearing between birth and 3-4 years of age is called congenital glaucoma. The incidence is 1 in 10,000 births. It is more common in boys and usually bilateral.

Types

- Congenital glaucoma (40%)—Present since birth
- Infantile glaucoma (55%)—Manifests prior to 2 years
- Juvenile glaucoma (5%)—Presents between 2-10 years

When it occurs before 3 years, eye ball usually enlarges and the term '*Buphthalmos*' is used.

Etiology

Due to failure in the development of tissues in the angle of anterior chamber:
- The angle remains closed by the persistent mesodermal tissues
- Canal of Schlemm is deficient or absent
- Absence of aqueous veins.

Symptoms

- Watering - First symptom
- Photophobia
- Blepharospasm
- Eye rubbing
- Corneal opacity.

Signs

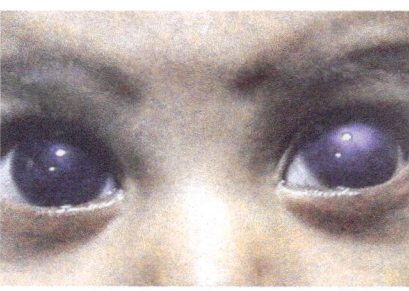
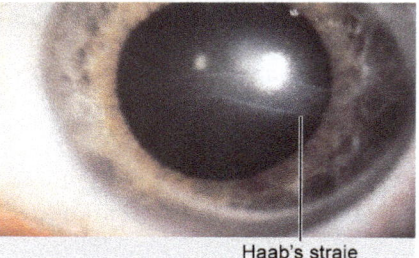

Fig. 11.9: Buphthalmos with corneal opacity left eye.

- Increased corneal diameter
  > 12 mm at birth
  > 13 mm after 2 years
  - Corneal edema–first sign
  - Haab's striae–horizontal splits in Descemet's layer
  - Deep anterior chamber
  - Increased IOP
  - Disc cupping.

Differential Diagnosis

- Cloudy cornea at birth: *(Mnemonic – STUMPED)*
  S - Sclerocornea
  T - Trauma
  U - Ulcer
  M - Mucopolysaccharidosis
  P - Peter's anomaly
  E - Congenital Hereditary Endothelial dystrophy
  D - Dermoid
- Large cornea:
  Megalocornea, keratoglobus, high myopia
- Watering:
  Congenital dacryocystitis.

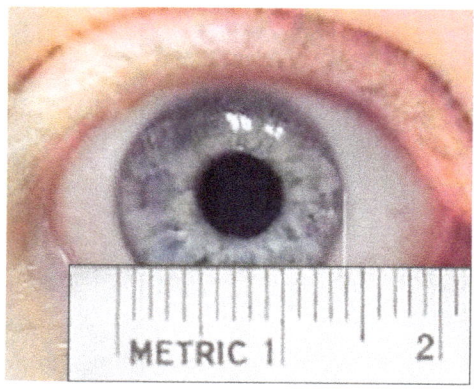

Fig. 11.10: Megalocornea.

Differences between buphthalmos and megalocornea.	
Buphthalmos	**Megalocornea**
Incidence is equal in both sexes	Common in males
Diminished vision	Normal vision
Corneal edema, tears in Descemet's membrane	Cornea clear
Abnormalities of angle of anterior chamber	No abnormalities
Raised intraocular pressure	Normal intraocular pressure
Glaucomatous cupping	Physiological cupping

Treatment

- **Medical**
  - Timolol maleate 0.5% or Dorzolamide 2% eye drops
  - Tab. Acetazolamide 5-10 mg/kg body weight
- **Surgical**—usually indicated
  - Goniotomy—Consists of incising the abnormal tissue by the goniotomy knife introduced through the opposite limbus
  - Trabeculotomy—The inner wall of Schlemm's canal is broken by trabeculotome.
  - Aqueous from anterior chamber then drains into Schlemm canal
  - Trabeculectomy
  - Combination of trabeculectomy with trabeculotomy.

10. Discuss the clinical features, investigations and treatment of primary open angle glaucoma.

Incidence: 1 in 200.

Symptoms

- Painless progressive loss of vision
- Mild headache and eye pain
- Increasing difficulty in near work
- Frequent change of presbyopic glasses
- Delayed dark adaptation.

Signs

- Raised IOP > 21 mm Hg
- Optic nerve head changes—occur before visual field loss:
  - Asymmetry of the cup disc ratio (>0.2) between the two eyes
  - Localized notch or thinning of neuroretinal rim
  - Enlarged cup: Disc ratio > 0.5, especially if in the vertical axis
  - Pallor of neuroretinal rim
  - Superficial disc hemorrhages
  - Bayonetting sign-double angulation or kinking of blood vessels at cup margin- retinal vessels appear to be broken at the margin of cup
  - ISNT rule violation- Normally the thickness of neuroretinal rim is in the following decreasing order (I) Inferior (S) Superior (N)Nasal (T) Temporal. In Glaucoma this ISNT rule is violated – inferior or superior rim is thinner than others.
  - Peripapillary atrophy
  - Laminar dot sign—slit like openings of lamina cribrosa due to degeneration of nerve fiber

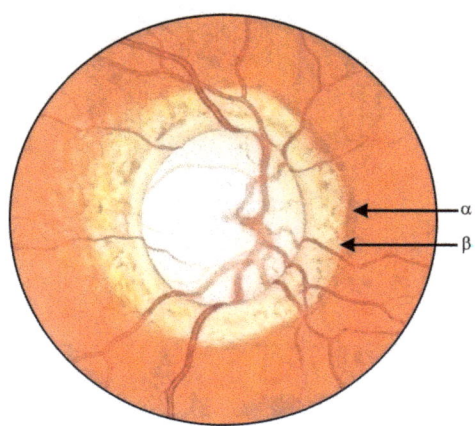

Fig. 11.11: Advanced cupping with parapapillary changes, where α denotes peripheral alpha zone of hyperpigmentation and hypopigmentation, and β denotes central beta zone of chorioretinal atrophy.

- Visual field defects:
  - Bjerrum's paracentral scotoma—10-20°
  - Seidel sign—vertical elongation of blind spot
  - Arcuate scotoma—Ronne's nasal step
  - Double arcuate scotoma
  - Temporal central island
  - Tubular vision.

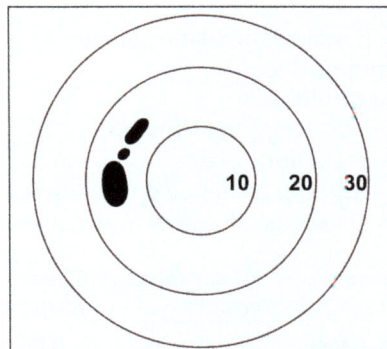

Fig. 11.12: Paracentral scotoma.

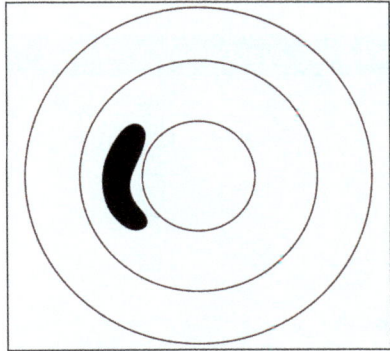

Fig. 11.13: Seidel's sign.

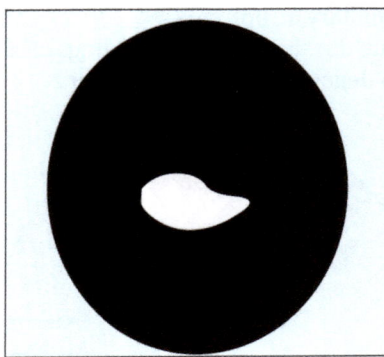

Fig. 11.14: Tubular vision.

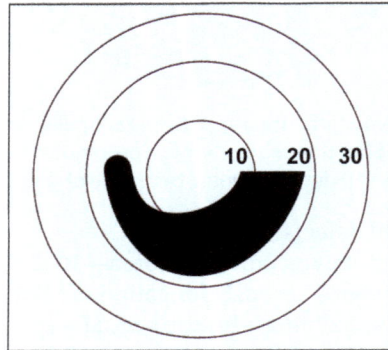

Fig. 11.15: Arcuate or Bjerrum's scotoma.

Differential Diagnosis

- Low tension or normotension glaucoma
- Ocular hypertension
- Mimicking conditions:
  - Physiological cupping—myopia
  - Coloboma of optic disc
  - AION—Anterior ischemic optic neuropathy
  - Chiasmal lesions—Primary optic atrophy.

	Physiological cupping	*Primary optic atrophy*	*Glaucomatous optic atrophy*
CUP	Tunnel shaped sloping edge	Saucer shaped	Cup disc ratio raised
DISC	Pink	White	Thinning of neuroretinal rim

Magnification for disc evaluation.

Lens	Magnification
Superfield	1.5X
90 D	1.3X
78 D	1.1X
60 D	1.0X

Investigations

- IOP
- Fundus
- Gonioscopy
- Perimetry
- Water drinking test
- Confocal scanning laser topography
- Nerve fiber layer analyzer
- Optic nerve head analyzer:
  - Confocal scanning laser ophthalmoscopy (CSLO)—Heidenberg retinal tomography (HRT)
    » Indirectly measures nerve fiber layer thickness
  - Optical coherence tomography (OCT)
    » Cross sectional image of RNFL
  - Scanning laser polarimetry (SLP)
    » Nerve fiber analyzer–GDX (Glaucoma diagnosis)
    » Quantitative analysis of RNFL thickness to detect early glaucomatous damage
  - Optic nerve blood flow measurement
    » Color Doppler imaging.

Treatment of Glaucoma

- Medical
- Laser
- Surgical

Medical

Guidelines recommended by American Association of Ophthalmologists (AAO)

- Ocular hypertension: Reduction of IOP by 20% from baseline
- In mild glaucomatous damage: Reduction of IOP by 20–30%
- In advanced glaucomatous damage: Reduction of IOP by 40% from baseline
- In normotension glaucoma: Reduction of IOP by 30% from baseline
- Usually the first line of treatment is either prostaglandin analogue or betablocker. The aim of the treatment is to achieve Target IOP, which is the optimum pressure that will not cause further optic nerve damage.

  i. **Parasympathomimetics (miotics):**
   - Pilocarpine 1%, 2%, 4% (q.i.d)
   - Carbachol 0.75% (q.i.d)
   - Decreases IOP by 15–25%
   - Side effects: Bradycardia, frontal headache, myopia, iris cysts, follicular conjunctivitis
   - Contraindications: Glaucomatocyclitic crisis, aphakic glaucoma, buphthalmos, spherophakia, inflammatory glaucoma

  ii. **Beta adrenergic receptor antagonists (β-blockers):**
   - Timolol maleate 0.5%—nonselective beta-blockers
   - Levobunolol 0.5%—nonselective beta-blockers
   - Betaxolol 0.25%—cardioselective
   - Decreases IOP by 20–30%

   Indications: POAG and secondary glaucoma, good synergic effect with miotics.

   Side effects: Hyperemia, superficial punctate keratitis, corneal anesthesia, bradycardia, arrhythmia, bronchospasm in asthmatics.

  iii. **Alpha-2 adrenergic receptor agonists (sympathomimetics):**
   - Nonselective—Epinefrin and dipivefrin

- Selective—Brimonidine 0.2%, 0.15% b.d.
- Apraclonidine 0.5% BD
- Action: Increases uveoscleral outflow, decreases aqueous production. Decreases IOP 15–30%
- Side effects: Allergy, drowsiness due to CNS depression
- Contraindication: Buphthalmos

iv. **Prostaglandin analogues:**
- Latanoprost 0.005%—once daily at night
- Also useful in normotension glaucoma
- Takes a week to act
- Bimatoprost 0.03%—< a week to act
- Travoprost 0.004%—1 or 2 weeks to act
- Tafluprost 0.0015%
- Decreases IOP by 25–35%
- Action: increases uveoscleral outflow, potent IOP lowering and good control of diurnal fluctuation
- No systemic side effects

To be avoided in keratitis, uveitis and cystoid macular edema

v. **Neuroprotective drugs:**
These drugs enhance the vascular supply of optic nerve head and decrease the pro-apoptic factors.
- Betaxolol
- Brimonidine
- Latanoprost
- Bimatoprost
- Travoprost
- Tafluprost

vi. **Carbonic anhydrase inhibitors**: Topical-Decreases IOP by 15–20%
- Dorzolamide 2% tds
- Brinzolamide 1%
- Acetazolamide 5%
- Systemic acetazolamide—250 mg qid. in all acute glaucoma—decreases IOP by 30%
- Side effects—paresthesia, tingling and numbness, fatigue, depression, diarrhea, renal calculi, Stevens-Johnson syndrome, bone marrow depression

vii. **Hyperosmotic agents:**
- Increase osmolarity of blood
- Oral glycerol 1–1.5 g/kg 50% solution
- 20% Mannitol 1–2 g/kg
- Hypotensive effect peaks in 30 minutes, lasts for 5 hours
- Side effects: Cardiovascular overload, headache, nausea.

viii. **Rho kinase inhibitor:** Recent drug which increases trabecular outflow—Ripasudil 0.4% eye drops twice daily.

Laser Therapy
- **Argon laser trabeculoplasty (ALT)**
  - Shrinkage of collagen
  - Junction of pigmented and non-pigmented region of trabeculum
  - Opens inter trabecular spaces and increases aqueous outflow due to widening of spaces
  - Decreases IOP 8–10 mm in 75% of cases, effect may diminish in time

- **Selective Laser Trabeculoplasty (SLT)**
  - Specifically targets fragmented cells in the trabecular meshwork without affecting the surrounding tissue.
  - Produces less tissue destruction than ALT and is repeatable.

Surgical
- Trabeculectomy:
  - Viscocanalostomy
  - Artificial drainage shunts

Trabeculectomy
- Lowers IOP by creating a fistula which allows aqueous outflow from anterior chamber to sub-Tenon's space
- Fistula is covered by superficial scleral flap
- Limbal or fornix based conjunctival flap
- Lamellar scleral flap of 2/3rd thickness (3 × 4 mm)
- Anterior chamber entered along entire width of scleral flap
- Block of deep scleral flap 1.5 × 2 mm excised with knife or Kelly's punch
- Peripheral iridectomy done
- Superficial scleral flap sutured
- 5-fluorouracil 50 μg/mL or mitomycin C 0.2–0.5 mg/mL may be used to improve long term control of IOP
- Instead of above mentioned antimetabolites, Ologen, a collagen matrix can also be used to improve the success of trabeculectomy.

Artificial Drainage Shunts
- Plastic devices which create a communication between anterior chamber and sub conjunctival space
- Shunts are attached to posterior episcleral implant
- Implant types:
  - Nonvalve—Molteno, Baerveldt
  - Valve—Krupin, Ahmed.

11. Discuss the stages, clinical features and treatment of primary angle closure glaucoma (PACG). What are the recent drugs in the management of glaucoma?

Incidence: Male:Female—1:4

Precipitating Factors
- Dim illumination
- Emotional stress
- Use of mydriatics.

Stages
- Primary angle closure glaucoma suspect (prodromal stage)
- Subacute or intermittent PACG (phase of constant instability)
- Acute primary angle closure glaucoma
- Chronic primary angle closure glaucoma
- Absolute glaucoma.

Primary Angle Closure Glaucoma Suspect (Prodromal Stage)
- Intermittent attacks of increased IOP
- Transient blurring of vision
- Colored halos around light

- Mild headache
- Provocative tests:
  - Prone test
  - Dark room test
  - Mydriatic test.
  (Positive if 8 mm rise occurs within one hour)
- **Treatment:**
  - Laser iridotomy
  - Surgical peripheral iridectomy.

Subacute or Intermittent PACG (Phase of Constant Instability)

- Increase in IOP becomes more frequent
- Attack lasts from few minutes up to 1 to 2 hours
- Mild headache, colored halos.

Treatment

- Same as primary angle closure glaucoma suspect stage
- If occludable angle after medical control of IOP, YAG-laser iridotomy is to be done
- In dim illumination, watching cinema may precipitate pupillary block–relieved by rest due to meiosis.

Acute Primary Angle Closure Glaucoma

- Sudden rise in IOP due to total angle closure
- Symptoms:
  - Pain radiates along branches of trigeminal nerve, so nausea, vomiting, prostration, marked redness, defective vision, colored halos, and photophobia.

Signs:
- Lid edema
- Circumciliary congestion
- Corneal edema
- Mid dilated vertically oval pupil
- Shallow AC
- Markedly increased IOP.

Differential Diagnosis
- Acute iridocyclitis
- Conjunctivitis
- Phacolytic glaucoma
- Phacomorphic glaucoma
- Glaucomatocyclitic crisis.

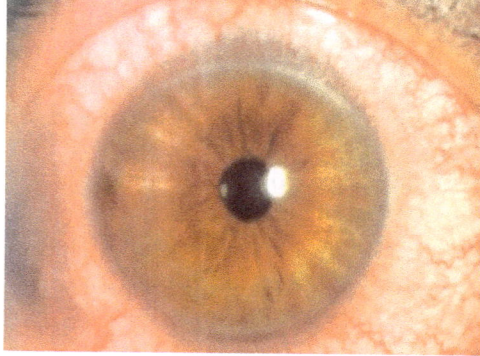

Fig. 11.16: Acute congestive phase of primary angle closure glaucoma.

Treatment

Medical:
- Acetazolamide–250 mg QID
- Hyperosmotic agents:
  - 20% mannitol IV drip (1–2 gm/kg) in 45 minutes
  - 50% oral glycerol (1 g/kg)
- 2% pilocarpine—initially every 30 minutes for 2 hours and later hourly till maximum meiosis is achieved
- Analgesics.

Surgical:
- If peripheral anterior synechiae (PAS)
  - < 50% of angle–peripheral iridectomy or YAG laser iridotomy
  - > 50% of angle–trabeculectomy for affected eye, peripheral iridectomy or laser iridotomy of fellow eye
- Chronic primary angle closure glaucoma:
  - Evidence of past acute attack-indicated by Vogt's triad

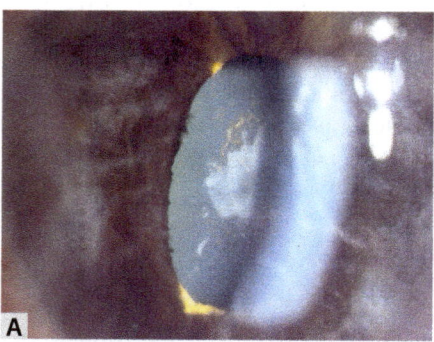

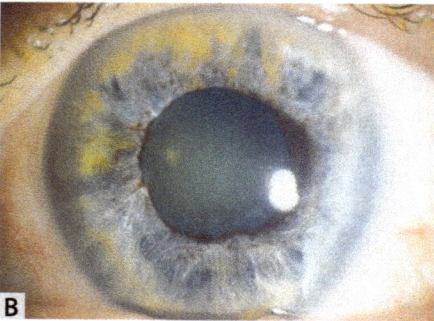

Figs. 11.17A and B: Vogt's triad: (A) Glaucoma flecken; and (B) Iris atrophic patches.

- **Vogt's triad comprises of:**
  i. Glaucoma flecken—anterior subcapsular lenticular opacity
  ii. Patches of iris atrophy
  iii. Dilated nonreactive pupil—due to sphincter atrophy
  - Chronic congestive phase due to repeated acute attacks
  - Creeping angle closure
  - IOP—constantly raised
  - Disc cupping
  - Field defects—similar to POAG. Treatment: Trabeculectomy after lowering IOP.
- Absolute glaucoma:
  - End stage
  - Painful blind eye

- No Perception of Light (PL) – IOP very high
- Cornea—bullous keratopathy
- Pupil—fixed and dilated.

Treatment
- Cyclocryotherapy
- Enucleation of painful blind eye.

Recent drugs in the management of glaucoma:
- Alpha-2 adrenergic receptor agonists such as Brimonidine
- Prostaglandin analogues such as Latanoprost, Bimatoprost, Travoprost and Tafluprost
- Rho kinase inhibitor—Ripasudil.

12. Enumerate the types, clinical features and treatment of secondary glaucoma.

Definition
Secondary glaucoma occurs due to a specific anomaly or disease of the eye.

Features of Secondary Glaucoma
- Usually unilateral
- Can occur at any age
- Usually acute in onset and rapid in progression
- The pathology may be anywhere in the eye
- Management depends on the control of underlying cause.

Classification
Depending on the cause, classified as follows:
- Inflammatory and postinflammatory
- Lens induced
- Pigmentary
- Neovascular
- Associated with intraocular tumors
- Pseudoexfoliation syndrome.
- Glaucoma in aphakia
- Steroid induced glaucoma
- Ciliary block glaucoma (malignant glaucoma)
- Associated with intraocular hemorrhage.

Inflammatory and Postinflammatory
- Mainly due to uveitis
- Clogging of trabecular meshwork
  - By inflammatory material and associated trabeculitis
- Post-inflammatory glaucoma
  - From annular synechia, seclusio pupilla, occlusio pupilla - angle closure following iris bombe or due to organization of inflammatory debris
- Specific hypertensive uveitis syndromes
  - Fuch's uveitis syndrome
  - Glaucomatocyclitic crisis.

Lens Induced
- **Phacomorphic**
  - Secondary angle closure and/or pupil block by lens intumescence
- **Phacolytic**
  - Acute secondary open angle glaucoma due to clogging of trabecular meshwork by macrophages laden with lens proteins in Morgagnian cataract
- **Lens particle glaucoma**
  - Trabecular blockage by lens particles
- **Phacoanaphylactic**
  - Sensitization of same or fellow eye to lens proteins
  - Clogging of trabeculum by inflammatory material.

Pigmentary Glaucoma
- Occurs in 35% of patients with pigment dispersion syndrome
- Common in young myopic males

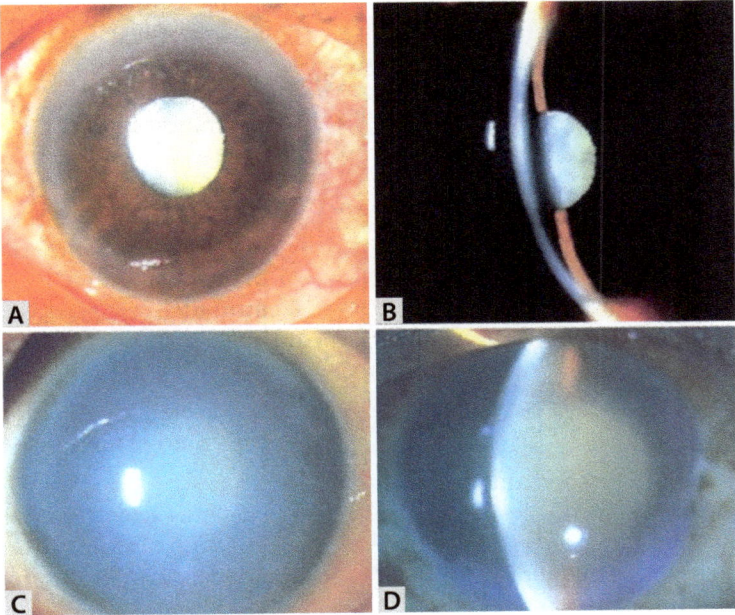

Figs. 11.18A to D: Phacomorphic and phacolytic glaucoma: (A) Phacomorphic glaucoma; (B) Slit-lamp appearance—phacomorphic glaucoma; (C) Phacolytic glaucoma; and (D) Slit-lamp appearance—phacolytic glaucoma.

- Krukenberg's spindle is seen: Pigment deposition on corneal endothelium also on trabecula, lens and zonules
- Pigment deposition above Schwalbe's line in angle of anterior chamber
- Treatment similar to POAG.

Neovascular Glaucoma
- Formation of neovascular membrane at the angle of anterior chamber
- Stimulus to new vessel formation in retinal ischemia

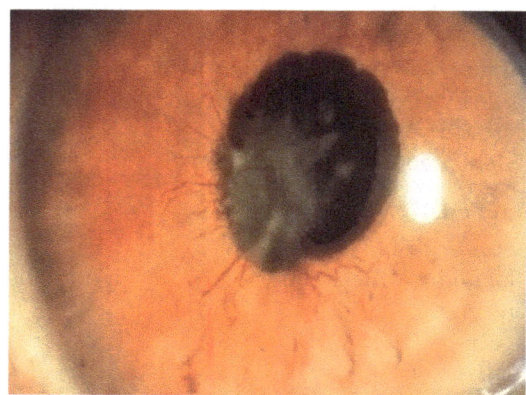

Fig. 11.19: Neovascular glaucoma.

- **Causes:**
  - Central retinal vein occlusion (CRVO)
  - Eales disease
  - Chronic uveitis
  - Central retinal artery occlusion (CRAO)
  - Intraocular tumors.

Treatment
- Pan retinal photocoagulation (PRP) to prevent new vessel formation
- Intravitreal injection of antivascular endothelial growth factor:
  - Lucentis (ranibizumab)
  - Macugen (pegaptanib)
  - Avastin (bevacizumab)
- Implant operation (triamcinolone)
- Cyclocryotherapy.

Associated with Intraocular Tumors
- Retinoblastoma or malignant melanoma
- Raised IOP by:
  - Trabecular block by tumor cells
  - Neovascularization of the angle
  - Venous stasis following obstruction to vortex veins
- Treatment—enucleation of the eyeball.

Pseudoexfoliation Glaucoma
- Secondary open angle glaucoma
- Amyloid like deposits on pupillary border, anterior lens surface, posterior surface of iris zonules and ciliary processes
- Occurs in 70% of cases with pseudoexfoliation
- Other features and treatment similar to POAG

- Sampolesi's line—pigment dispersion anterior to Schwalbe's line in angle of anterior chamber.

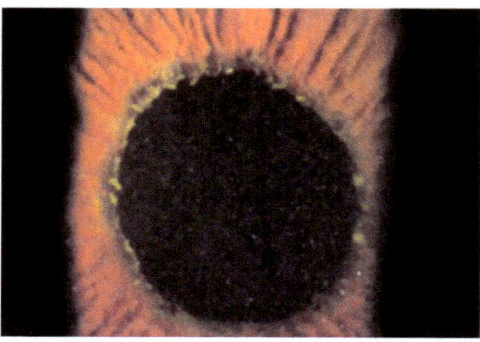

Fig. 11.20: Pseudoexfoliation in pupillary border.

Glaucoma in Aphakia/Pseudophakia
Causes:
- Vitreous filling the AC
- Angle closure due to flat AC
- Pupil block
- Pre-existing POAG
- Epithelial in growth into the angle of AC.

Steroid-induced Glaucoma
- Usually occur after 6 weeks of steroid therapy
- 5% high steroid responders
- 35% moderate responders
- 60% non-responders
- **Cause:**
  Mucopolysaccharides are deposited in trabecular meshwork
  - Features: Similar to POAG
  - **Treatment:**
    » Normalizes in 2–4 weeks after cessation of steroids
    » 0.5% timolol BID
    » Filtration surgery in intractable cases.

Ciliary Block Glaucoma (Malignant Glaucoma)
- After filtration surgery for PACG or after cataract surgery
- **Causes:**
  - Misdirection of aqueous into the vitreous pushing the iris lens diaphragm forwards
  - Flat anterior chamber with negative Seidel's test
  - Markedly raised IOP
- **Treatment:**

Medical:
- 1% atropine eye drops TDS
- Acetazolamide 250 mg TDS
- 0.5% timolol maleate BID

Surgical:
- Posterior sclerotomy with vitreous aspiration
- Injection of air into AC
- Anterior hyaloidotomy by laser or laser peripheral iridoplasty.

Associated with Intraocular Hemorrhage

- Hemolytic glaucoma
  - Obstruction of trabecular meshwork by macrophages filled with lysed red blood cell (RBC) debris after hyphema
- Ghost cell glaucoma
  - In vitreous hemorrhage, RBCs converted into khaki-colored ghost cells block trabecular meshwork
- Red cell glaucoma
  - Blockade of trabecular meshwork by RBCs following massive hyphema
- Hemosiderotic glaucoma
  - Due to sclerotic changes in trabecular meshwork induced by iron from hemoglobin.

Treatment

- Beta-blockers, steroids and mydriatic
- In massive hyphema, if IOP is > 50 mm of Hg for 2 days or > 35 mm of Hg for 5 days. Surgical evacuation of blood with or without trabeculectomy.

CHAPTER 12

Vitreous

1. Describe the anatomy of vitreous.

Vitreous is a transparent, colorless gelatinous mass occupying the posterior segment of the eyeball. It is attached to the edges of the optic disc, macula and a zone near the ora serrata.
- Its volume is 4–4.5 mL.
- It is hydrophilic gel consisting of:
    - Water (99%)
    - Hyaluronic acid
    - Collagen fibrils
    - Hyalocytes
    - Mucopolysaccharides.

The interaction between hyaluronic acid and collagen fibrils is responsible for the gel form of vitreous body.

2. What are the diseases of vitreous?

The diseases of vitreous are:
- Degeneration of vitreous
- Opacities of vitreous
- Vitreous bands and membrane
- Persistent hyperplastic primary vitreous
- Detachment of vitreous
- Vitreous hemorrhage.

3. Discuss the degenerations of vitreous.

- **Synchysis:** Liquefaction of vitreous
    - Most common
    May be associated with syneresis.

Causes
- Injury due to diathermy or cryotherapy
- Radiation
- Postinflammatory
    - Vitreous loses its normal fibrillar structure and liquefaction pockets are formed.
- **Synersis:** Collapse of vitreous
    - Vitreous become completely fluid so that strands or membrane appear to be freely floating on it.

4. Discuss the degenerative opacities of vitreous.

- Asteroid hyalosis
- Synchysis scintillans
- Amyloid degeneration.

Asteroid Hyalosis

- Unilateral disorder
- Occur in patients over 60
- Twice as common in men as women
- Seen as small calcium laden lipids
- Presents as similar to stars in the night sky on eye movement, the asteroid bodies move within the vitreous but return to their original position
- Does not cause vision loss.

Synchysis Scintillans

Vitreous is laden with small white angular and crystalline bodies formed of cholesterol. It affects damaged eyes which have suffered from trauma, vitreous hemorrhage, or inflammatory diseases.

In this condition vitreous is liquid and so the crystals sink to the bottom. These crystals are stirred up with every movement of eyeball to settle down again.

Beautiful shower of golden rain is seen on ophthalmoscopic examination and hence the term synchysis scintillans.

Cholesterol crystal in the vitreous since they are not attached to vitreous framework, they settle out inferiorly after eye movement.

	Asteroid hyalosis	Synchysis scintillans
Laterality	Unilateral	Bilateral
Composition	Calicium containing phospholipids	Cholesterol crystals
Symptoms	Symptom free	Golden crystals may be seen before the eye
State of vitreous	Gel	Fluid
Attachment to vitreous	Attached	Free
Effect of gravity	Unaffected	Affected Settles at bottom

Amyloidosis

- Occur after 40 years
- Bilateral granular, strand like opacities, within the central vitreous.

Treatment
- Pars plana vitrectomy.

5. What is epiretinal membrane?

- Epiretinal membrane or preretinal membrane
- Pathological membrane lining the inner surface of retina

- These membrane are formed by
  - Fibrocytes
  - Hyalocytes
  - Retinal pigment epithelium
  - Endothelial cells of capillaries when the membrane contracts the retina also wrinkles resulting in wrinkling of macula(macular pucker).

Treatment

Membrane stripping to be done during pars plana vitrectomy. Retinal tear may follow if untreated.

6. Write short notes on persistent hyperplastic primary vitreous.

The hyaloid vascular system usually atrophies by 8th month of gestation. Sometimes the hyaloid artery fails to degenerate. This along with hyperplasia of posterior part of vascular network leads to persistent hyperplastic primary vitreous.
- Usually unilateral.
- Presence of a retrolental mass with long extended ciliary process is characteristic.
- Typically presents as a white reflex in the pupil.
- Associated lesions:
  - Congenital cataract and glaucoma
  - Microphthaloms.
- CT and ultrasonography will clinch the diagnosis.

Treatment
- Aspirate the lens
- Excise the retrolental membrane
- Vitrectomy.

7. Write short notes on posterior vitreous detachment.

Ageing causes reduction in hyaluronic acid which results in less support to the collagen. This induces detachment of the posterior hyaloid face from the optic disc resulting in vitreous detachment. On ophthalmoscopy, it appears as an annulus floating in the vitreous over the posterior pole which is known as Weiss ring.

8. Write short notes on vitreous hemorrhage.

Extravasation of blood within and around the vitreous body.

Etiology
- Trauma – blunt or penetrating
- Proliferative retinopathy:
  - Diabetic retinopathy
  - Retinal vein occlusion
  - Eales disease
  - Sickle cell retinopathy.
- Blood dyscrasias—hemophilia, purpura.
- Posterior vitreous detachment with collapse.
- Retinal breaks with or without detachment.

Clinical Features

The vitreous hemorrhage may be found either in subhyaloid space or in vitreous cavity or in both.

The subhyaloid blood moves with gravity and appears boat shaped because it remains unclotted for a long time.

When the blood in vitreous cavity clots, it becomes a white opaque mass.

Symptoms
- Sudden onset of floaters
- Diminution of vision.

Examination
- Indirect ophthalmoscopy
- Ultrasonography.

Complications
- Recurrent vitreous hemorrhage may lead to degeneration of vitreous
- Tractional retinal detachment
- Ghost cell glaucoma
- Hemosiderosis bulbi.

Treatment

Bed rest, eye patching, elevation of head end of bed.

If the blood does not absorb by 6 months and the patient vision is less than 6/60 or if associated with retinal detachment, vitrectomy is indicated.

Vitrectomy

Surgical removal and replacement of the vitreous is called vitrectomy.

Three Types:
i. Anterior vitrectomy: Anterior vitreous is removed
ii. Core vitrectomy: Central bulk is removed
iii. Total vitrectomy: Entire vitreous is removed.

Anterior vitrectomy is by open sky technique.
Anterior vitrectomy is usually done during:
- Cataract surgery when vitreous loss has occurred
- Perforating injury
- Dislocation or subluxation of lens
- Vitreous touch syndrome.
- *Core, subtotal and total vitrectomy* is by **pars plana approach.**

Indications of Pars Plana Vitrectomy
- Dropped nucleus or dropped IOL removal
- Retinopathy of prematurity
- Intraocular foreign bodies
- Persistent hyperplastic primary vitreous
- Endophthalmitis
- Vitreous hemorrhage and vitreous membrane
- Eales disease
- Retinal detachment with giant tears and vitreous traction.

Treatment:
- Three incisions are given in the pars plana region
- Three probes are introduced through three incisions:
  - 1st probe – Cutting and aspiration
  - 2nd probe – Illumination
  - 3rd probe – Infusion through cannula.

CHAPTER 13

Retina

INTRODUCTION

Retina forms part of the posterior segment which also includes vitreous, choroid, posterior sclera and optic disk.

1. Describe the structure and functions of retina.

Structure of Retina

- Innermost layer of the eye
- Development from neuroectoderm
- Thickness of retina
- Near optic disk – 0.5 mm
- At equator – 0.2 mm
- Anteriorly – 0.1 mm

Layers of the Retina

- Pigment epithelium
- Layer of photoreceptors

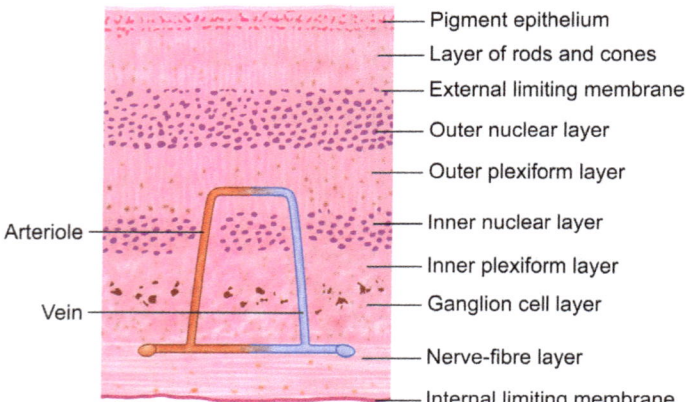

Fig. 13.1: Structure of retina.

- External limiting membrane (ELM)
- Outer nuclear layer: Consists of nuclei of rods and cones
- Outer plexiform layer
- Inner nuclear layer: Consists of bipolar cells, horizontal cells, amacrine cells and Muller cells which connect different cells together
- Inner plexiform layer
- Ganglion cell layer
- Nerve fiber layer
- Internal limiting membrane (ILM): Footplates of Muller cells end in the internal limiting membrane.

Muller Cells

- Muller cells: Modified astrocytes extend from ILM to ELM.

Peripheral Retina

- Extends from macula to ora serrata
- Have a single layer of ganglion cells
- 120 million rods
- 6 million cones of which 50% are in the macula.

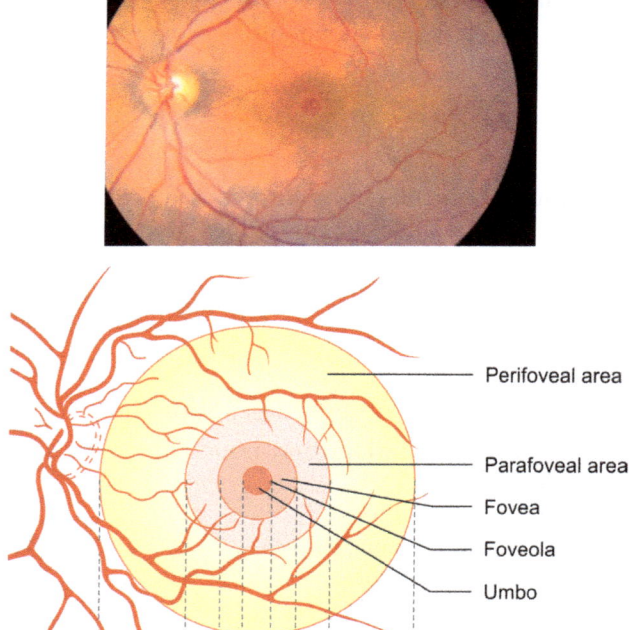

Fig. 13.2: Normal fundus.

Macula

- Outer plexiform layer in the macula is called Henle's fiber layer
- Radial orientation of fibers: Responsible for macular star formation

- Macula: Area of the retina with more than one ganglion cell layer
- Fovea: Central depression of inner retinal surface – avascular zone
- Foveola: Absence of ganglion and other nucleated cells.

Diameters

- Macula – 5.5 mm
- Fovea – 1.5 mm
- Foveola – 350 micrometer
- Umbo – 150 micrometer
- Avascular zone – 450 micrometer
- Ratio of Macula:Fovea:Foveola = 16:5:1.

Blood Supply

- Choriocapillaries supply outer four layers
- Central retinal artery supplies inner six layers.

Venous Drainage

- Outer four layers drained by vortex veins through choriocapillaries
- Inner six layers drained by central retinal vein.

Functions of Retina

- Central part—the macula—cones:
  - Color vision
  - Sharp vision—distant and near
- Peripheral part—mainly of rods:
  - Night vision
  - Dark adaptation
  - Field of vision
- In the outer segment of the retina conversion of light energy to electrical energy takes place
- Pigment epithelium—services and maintains overlying photoreceptors cells
- Functions of retinal pigment epithelium (RPE)
  - Absorbs strong light
  - Actively transports metabolites
  - Forms outer blood-retinal barrier
  - Helps in regeneration of visual pigments.

2. Describe the methods of examination of retina.

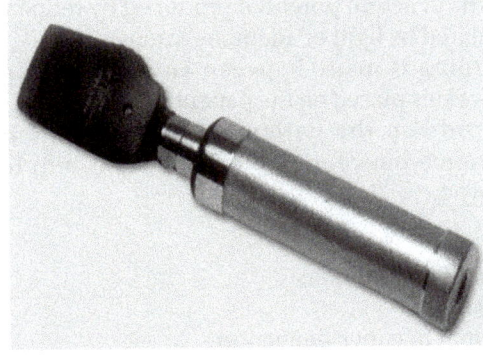

Fig. 13.3: Direct ophthalmoscope.

- Direct ophthalmoscope
- Indirect ophthalmoscope
- Slit-lamp biomicroscope with special lenses
- Fluorescein angiography
- Indocyanine green angiography
- Ultrasonography.

Direct Ophthalmoscopy

Invented by Babbage–1848
Popularized by Von Helmholtz–1850.

Distant Direct Ophthalmoscopy: +20 D lens in ophthalmoscope at 20–25 cm.

Uses

- To diagnose opacities in media
- To recognize the subluxation of the lens
- To recognize detached retina
- To differentiate between a mole and hole in the iris
  - Portable, battery-operated, self-illuminated, handheld instrument
  - Extent of field seen-from posterior pole to equator
  - Area of visualization increases as the eye is approached
  - Magnification—15 times in emmetrope
  - Less in hypermetrope and more in myopes
  - Real and erect image.

Indirect Ophthalmoscopy

- Invented by Nagel in 1864.

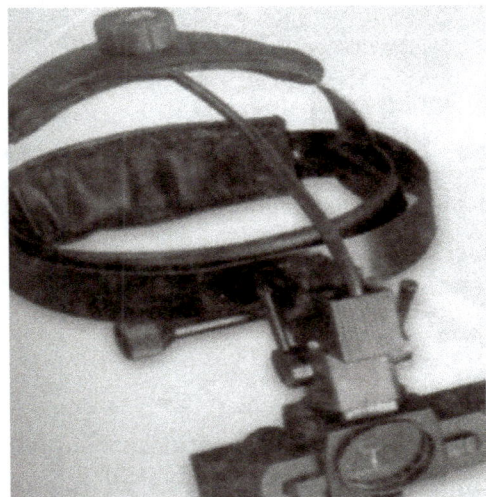

Fig. 13.4: Indirect ophthalmoscopy.

Principle

Makes the observed eye myopic irrespective of its refraction by placing strong convex lens (+20 D) in front of the eye:
- Real inverted image is formed
- Lenses used +28 D, +20D, +13D
- +13 D gives 5 times magnification
- +20D gives 3 times magnification

Advantages

- Large field of view
- Allows examination in hazy media
- Stereoscopic view.

Disadvantage
- Image inverted vertically and laterally

	Direct ophthalmoscope	Indirect ophthalmoscope
Magnification	15X	3–5X
Static field of view	10 degrees	46 degrees (with +20 D)
Dynamic field of view	Up to equator	Up to ora serrata
Technique	Easy	Difficult
Illumination	Good	Excellent, fundus can be seen through hazy media
Stereopsis	Absent	Present

Contact Lenses
- Goldman three mirror contact lens
- Panfundoscopic lens
- Nullify the power of the cornea

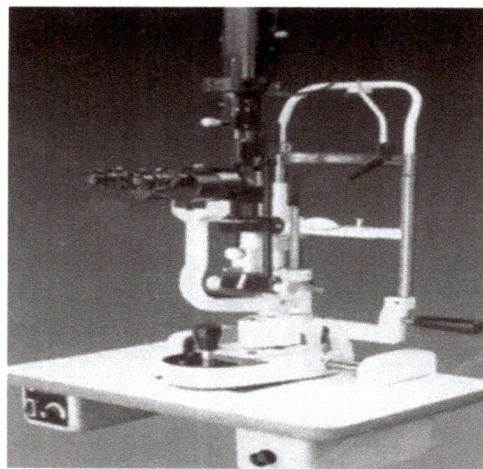

Fig. 13.5: Slit-lamp biomicroscopy with special lenses.

Noncontact Lenses
- Hruby lens –55 D
- +78 D
- +90 D

Goldmann three-mirror Lens
- Three mirrors placed in different inclinations—73°, 67°, 59°
- Central lens for disk and posterior pole
  - 59° mirror—gonioscopy mirror: Smallest tongue shaped to view the angle of anterior chamber
  - 67° middle sized bigger mirror—to view central retina to mid periphery
  - 73° largest mirror—to view from mid periphery to periphery.

Other Lenses
- Pan fundoscopic lens
  - Whole retina can be seen
  - High plus lens can be used to give laser burns
- +78 D lens–1.3X + 90 D lens–1.1X
- Image inverted laterally and vertically
- –55 D lens—small field.

Fluorescein Angiography

[Discussed in Miscellaneous chapter]

Indocyanine Green Angiography (ICG)
- 1–2 mL of ICG 25 mg/mL
- Late exposure up to 30–60 minutes post injection is taken
- Absorbs light at 805 nm and emits light at 835 nm (near-infrared).

Advantages of ICG

To visualize
- Choroidal neovascular membranes
- Choroidal tumors
- Choroidal vasculature.

Ultrasonography
- Ultrasonic frequencies in the range of 10 MHz or 10 million cycles per second are used for ophthalmic diagnosis
- Body scanning probe frequency is only 2.5–5 MHz.

Principle of Ultrasonography
- The transducer transforms electrical energy to sound energy which is directed in the tissues
- Reflected sound waves are received by ceramic plates which convert sound energy into electrical energy.

A scan is time amplitude:
- One dimensional display—horizontal dimension is proportionate to time
- Vertical deflection—denotes position of echo.

B scan – intensity modulated:
- 2-dimensional display—horizontal dimension is proportional to time and distance
- Vertical echoes—represented as bright intensity modulated dots
- By judging the bright dots and space, it can be interpreted.

3. Describe the investigations of retinal function.
- Electroretinography
- Electrooculogram
- Dark adaptometry
- Color vision tests
- Methods of retinal nerve fiber layer assessment.

Electroretinography

Measures function of outer retinal layers.
- Records of action potential produced by retina when it is stimulated by light of adequate intensity
- Recording is made between an active electrode in a contact lens placed on the patient's cornea and a reference electrode on the patient's forehead—the potential difference between two electrodes is amplified and deployed.

ERG
- Normal ERG is biphasic
- A wave:
  - Initial negative deflection
  - Arises from photoreceptors

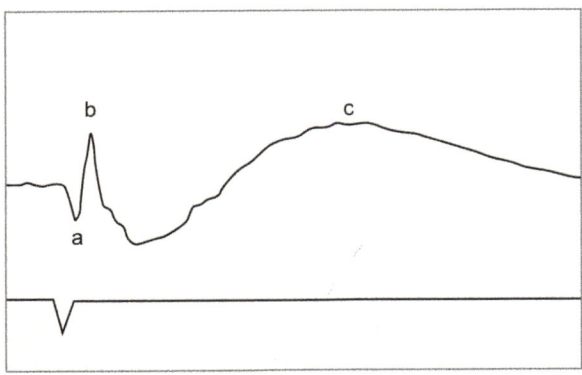

Fig. 13.6: Electroretinography.

- B wave:
    - Positive deflection
    - Elicited by Muller and bipolar cells

Oscillatory potentials: Small wavelets on ascending limb of B wave produced by amacrine cells.

- C wave:
    - Positive wave of RPE seen only in dark adapted eye
    - ERG measures mass retinal response.

Indications:
- To diagnose generalized retinal degeneration—retinitis pigmentosa, congenital night blindness
- Amplitude of B wave decreased in anoxic conditions like CRAO and ischemic CRVO.

Electrooculogram (EOG)

- Measures standing potential between electrically +ve cornea and –ve back of eye
- Reflects activity of RPE and photoreceptors:
    - Electrodes are attached to skin near medial and lateral canthi
    - Patient asked to move eyes from side to side
    - When the eyes move, cornea near electrode becomes +ve with respect to other
    - Potential difference between the electrodes amplified and measured.

Uses

- To diagnose Best's disease and carriers:
    - Where ERG is normal but EOG is abnormal. EOG is more sensitive than ERG in diagnosis of retinitis pigmentosa
- To diagnose chloroquine toxicity.

Dark Adaptometry

- Ability to adapt to decreased illumination is measured
- Useful to diagnose night blindness.

Abnormal in:
- Pigmentary dystrophies of the retina
- Vitamin A deficiency
    - Glaucoma

After 5 minutes of light adaptation, the patient is seated in dark. Spots of increasing luminance are presented until seen by the patient.

- Dark adaptation curve increases in sensitivity after 5-10 minutes
- Reaches plateau by 20 minutes.

Color Vision Tests

- Lantern test
- Holmgren wool test
- Farnsworth-Munsell 100-hue test
- Ishihara pseudoisochromatic charts
- Nagel anomaloscope.

Methods of Retinal Nerve Fiber Layer (RNFL) Assessment

- Red free filter indirect ophthalmoscope
- Fundus photography of RNFL
- **Newer methods**
    - GDx vcc – scanning laser polarimetry
    - HRT
        » Heidelberg retinal tomograph
        » Confocal scanning laser ophthalmoscopy
    - Optical coherence tomography (OCT).

GDx vcc

- Measures thickness of RNFL in the peripapillary area
- Resolution up to 5 microns
- Can be used in undilated pupil
- Short test time – 3 minutes
- Used mainly in glaucoma.

HRT

- Analyses 3-dimensional images of optic nerve head and retina
- Pupil dilatation is necessary
- Test time –15 minutes
- Resolution –15 microns.

Optical Coherence Tomography

- Works similar to ultrasound but uses light waves instead of sound waves
- Gives cross image of the retina, adding third dimension viz. depth
- Clear media and pupillary dilation are necessary
- Test time – 15 minutes. Resolution – 10 microns.

Macular Hole with Vitreous Traction:

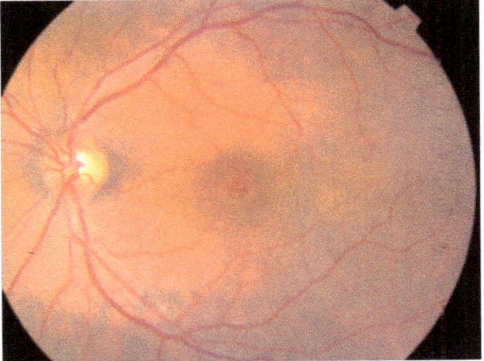

Fig. 13.7: Fundus picture of macular hole.

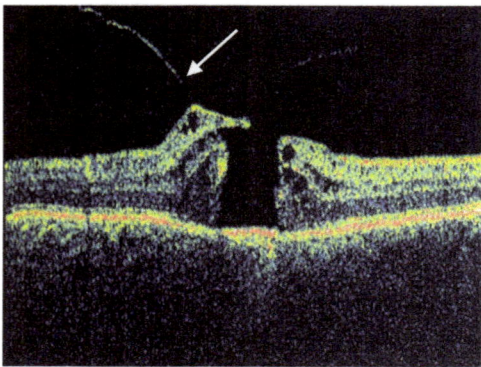

Fig. 13.8: Optical coherence tomography.

Uses
- To assess RNFL thickness in glaucoma
- To diagnose macular diseases such as:
  - Central serous retinopathy
  - Epimacular membrane
  - ARMD and macular hole.

4. Write short notes on retinal hemorrhages.

These are of two types:
  i. **Superficial retinal hemorrhages:** Striate or flame shaped because they are situated in the nerve fiber layer. They are bright red and obscure retinal vessels. They are seen in:
     - Hypertensive retinopathy
     - Diabetic retinopathy
     - Central vein occlusion
     - Anemia
     - Leukemia
     - AIDS.
  ii. **Deep retinal hemorrhages:** These are rounded because they are situated in the outer plexiform layer. They are deep red and retinal vessels course over the hemorrhage. They are seen in diabetic retinopathy.

5. What are soft exudates (cotton wool spots)?

These are fluffy deposits with feathery edges lying in the nerve fiber layer. They obscure retinal vessels. It is due to ischemia and anoxia of the nerve fiber layer following occlusion of small vessels. Usually, disappear within 6–8 weeks. They are seen in:
- Hypertensive retinopathy
- Toxemia of pregnancy
- Papillitis and papilledema
- Anemia
- Leukemia
- AIDS.

6. What are hard exudates?

These are discrete yellowish-white plaques with a clear-cut margin. These are the result of a leak of plasma from capillaries with the absorption of fluid leaving behind the lipid material in the outer plexiform layer. These last some years. They are seen in:
- Diabetic retinopathy
- Coat's disease
- Circinate retinopathy
- Hypertensive retinopathy.

7. Describe the risk factors, pathogenesis, classification, clinical features, and man-agement of diabetic retinopathy.

Retinal changes occurring due to diabetes mellitus.

Risk Factors
- Duration of diabetes
  - 50% of patients develop retinopathy after 10 years
  - 70% of patients develop retinopathy after 20 years
  - 90% of patients develop retinopathy after 30 years
- Poor metabolic control
- Pregnancy
- Hypertension
- Nephropathy.

Local Protective Factors
- High myopia
- Chorioretinal scarring
- Glaucoma

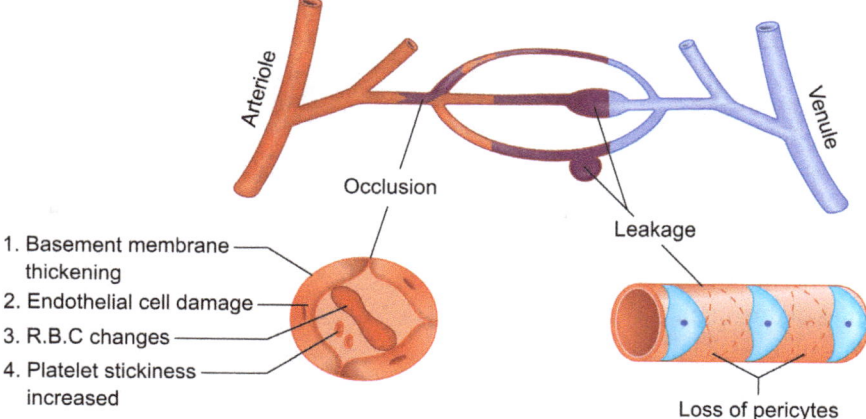

Fig. 13.9: Pathogenesis of diabetic retinopathy (DR).

- Optic atrophy
- Retinitis pigmentosa

It is due to decreased retinal metabolic demand.

Pathogenesis

Microangiopathy
- Two important factors:
  - Microvascular occlusion
  - Microvascular leakage.

Microvascular Occlusion

- Capillary changes
  - Loss of pericytes
  - Thickening of basement membrane
  - Proliferation of endothelial cells
  - Resulting in microaneurysms
- Hematological
  Deformation and aggregation of RBC and platelets resulting in decreased oxygen transport
  - Retinal hypoxia results in:
    » Arteriovenous shunts
    » Intraretinal microvascular abnormalities (IRMA). IRMA-shunts from arterioles to venules.

Neovascularization

- Liberation of vascular endothelial growth factor (VEGF) by the hypoxic retina
- Promotes neovascularization of the retina and optic nerve head
- Consequences of retinal ischemia.

Microvascular Leakage

- Breakdown of inner blood-retinal barrier
- Microaneurysms—weakening of capillary walls
- Increased vascular permeability resulting in focal or diffuse retinal edema—Hard exudates may occur in a circinate pattern.

Classification

- Eva Kohner's
- Early treatment diabetic retinopathy study (ETDRS).

Eva Kohner's Classification

- Background retinopathy
- Preproliferative retinopathy
- Proliferative retinopathy.

ETDRS Classification

- Background or nonproliferative:
  - Mild
  - Moderate
  - Severe
  - Very severe
- Maculopathy with or without clinically significant macular edema (CSME)
- Proliferative diabetic retinopathy (PDR)
  - Without high-risk characteristics (HRC)
  - With HRC. *Nonproliferative retinopathy.*

Mild
- Few microaneurysms (MA)
  - Retinal hemorrhages
  - Hard exudates
  - Seen in 1 quadrant.

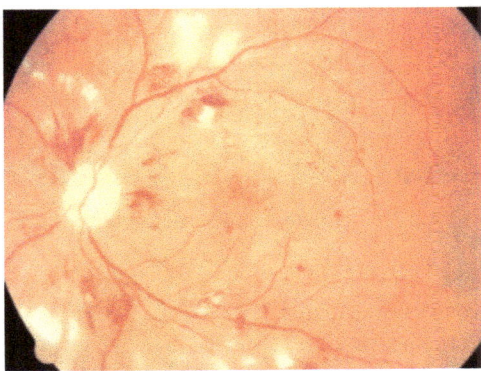

Fig. 13.10: Soft exudates.

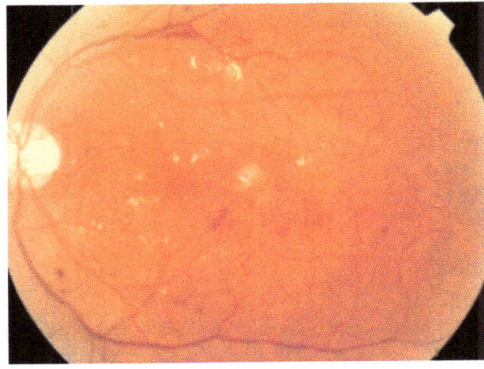

Fig. 13.11: Nonproliferative diabetic retinopathy—microaneurysms (MA) and dot and blot HGS.

Moderate
Above features are seen in 2 or 3 quadrants.

Severe (Preproliferative Retinopathy)
- 4-2-1 Rule
- Defined as anyone of the following:
  - 4 quadrants of hemorrhages/microaneurysms
  - 2 quadrants of venous beading
  - 1 quadrant of intraretinal microvascular abnormalities (IRMA).

Very Severe
- Defined as 2 or more of the above features.

Proliferative Diabetic Retinopathy
Neovascularization of disk or elsewhere, with or without following three high-risk characteristics:
  i. Neovascularization of disk (NVD) > 1/4 to 1/3 disk area
  ii. Any NVD with vitreous hemorrhage (VH)
  iii. Neovascularization elsewhere (NVE) > 1/2 disk area with VH.

PDR—High-risk

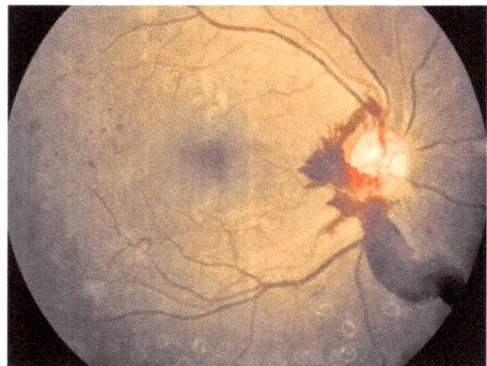

Fig. 13.12: Proliferative diabetic retinopathy—high-risk.

Proliferative DR
- New vessels on the disk (NVD)
- New vessels elsewhere (NVE).

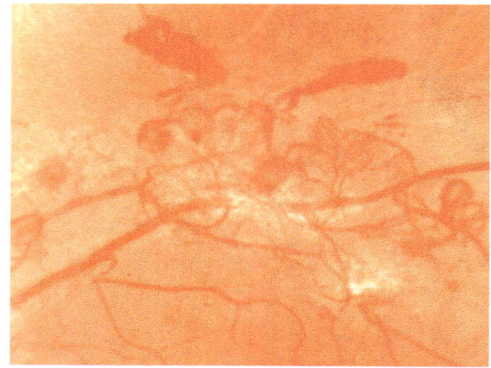

Fig. 13.13: New vessels on the retina with hemorrhages.

Maculopathy
- Clinically significant macular edema (CSME)
- Edema involving the center of the macula
- Seen with SL examination with +90 D lens:
  i. Thickening of the retina within 500 µ of foveal avascular zone (FAZ)
  ii. Hard exudates within 500 µ of FAZ with associated thickening of the adjacent retina
  iii. Zone of retinal thickening 1 disk area or larger any part of it is within 1 DD of the foveal center.

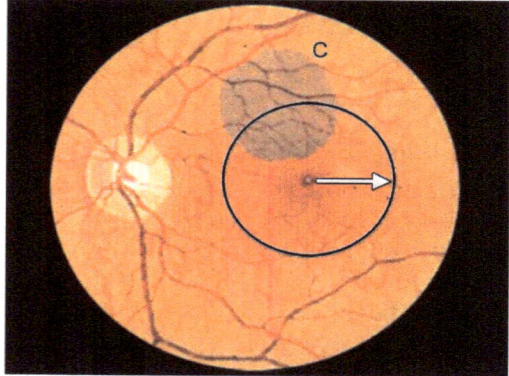

Fig. 13.14: Clinically significant macular edema.

Three Criteria

Criteria 1

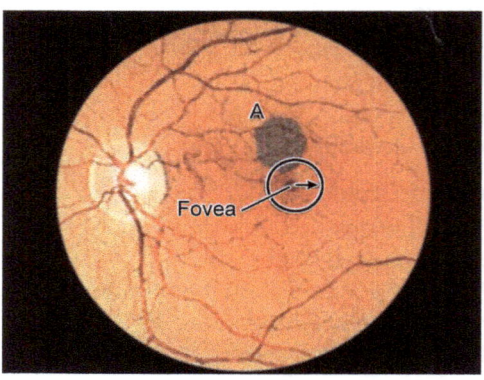

Fig. 13.15: Retinal thickening within 500 µ from the fovea.

Criteria 2

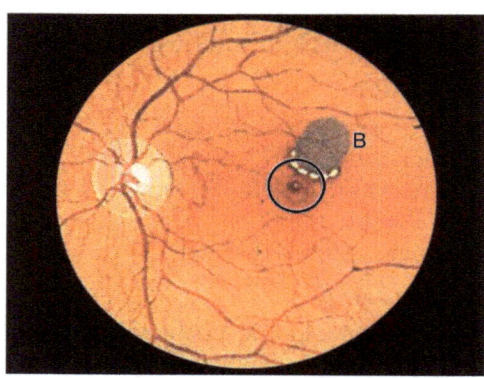

Fig. 13.16: Hard exudates within 500 m of fovea with adjacent retinal thickening.

Criteria 3

Retinal thickening of >1 DD even if partly within 1 DD of the foveal center.

NPDR–CSME

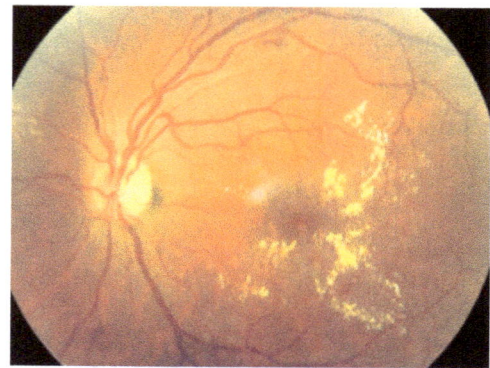

Fig. 13.17: Hard exudates in the macula with clinically significant macular edema in severe nonproliferative diabetic retinopathy.

Advanced Diabetes Eye Disease
- Persistent new vessels
- Tractional retinal detachment
- Neovascular glaucoma.

Advanced

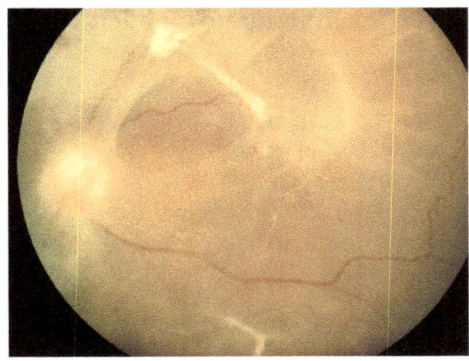

Fig. 13.18: Extensive avascular glial tissue and localized inferior retinal detachment in proliferative diabetic retinopathy.

Causes of Visual Loss
- In NPDR:
  - Macular edema or ischemia
- In PDR:
  - Tractional RD
  - Neovascular glaucoma
  - Vitreous hemorrhage.

Differential Diagnosis
- Hypertensive retinopathy
- Retinal vein occlusion
- Radiation retinopathy
- Ocular ischemic syndrome
- Anemia/leukemia.

Investigations
- Direct and indirect ophthalmoscopy
- Slit-lamp examination with 90 D lens
- Color fundus photography
- Fluorescein angiography
- Optical coherence tomography.

FFA – Indications
- All eyes with maculopathy
- Unexplained visual loss
- Asteroid hyalosis
- Doubtful diagnosis.

Treatment
- Control of diabetes
- Laser
- Intravitreal injection of triamcinolone
- Surgery
- Low vision aids.

Treatment of DR
Based on several studies
- Early Treatment Diabetic Retinopathy Study (ETDRS) – Role of focal laser
- Diabetic Retinopathy Study (DRS) – Role of PRP
- Diabetic Retinopathy Vitrectomy Study (DRVS) – Role of pars plana vitrectomy.
- Diabetic Control and Complications Trial (DCCT) – Control of DR in type I diabetes.
- United Kingdom Prospective Diabetes Study (UKPDS) – Control of DR in type II diabetes
- **Early treatment diabetic retinopathy study (ETDRS)**
  - Focal laser decreases vision loss from macular edema by 50%
  - No benefit from aspirin
- **Diabetic retinopathy study (DRS)**
  - Pan retinal photocoagulation (PRP) reduces the incidence of severe vision loss in high-risk PDR by 60%
- **Diabetic retinopathy vitrectomy study (DRVS)**
  - Early vitrectomy of vitreous hemorrhage in type I diabetic is advised
  - Can be deferred in type II diabetic
- **Diabetic control and complication trial (DCCT)**
  - In type I diabetics tight control of blood sugar decreases progression of retinopathy and macular edema
  - HbA1c < 8% – reduced risk of retinopathy
  - Rapid normalization and tight control of blood sugar after a period of prolonged hyperglycemia can lead to worsening of retinopathy
- **United Kingdom prospective diabetes study (UKPDS)**
  - Tight control of blood sugar and blood pressure slows progression of retinopathy and development of macular edema in type II diabetic patients.

Control of Diabetes
- DCCT for IDDM
- UKPDS for NIDDM.

Important Studies in DR
- DRS: Role of PRP
- DRVS: Role of PPV (pars plana vitrectomy)
- ETDRS: Role of focal laser- CSME.

For CSME
- Focal laser
  - Argon green is preferred
  - Yellow laser can also be used.

For PDR
- Pan retinal photocoagulation (PRP) – Spot size 500 μ, duration 0.15 sec, number of burns 1,200–1,600, burns of moderate intensity placed ½ to 1 burn apart
- Panretinal photocoagulation
- Criteria – high-risk characteristics in PDR.

Intravitreal Injections
- *Steroids:* IV Triamcinolone/Ozurdex
- Antivascular endothelial growth factors (anti-VEGF):
  - Bevacizumab (Avastin)
  - Ranibizumab (Lucentis)
  - Aflibercept (Eylea).

Surgical Treatment
- Vitreoretinal surgery
- Pars plana vitrectomy

- Endolaser photocoagulation
- Release of tractional bands
- Removal of subretinal neovascular membrane
- Treatment of retinal detachment (RD).

Surgery: Pars Plana Vitrectomy (PPV)
- Non-clearing vitreous hemorrhage
- Tractional RD affecting fovea
- Combined RD (with hole and traction)
- Taut posterior hyaloid
- Persistent macular edema
- Vitreomacular traction
- Removal of membranes: segmentation/delamination
- **Laser:** PRP or tamponade only for breaks.

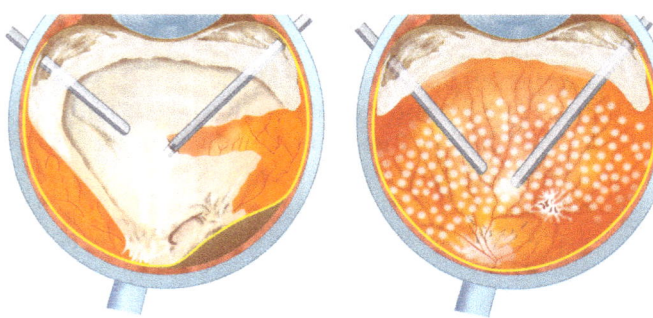

Fig. 13.19: Removal of tractional membrane and endolaser photocoagulation.

Diabetic Retinopathy: Treatment Guidelines
- Background:
  - Control of diabetics
  - Regular review
- Maculopathy:
  - CSME
  - Focal leak
  - Circinate retinopathy—focal photocoagulation
  - Diffuse leak around macula—grid laser
- Pre-proliferative retinopathy—frequent review
- Proliferative retinopathy—PRP
- Advanced diabetic eye disease—vitreoretinal surgery and photocoagulation.

Diabetic Retinopathy Screening: Guidelines by AAO* and AADA**.		
	First examination	Review
➢ Type I diabetic	5 years after onset of diabetes	Every year
➢ Type II diabetic	At the time of diagnosis	Every year
➢ During pregnancy women with Diabetic	First trimester	3 Monthly

*AAO**: American Academy of Ophthalmologists; AADA****: American Academy of Diabetic Association.

Review of Patients with Diabetic Retinopathy.	
Mild NPDR	12 Months
Moderate NPDR without macular edema	6–12 months
Moderate NPDR with non CSME	4–6 months
NPDR with CSME PDR	3–4 months

8. Discuss the pathogenesis, classification, clinical features and complications of hypertensive retinopathy.

Introduction
Retinal changes occurring due to hypertension.

Predisposing Factors
- Severity of hypertension
- Duration
- Age of patient:
  - In young—narrowing of retinal arterioles due to spasm
  - In aged—depends on pre-existing involutional sclerosis.

Pathogenesis
Results from 3 changes:
 i. Vasoconstriction
 ii. Atherosclerotic changes
 iii. Increased vascular permeability

Vasoconstriction
- Primary response of retinal arterioles is narrowing:
  - In pure form—seen in young
  - In aged people
- Narrowing modified by rigidity of arterioles from involutional sclerosis.

Atherosclerotic Changes
- Manifests as changes in arteriolar reflex and AV crossing changes
- Thickening of vessel wall due to involutional sclerosis.

Increased Vascular Permeability
- Disruptions of inner blood-retinal barrier due to retinal hypoxia:
  - Narrowing of retinal arteriole
  - Retinal ischemia

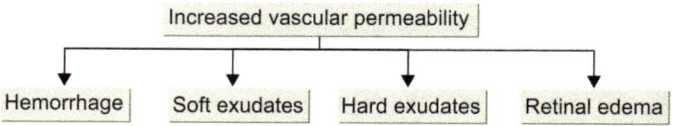

Phases of Retinopathy
- Vasoconstrictive phase
- Sclerotic phase
- Exudative phase
- Complication of sclerotic phase.

Phase: 1 and 2—asymptomatic
 3 and 4—vision is affected

Vasoconstrictive Phase
- Focal and diffuse constriction of arteries
- Occurs in 2nd and 3rd order arteries
- Common in young patients.

Sclerotic Phase: Sets in where BP Remains Elevated for Prolonged Period
- Narrowing of arteries
- AV crossing changes
- Sclerosis of vessel walls (copper/silver wiring)
- Vascular tortuosity
- Increased angle of branching of arterioles.

Exudative Phase
- Flame-shaped hemorrhages
- Cotton wool spots
- Hard exudates
  - Macular star
  - Circinate retinopathy.

Complications of Sclerotic Phase
- Central or branch vein occlusion
- Macular edema
- Neovascularization.

Classification
Depends of inter-relationship of arteriosclerotic and hypertensive changes
- Keith-Wagner-Barker
- Scheie.

Keith-Wagner-Barker Classification
Helps in assessing damage to heart, brain and kidneys.

Grades of HR	Fundus picture	Cardiorenal function
Grade 1 Mild	Mild to moderate narrowing or sclerosis of arteries	Normal
Grade 2 Moderate	Moderate to marked arteriolosclerosis and exaggeration of light reflex. Salus' sign	Satisfactory
Grade 3 High and sustained	Marked retinal arteriolar narrowing and focal constriction cotton wool exudate superficial hemorrhage. Gunn's sign and Bonnet's sign	Evidence of cardiorenal disease
Grade 4 Malignant	Grade 3 plus macular star and disk edema	Marked cardiorenal damage

Scheie's classification
Mainly based on arteriosclerosis:
- Grade 1:
  - Generalized arteriolar attenuation
  - Broadening of arteriolar light reflex
  - Concealment of vein at AV crossing.
- Grade 2:
  - Severe generalized and focal arteriolar constriction
  - Right angled deflection of veins—Salus' sign
- Grade 3:
  - Copper wiring of arterioles
  - Gunn's sign: Venous tapering on either side of crossing
  - Bonnet's sign: Banking of veins distal to AV crossings

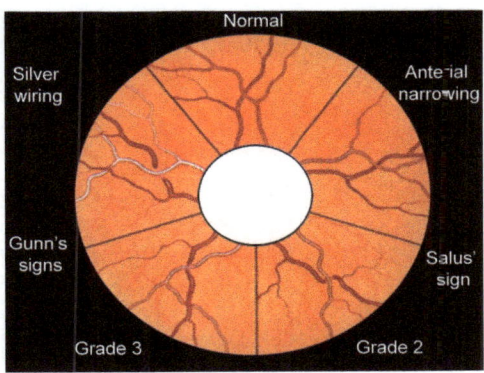

Fig. 13.20: Hypertensive retinopathy.

  - Flame-shaped hemorrhages
  - Cotton wool spots
  - Hard exudates
- Grade 4:
  - All changes in grade III with
  - Silver wiring of arterioles
  - Disk edema

Fundus Picture
- **Retinal changes:**
  - Arterial narrowing
  - Vascular leakage
  - Arteriosclerosis
- **Choroidal changes:**
  - Elschnig's spots
  - Siegrist streaks
  - Exudative RD.

Retinal Changes
- Arterial narrowing
  - Focal or generalized
  - Obstruction of precapillary arterioles
  - Cotton wool spots
- Vascular leakage:
  - Flame-shaped hemorrhages
  - Retinal edema
  - Macular star
  - Disk edema

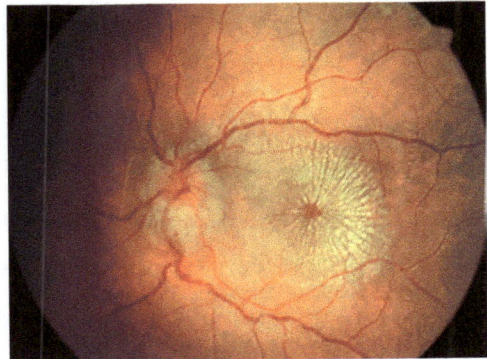

Fig. 13.21: Macular star.

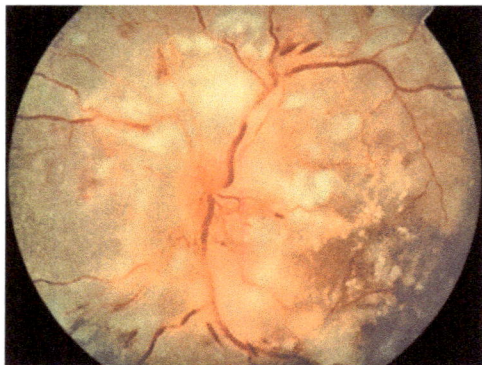

Fig. 13.22: Disk edema.

- Arteriosclerosis:
  - Thickening of vessel wall
  - Changes at AV crossing.

Grade 1: Generalized arteriolar attenuation,

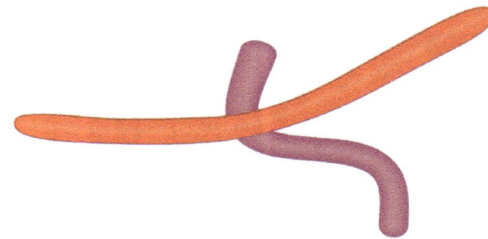

Fig. 13.23: Salus' sign—superficial artery deflects the course of underlying vein.

Grade 2: Broadening of arteriolar light reflex Deflection of vein at AV crossing – Salus' sign.

Salus' sign: Deflection in the course of the vein at arteriovenous crossings.

Grade 3:
- Copper wiring
  - Banking of veins distal to AV crossing—Bonnet's sign
  - Tapering of veins on either side of crossings—Gunn's sign.

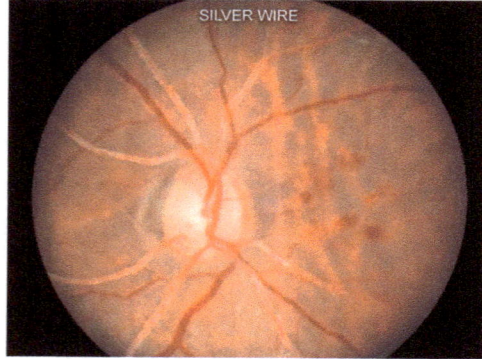

Fig. 13.24: Silver wiring of arterioles in grade 4 hypertensive retinopathy.

Grade 4:
- Grade 3 changes plus
- Silver wiring of arterioles.

Choroidal Changes

Rare: May occur due to acute hypertensive crisis in young adults.
- **Elschnig's spots:**
  - Focal choroidal infarcts
  - Small black spots surrounded by yellow halos
- **Siegrist's streaks:**
  - Due to fibrinoid necrosis seen in malignant hypertension
  - Seen as flecks arranged linearly along choroidal vessels
- Exudative retinal detachment seen in toxemia of pregnancy.

Complications of Hypertensive Retinopathy (HR)

- Retinal vein occlusion
- Retinal artery occlusion
- Retinal artery macroaneurysm
- Anterior ischemic optic neuropathy (AION)
- Ocular motor nerve palsy
- Aggravation of diabetic retinopathy.

Management of Hypertensive Retinopathy (HR)

Medical control of hypertension essential for good visual function and long-term survival of patients:
- BP to be lowered gradually
- General measures—weight control, sodium restriction, and exercise.

9. Describe the retinopathy of toxemia of pregnancy.
- Occurs in last trimester of pregnancy
- Consists of triad of hypertension, proteinuria and edema—preeclampsia
- Headache, vomiting, convulsion, eclampsia.

Fundus Picture

Three Stages:
  i. Stage of angiospasm
 ii. Stage of sclerosis of vessels
iii. Stage of retinopathy
  - Retinal changes run parallel with severity of hypertension.

Stage of Angiospasm
- Due to liberation of toxin
- Attenuation of retinal arteriole—starts in nasal periphery
- May become generalized due to spasm.

Stage of Sclerosis

Arteriovenous crossing signs occur:
- Salus' sign
- Gunn's sign
- Bonnet's sign.

Stage of Retinopathy
- Superficial and deep hemorrhages
- Retinal edema
- Exudative retinal detachment.

Complications
- Complete loss of vision
- Loss of life of mother and fetus.

Treatment

- Prevention—adequate antenatal care
- Control of high BP—rest, sedation and salt restriction
- Diuretics and antihypertensives.

Role of Ophthalmologist

- Diagnosis of early retinopathy
- Advised termination of pregnancy to avoid maternal mortality
- Prognosis—good for life and vision following termination of pregnancy.

10. What are the types of obstruction of retinal vessels?

- **Retinal artery occlusion:**
  - Central retinal artery occlusion
  - Branch retinal artery occlusion
  - Cilioretinal artery occlusion
- **Retinal vein occlusion:**
  - Central retinal vein occlusion (CRVO)
  - Branch retinal vein occlusion (BRVO)
  - Hemi-retinal vein occlusion.

11. Discuss the causes, clinical features, differential diagnosis and treatment of central retinal artery occlusion (CRAO).

Causes of CRAO

- Spasm of vessels
- Atherosclerosis
- Carotid embolism
- Cardiac embolism
- Giant cell arteritis
- Periarteritis.

Spasm of Vessels Occurs in Young

For example: Toxemia of pregnancy and quinine toxicity.

Atherosclerosis Related Thrombosis—80%

- Carotid artery atherosclerosis is the most common cause of CRAO
- Occurs at the level of lamina cribrosa
- Occurs in older age when they have hypertension.

Carotid Embolism

- Most common cause of branch retinal artery occlusion (BRAO).
- Cholesterol embolic (Hollenhorst plaques) located at arteriolar bifurcation—bright refractile golden to yellow orange crystals
- Fibrin-platelet emboli:
  - Dull gray elongated particles fill the lumen
  - Transient ischemic attacks
  - Amaurosis fugax
- Calcific emboli:
  - From atheromatous plaques
  - Often close to disk
  - May causes permanent occlusion of CRA or its branches.

Cardiac Embolism

The ophthalmic artery is the first branch of internal carotid artery. Hence embolic material from the heart and carotid arteries has a fairly direct route to the eye.

- 20% of retinal occlusion
- Calcification
- Vegetation
- Thrombus.

Giant Cell Arteritis

Periarteritis

- Connective tissue disorders

Symptoms: Painless sudden loss of vision

Signs: In complete block

- Amaurotic pupil
- Fundus: Attenuation of artery
- Appear extremely thin and thread like
- Veins: Usually normal
- *Cherry-red spot*:
  - Striking cherry-red spot at the macula
  - Retina becomes edematous and milky white
  - Choriocapillaris shine against white background of macula.

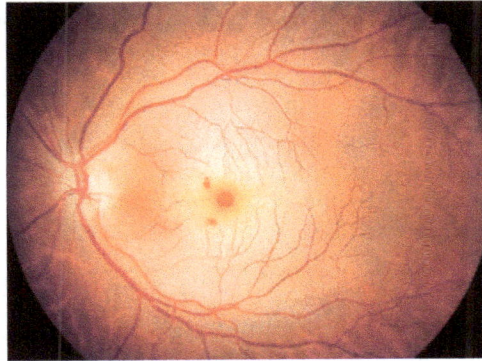

Fig. 13.25: Cherry-red spot.

Partial Occlusion of CRA

- Column of venous blood break into red beads
- Separated by clear interspaces which moves to and fro by gentle pressure on eyeball
  - Cattle truck appearance.

Cilioretinal Obstruction

- Cilioretinal artery present in 20% of population
- Arises from posterior ciliary artery circulation
- Supplies macula and papillomacular bundle.

Complications of CRAO

- Optic atrophy
- Rubeosis iridis.

Differential Diagnosis – CRAO

Sudden Painless Loss of Vision

- CRAO and CRVO
- Retinal detachment

- Vitreous hemorrhage
- Methyl alcohol poisoning
- Occipital lobe infarction
- Hysteria and malingering
- AION – nonarteritic type.

Causes of Cherry-red Spot

- CRAO
- Tay-Sachs disease
- Niemann-Pick disease
- Sandhoff's disease
- Gaucher's disease
- Quinine toxicity
- Berlin's edema
- Macular hole.

Treatment of CRAO

Ocular emergency—to be started within 90 minutes.
- Patient to lie flat
- Firm ocular massage—intermittent pressure for 15 minutes
- Sublingual isosorbide dinitrate—for dilatation
- Lowering of IOP—IV acetazolamide 500 mg followed by 20% mannitol
- Inhalation of carbogen (95% oxygen and 5% carbon dioxide mixture)
- Anterior chamber paracentesis
- IV streptokinase 7,50,000 units to disintegrate fibrin emboli along with IV methyl prednisolone 500 mg, to reduce allergy to streptokinase
- Retrobulbar (RB) injection of tolazoline 50 mg to decrease RB resistance to flow.

12. What are the types of retinal vein occlusions?

- Central retinal vein occlusion (CRVO)
- Branch retinal vein occlusion
- Hemiretinal vein occlusion.

13. Discuss the pathogenesis, clinical features, complication, and treatment of central retinal vein occlusion.

Pathogenesis

Atherosclerosis of retinal artery or arteriole important factor in CRVO and BRVO due to sharing of common adventitial sheath.

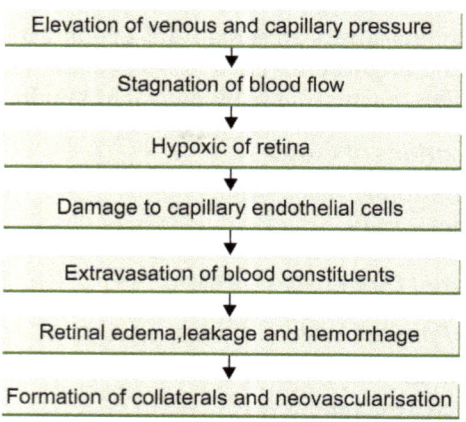

Thickness of artery compresses vein—precipitates CRVO or BRVO.

Risk Factors of CRVO

- Advancing age
- Systemic conditions
  - Hypertension, hyperlipidemia, diabetes
- Raised IOP
  - POAG
  - Ocular hypertension
- Inflammatory diseases
  - Sarcoidosis
  - Behcet's disease
- Hyperviscosity
  - Polycythemia, macroglobulinemia
- Acquired thrombophilic disorders
  - Hyperhomocysteinemia
- Inherited thrombophilic disorders
  - Increased level of clotting factors 7 and 11
  - Deficiencies of anticoagulants.

Types of CRVO

- Nonischemic
- Ischemic.

Features	Nonischemic CRVO	Ischemic CRVO
Incidence	70%	30%
Vision	> 6/60	< 6/60
Pupil	Relatively normal	RAPD
Hemorrhages	Dot and blot	Flame shaped
Cotton wool spots	Few	Numerous
Retina	Relatively normal	Edematous retina
Retinal nonperfusion	< 10 disk diopters	> 10 disk diopters
Risk for neovascularization	Low	High
Prognosis	Good	Bad

Complications

- Iris neovascularization
  - More common than NVD or NVE
- Neovascular glaucoma
- Tractional retinal detachment
- Vitreous hemorrhage
- Macular edema.

Treatment of CRVO

- Treat the underlying cause, manage IOP
- Intravitreal anti-VEGF
- Monthly follow up with gonioscopy during first 6 months after CRVO
- PRP for ischemic CRVO when 2 clock hours of neovascularization iris (NVI) or any angle NV is present.

14. Write short notes on branch retinal vein occlusion.

- Major branch vein occlusion
- Minor branch vein occlusion
- Peripheral branch vein occlusion.

Types of Branch Retinal Vein Occlusion

- Nonischemic
  - < 5 DD of capillary nonperfusion
- Ischemic
  - > 5 DD of capillary nonperfusion.

Features of Branch Retinal Vein Occlusion

- Flame-shaped and dot-blot hemorrhages
- Retinal edema
- Cotton wool spots.

Fluorescein Angiogram (FA)

- *Early phase:* Hypofluorescence due to blockage of choroidal fluorescence by hemorrhages
  - *Late phase:* Hyperfluorescence due to leakage.

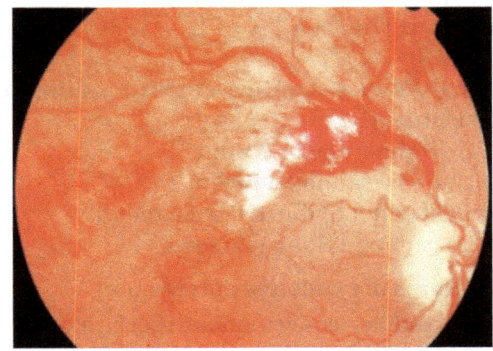

Fig. 13.26: Superotemporal branch retinal vein occlusion.

Prognosis

- Usually good
- Within 6 months, 50% of eyes develop collaterals and vision returns.

Complications

- Chronic macular edema
- Neovascularization:
  - NVD – 10%
  - NVE – 20–30%.

Treatment

- Macular edema and vision < 6/12 for 3 months
  - Grid laser photocoagulation
- Neovascularization—scatter laser
  - > 5DD of non-perfusion—PRP.

15. Write short notes on hemiretinal vein occlusion.

- Less common than CRVO or BRVO
- Involves occlusion of superior or inferior branch of CRVO
- Treatment—depends on severity of ischemia
- Similar to ischemic CRVO.

16. Discuss the pathogenesis, clinical features, differential diagnosis, and treatment of retinal detachment (RD).

Definition

Separation of sensory retina from retinal pigment epithelium by subretinal fluid (SRF).

Classification

- Rhegmatogenous
- Nonrhegmatogenous:
  - Tractional
  - Exudative.

Rhegmatogenous RD

- Occurs due to full thickness defect in sensory retina
- SRF from liquefied vitreous enters subretinal space
- Prevalence—1 in 10,000 eyes
- More common in myopia.

Tractional RD

Sensory retina pulled away from RPE by contracting vitreoretinal membrane.

Causes

- Proliferative diabetic retinopathy
- Retinopathy of prematurity
- Sickle-cell retinopathy
- Penetrating posterior segment trauma.

Exudative RD

- Fluid derived from choriocapillaris
- Gain access to subretinal space through damaged RPE.

Causes

- Choroidal tumors
- Exophytic retinoblastoma
- Harada's disease
- Toxemia of pregnancy
- Posterior scleritis
- Subretinal neovascularization.

Pathogenesis

Rhegmatogenous detachment.

Underlying mechanism:

- Retinal breaks
- Vitreous traction
- Retinal breaks occur in 5–10% of population
- 70% of breaks are located superiorly between 10 o'clock and 2 o'clock position.

Mechanism of Rhegmatogenous Detachment

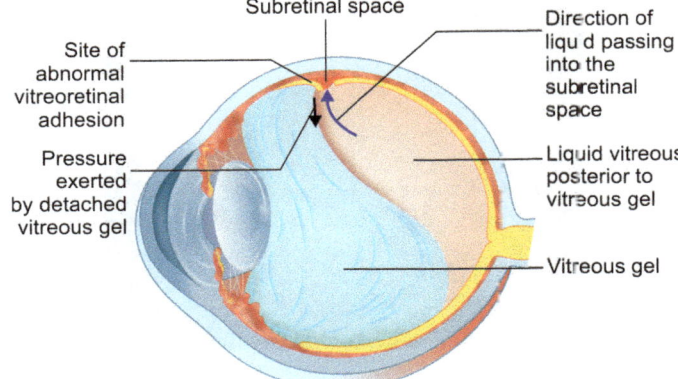

Fig. 13.27: Mechanism of rhegmatogenous retinal detachment.

- Liquefied vitreous
- Posterior vitreous detachment
- Retinal breaks
- Failure of RPE pump.

Tractional Detachment
- Vitreous traction tears the retina
- Formation of vitreous membrane
- Contraction of fibrous bands
- Bleeding induces fibroblastic proliferation
- Bands pull the retina
- Traction detachment sets in.

Exudative Detachment
- Causes—tumors of retina and inflammatory diseases
- Due to damage to RPE allowing fluid to leak into subretinal space.

Examination Techniques
- Direct ophthalmoscopy
- Indirect ophthalmoscopy
- Goldmann 3 mirror examination
- Slit-lamp examination with +78 D lens or +90 D lens
- B scan.

Clinical Features

Rhegmatogenous detachment.

Symptoms
- Variable
- Photopsia (seeing flashes of light)
- Metamorphopsia (seeing distorted images)
- Showers of black spots
- Cloudy vision.

Signs

Schaeffer's sign: Slit-lamp examination showing fine pigmented cells or tobacco dusting on anterior face of vitreous or in anterior chamber, with no previous eye disease, trauma, surgery or inflammation.

Diagnostic of retinal break:
- Detached retina presents as white or gray discoloration with folds, which oscillates on ocular movement.
- Retinal vessels crossing over detached retina look darker

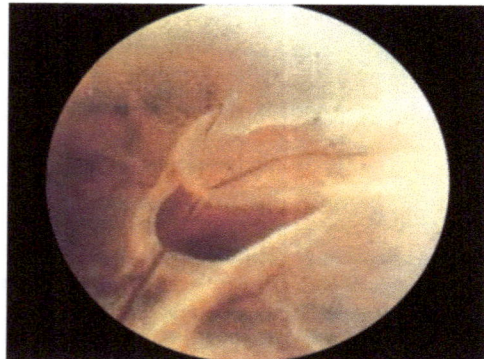

Fig. 13.28: Horseshoe tear.

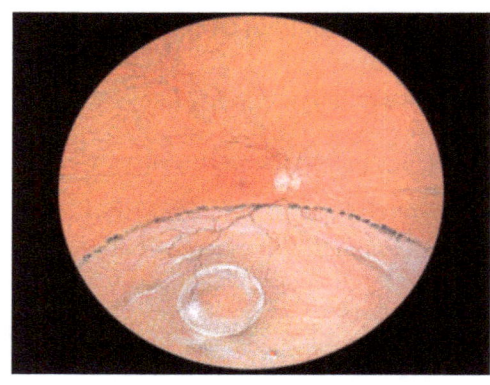

Fig. 13.29: Old retinal detachment.

Peripheral lesions require scleral indentation:
- Breaks will be seen
- Low IOP
- Visual fields—scotoma corresponding to area of detachment
- ERG—subnormal or absent
- B scan—reveals detachment

Shows marked pallor of the detached retina.
There is a subretinal vacuole seen.

Clinical features of exudative detachment
- Detached retina—convex smooth surface
- No retinal break
- Shifting of SRF on head movements
- Diminution of vision
- Black floaters
- No photopsia
- Fundus
  - Smooth convex gray discoloration
  - No retinal breaks
- Raised IOP if associated with tumors
- Visual fields—scotoma
- Transillumination—negative if due to tumors.

Clinical features of tractional detachment
- Smooth surface, usually taut, and immobile
- Concave towards the front of eye
- Usually limited to posterior fundus
- Breaks are usually absent.
  - To differentiate various types of RD see Table in Question no. 17.

Differential diagnosis
- Senile retinoschisis
- Choroidal detachment.

Senile retinoschisis

Separation at the level of Outer Plexiform Layer (In Congenital retinoschisis separation occurs at the nerve fibre layer). Common in lower temporal, bilateral smooth, thin convex elevation, immobile, and transparent inner retinal layer
- Sheathing of vessels
- No demarcation line
- Absolute field defect.

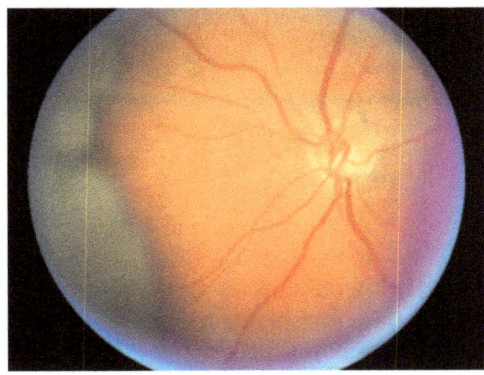

Fig. 13.30: Choroidal detachment.

Choroidal detachment

Separation between RPE and choroid due to fluid or blood in suprachoroidal space:
- Smooth, brown, dome shaped elevation, and bullous
- Very low IOP
- Ora serrata can be seen with scleral depression

Difference between retinal detachment and choroidal detachment.		
	Retinal detachment	*Choroidal detachment*
Color	Pale	Darker/normal color
Dome	Convex corrugated	Convex smooth
Breaks	Present	Absent
Ora serrata	Visible with indentation	Easily visible
Maximal extent	Anterior: Ora serrata Posterior: Unlimited	Anterior: Ciliary body Posterior: Vortex veins

Goals of Treatment

- Identify all retinal breaks
- Close all breaks
- Place scleral buckle to support all retina breaks
- Retinal tears should be flat on buckle.

Treatment of Rhegmatogenous RD

Rhegmatogenous detachment:
- Seal and support the break
- Sealing can be done by cryopexy, photocoagulation or diathermy
- Scleral buckle supports the break by reducing the vitreoretinal traction as well as apposing RPE to the sensory retina
- Retinal detachment with vitreoretinal traction or proliferative vitreoretinopathy require pars plana vitrectomy
- Prophylactic photocoagulation or cryopexy is recommended in high myopia with lattice degeneration or holes in ora serrata.

Treatment

- Scleral buckling
- Drainage of subretinal fluid
- Intravitreal injections
- Pneumatic retinopexy
- Pars plana vitrectomy.

Scleral Buckling

- It is a surgical technique for creating an inward indentation of the sclera
- Explant is the material directly sutured to the sclera to create a buckle.

Types of explants

- Radial explant—placed at right angles to the limbus
- Circumferential explant:
  - Segmental
  - Encircling

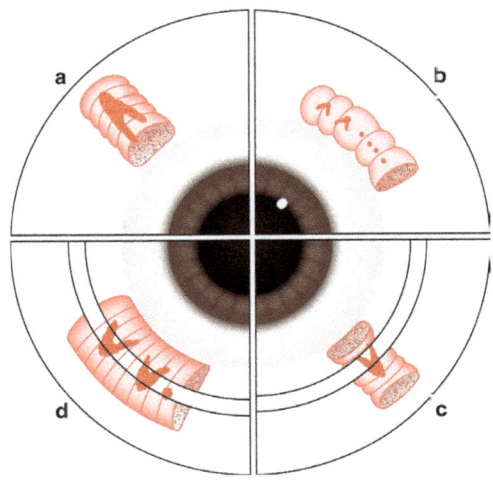

Fig. 13.31: Types of scleral buckling.

- Silicone sponges:
  - Hard and soft
  a. Radial sponge
  b. Circumferential sponge
  c. Encirclement with radial sponge
  d. Encirclement with solid silicone tyre.

Intravitreal Injections

- Air
- Saline
- Expanding gases
- Silicone oil
- Perfluorocarbons.

Pars Plana Vitrectomy

Indications
- Tractional RD involving fovea
- Selective rhegmatogenous RD with breaks which cannot be closed by conventional methods.

Treatment of Exudative Detachment

- May undergo spontaneous resolution following absorption of fluid
- Treatment of ocular inflammation or neoplasm.

Treatment of Tractional RD

- Tractional pull is relieved by segmentation or delamination
- The epiretinal membrane can be removed by peeling during pars plana vitrectomy with prophylactic encirclage.

17. Differentiate various types of retinal detachment.

Characteristics	Rhegmatogenous RD	Tractional RD	Exudative RD
History (ocular and systemic)	Photopsia, floaters, field defect, pseudophakia, myopia, blunt trauma	Diabetes, prematurity, penetrating trauma, venous occlusions	Malignant hypertension, eclampsia, renal failure
Retinal break	Seen	No primary break; may develop secondary break	No break
Extent of detachment	Extends to Ora	Frequently does not extend to Ora	Variable
Retinal mobility	Undulating folds	Taut retina, concave borders	Smooth elevated bullae
Configuration	Convex	Concave	Convex
Vitreous pigmentation	Present	Present in trauma	Absent
Vitreous changes	Posterior vitreous detachment	Vitreoretinal traction	Not present
Causes	Retinal break	Proliferative diabetic retinopathy, vasculitis, retinopathy of prematurity	Uveitis, choroidal melanoma or hemangioma VKH syndrome, retinoblastoma

18. Describe the inheritance, pathogenesis, clinical features, differential diagnosis, and treatment of retinitis pigmentosa.

Definition
Slow degenerative disease of retina particularly the rods. It is diffuse retinal dystrophy due to mutation of *Rhodopsine* gene.

Inheritance
- Sporadic—45%—No family history
- Autosomal dominance—25%—better prognosis
- Autosomal recessive—20% —associated with systemic syndromes
- X linked recessive—8%—worst prognosis.

Pathogenesis
- Retinal pigment epithelium proliferates and migrates into anterior retina
- Melanin deposits in and around retinal arterioles
- Bone spicules pattern of pigmentation
- Hyalinization of walls of arterioles.

Symptoms
- Night blindness
- Usually begins in 2nd decade of life
- Peripheral vision affected first.

Signs
- Usually bilateral and symmetrical fundus picture
- Diagnosis based on triad of:
  - Arteriolar attenuation
  - Pigmentary bone spicules
  - Waxy pallor of optic disk
  - Field defect:
    » Pigments are more prominent in mid periphery or around blood vessels
    » Results in ring like scotoma in the visual field
    » In advanced case only tubular vision presents
  - Delayed dark adaptation
  - ERG – reduced B wave
  - EOG – absence of light rise

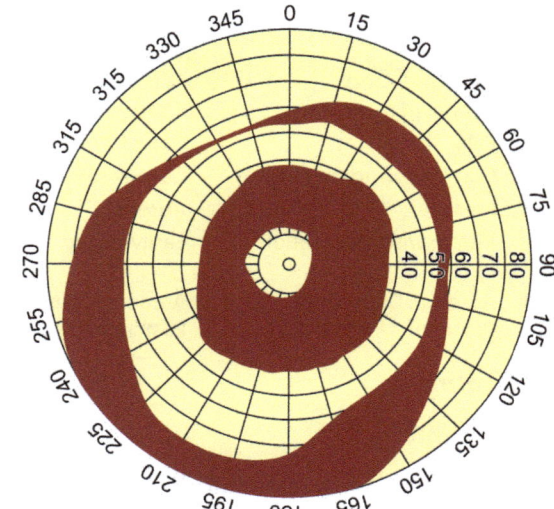

Fig. 13.32: Rings scotoma.

Differential Diagnosis
- Other causes of night blindness (Nyctalopia):
  - Congenital
  - Vitamin A deficiency
  - Extensive chorioretinitis
  - Gyrate atrophy—increased ornithine level in blood
  - Oguchi's disease—yellow metallic sheen of posterior pole
    » Returns to normal after dark adaptation
- Disorder mimicking fundus picture of RP:
  - End stage phenothiazine toxicity
  - End stage chloroquine retinopathy
  - Late stage of syphilis
  - Congenital rubella
  - Retinochoroidal atrophy
    » Pigmented paravenous type.

Types of RP
- Unilateral RP
- Sector RP
- Retinitis punctata albescence
- Retinitis pigmentosa sine pigmento
  - No visible pigment deposits.

Syndromes associated with RP
- Laurence-Moon-Bardet-Biedl syndrome
  - Obesity, hypogenitalism, mental retardation, polydactyly
- Usher's syndrome
  - Deafness and blindness
- Refsum syndrome - Increased phytanic acid level
  - Ataxia, deafness
- Bassen-Kornzweig syndrome
  - Abetalipoproteinemia, fat intolerance, diarrhea
- Kearns–Sayre syndrome
  - Ocular myopathy, heart block.

Treatment of RP
- Vitamin A oral 15,000 units daily
- Vitamin B6 for gyrate atrophy
- Restrict milk and leafy vegetable
  - In Refsum syndrome
- For associated macular edema
  - Grid laser photocoagulation
- Low vision aids
  - Near vision—hand and stand magnifier
  - Telescopic aid for distant vision
  - Closed circuit television
- Genetic counseling—avoid consanguineous marriage.
- Bionic eye—visual device to restore functional vision in blindness.

19. Write short notes on age-related macular degeneration (ARMD).

Definition
Age related bilateral nonhereditary degeneration of macula characterized by loss of central vision.

Prevalence
Most common cases of irreversible visual loss over 50 years of age.

Risk Factors
- Age > 50 years
- Hypermetropia
- Sunlight
- Smoking
- Malnutrition
- Cardiovascular diseases.

Types
- Atrophic or dry type—90%
  - Slowly progressive disease characterized by Drusen and geographical atrophy of retinal pigment epithelium (RPE)
- Exudative or wet type—10%
  - Rapidly progressive characterized by choroidal neovascularization (CNV) and subretinal scarring.

Pathogenesis
Normal aging produce histological changes in RPE, Bruch's membrane and choriocapillaries
- Thickening, hyalinization of Bruch's membrane, fine granular deposits beneath RPE
- *Drusen:* Deposition of hyaline material between RPE and Bruch's membrane. These are accumulation of secretions of undigested material from RPE into inner layer of Bruch's membrane.

Clinical Features
Dry ARMD: Mild-to-moderate loss of Vision over Several Months
- Loss of foveal reflex
- Focal hyper pigmentation of RPE
- Sharply circular areas in RPE atrophy-focal atrophy
- Drusen—yellowish-white spots
- Geographical atrophy
  - Amsler grid—shows central or paracentral scotoma
  - Fundus fluorescein angiography (FFA): Hyperfluorescence.

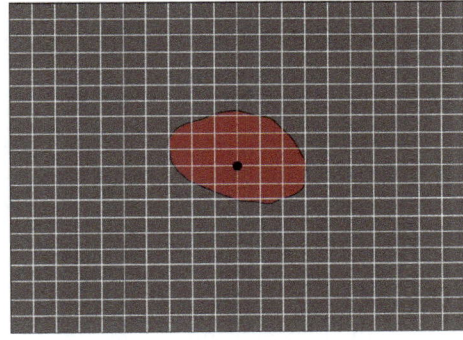

Fig. 13.33: Amsler grid.

Wet or Exudative ARMD
- Serous detachment of RPE
- Choroidal neovascular membrane (CNVM)
  - Appears as dirty gray membrane beneath retina—leaks blood and causes hemorrhagic detachment
  - End stage fibrovascular scar.

Clinical Features of Wet ARMD
- Symptoms:
  - Metamorphopsia
  - Distortion of lines or edges
  - Severe loss of vision
- Amsler grid—central or paracentral scotoma
- Fundus fluorescein angiography—Leakage into subretinal space
- Indocyanine green angiography—Visualizes CNVM better.

Treatment of ARMD
- Medical:
  - Antioxidants

- Lutein and zeaxanthin
- Oral zinc
- Low vision aids
- Photocoagulation
- Extrafoveal CNV: Argon blue green laser
- Subfoveal classic CNV: Photodynamic therapy
- Occult CNV: Transpupillary thermotherapy.

Photodynamic therapy (PDT)
- Nonthermal laser
- Applied to photosensitized CNV (by verteporfin) to produce photochemical reaction- damage to endothelium and causes vessel thrombosis
- Anti-vascular endothelial growth factor injection (Macugen, Avastin, Lucentis).

20. Write short notes on central serous retinopathy (CSR) or central serous chorioretinopathy (CSCR).

Definition
Sporadic, self-limited disease:
- Characterized by macular edema occurring in young adult males or middle aged
- Usually unilateral with history of emotional stress
- Common in type A personality
- Use of vasoconstrictive agents
- Age group 20–50 years.

Pathogenesis
- Focal disease of RPE
- Disruption of outer blood retinal barrier
- Fluid leaks from choriocapillaries through defect in RPE into subretinal space.

Symptoms of CSR
- Sudden onset of blurred vision in one eye
- Relative positive scotoma
- Micropsia and metamorphopsia.

Signs of CSR
- Vision reduced up to 6/18
- Vision can be improved by plus lenses
- Abnormal photostress test
- Fundus picture: Shallow round or oval elevation of sensory retina at posterior pole outlined by glistening reflex.

Investigations
- Amsler grid: Small central scotoma
- Slit-lamp biomicroscopy with +78 D or +90 D lens
- *Fundus fluorescein angiography of CSR:* Two patterns may be seen.
  i. **Smokestack appearance**:
     - Small hyperfluorescent spot appears.
     - Later it ascends vertically like smokestack
     - Then spreads laterally to form mushroom or umbrella configuration
  ii. **Ink-blot appearance:**
     - Hyperfluorescent spot increases in size

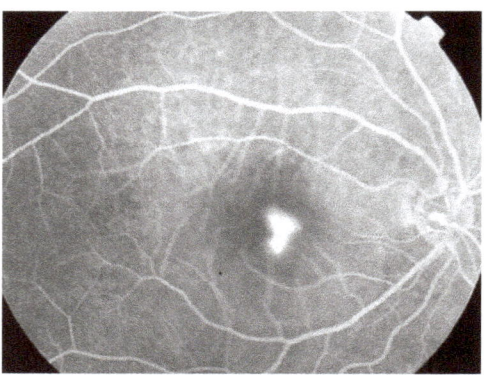

Fig. 13.34: Fundus fluorescein angiography—smokestack pattern in central serous retinopathy.

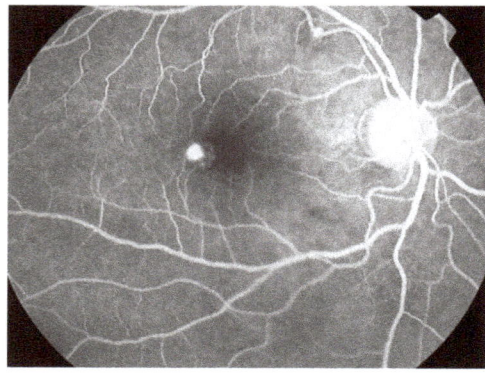

Fig. 13.35: Fundus fluorescein angiography—ink-blot pattern in central serous retinopathy.

Differential Diagnosis of CSR
- ARMD
- Optic pit
- Macular detachment
- Choroidal tumor
- Pigment epithelial detachment

Treatment of CSR
- Spontaneous resolution in 80% of cases within 1–6 months
- Potassium sparing diuretic- Eplerenone 25 mg b.d. for 4 weeks
- Ketaconazole 200 mg b.d. for 4 weeks

If Tuberculosis etiology is suspected, Rifampicin 600 mg o.d. for 4 weeks
- Laser photocoagulation—indicated in:
  - Persistence beyond 4–6 months
  - Recurrence
  - Visual defect in the other eye due to previous episode
- Intravitreal anti-VEGF for persistent CSR.

21. Write short notes on cystoid macular edema (CME).

Definition
Accumulation of fluid in outer plexiform and inner nuclear layers of retina centered about the foveola and the formation of fluid-filled cyst like changes.

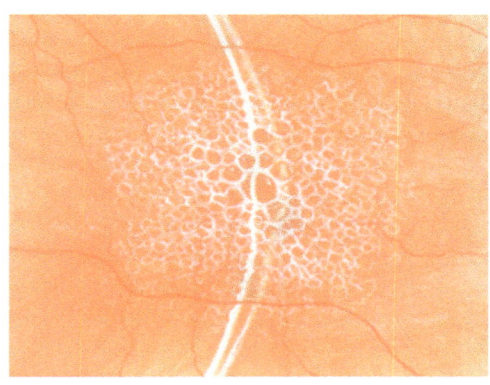

Fig. 13.36: Slit-lamp and +90 D lens examination showing multiple cystoid areas in cystoid macular edema.

Etiology of CME

- Diabetes
- Epinephrine
- Pars planitis
- Retinitis pigmentosa
- Irvine-Gass syndrome
- Venous occlusion
- Prostaglandin E2
- Nicotinic acid maculopathy
- UV radiation
- Phototoxicity from operating microscope.

Pathogenesis

- Disruption of inner blood-retinal barrier
- Abnormal perifoveal retinal capillary permeability.

Clinical Features

- Loss of foveal depression
- Thickening of retina
- Multiple cystoid areas in the sensory retina
- Yellow spot at foveola may be seen.
- Better seen with slit lamp and +90 D lens.

Investigations

- FFA—flower petal appearance due to accumulation of dye in microcystic spaces.
- Optical coherence tomography – cystic intraretinal spaces
    - Fundus picture of CME
    - Showing increasing leakage in FFA.

Treatment

- Depends on etiology
- Focal laser
- Topical steroids and NSAID
- Oral acetazolamide
- Sub-Tenon's steroid injection
- Preoperative use of anti-inflammatory agents.

22. What is photoretinitis?

It is also called solar retinopathy and eclipse blindness. It refers to retinal injury induced by direct or indirect sun viewing. It can also occur after exposure to the flash of short circuiting of electric current. The lesion is caused by infrared rays from sun which produces thermal damage on retinal pigment epithelium.

Symptoms

- Positive scotoma
- An afterimage which persists for a long time.
- Metamorphopsia—objects appear wavy and distorted.

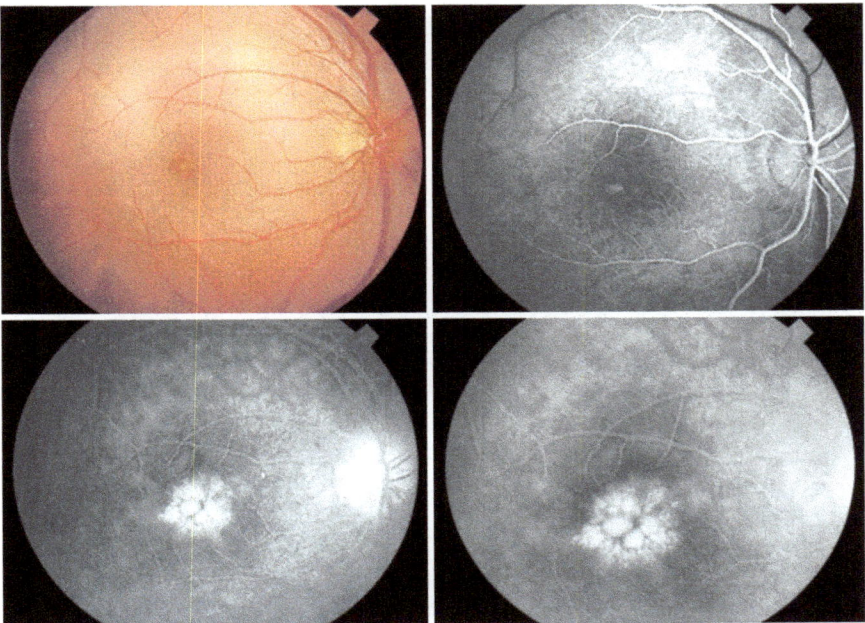

Fig. 13.37: Showing increased leakage in fundus fluorescein angiography to flower petal appearance.

Signs

Ophthalmoscopically, it appears as a bean or kidney-shaped pigmented spot with yellowish-white center in the foveal region. In worst cases, macular hole may appear.

Treatment

There is no effective treatment. Eclipse viewing is to be discouraged unless they wear protective glasses which absorb ultraviolet and infrared rays.

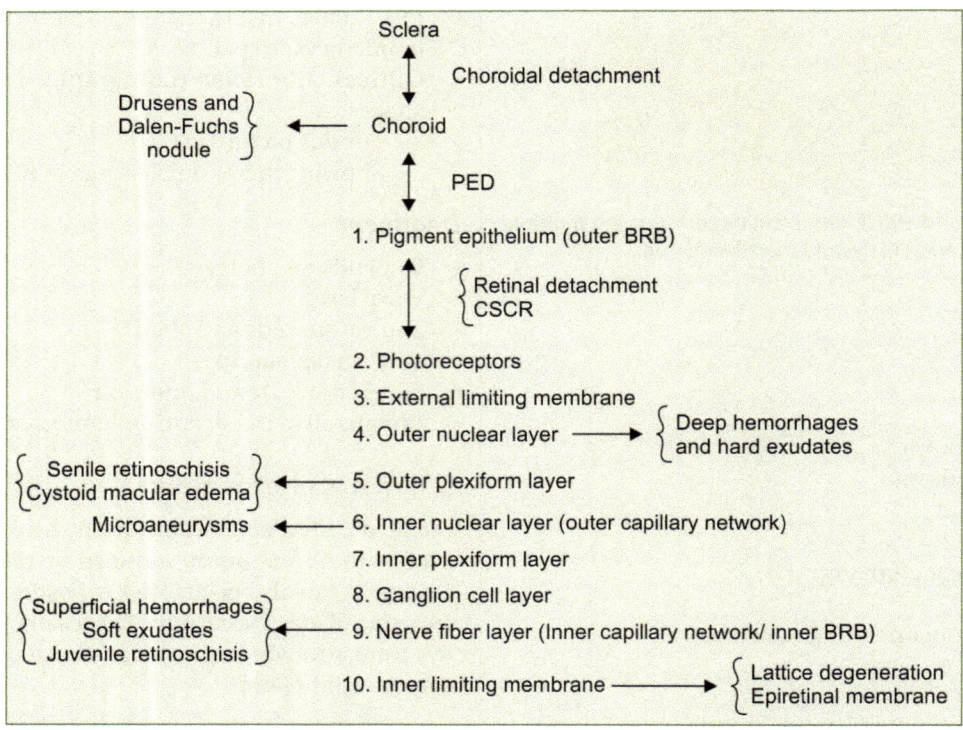

Fig. 13.38: Levels of lesions and corresponding diseases.

(BRB: blood retinal barrier; PED: pigment epithelial detachment; CSCR: central serous chorioretinopathy)

14. Intraocular Tumors

1. Classify intraocular tumors.

- Iris:
  - Malignant melanoma of iris
  - Nevus of the iris.
- Ciliary body:
  - Malignant melanoma of ciliary body.
- Choroid:
  - Nevus
  - Melanocytoma
  - Hemangioma
  - Malignant melanoma.
- Retina:
  - Retinoblastoma.

2. Discuss the genetics, pathology, clinical features, differential diagnosis, and management of retinoblastoma.

Retinoblastoma is a malignant transformation of primitive retinal cells before final differentiation. It is also called glioma of retina. It is usually present before 3 years of age.

- Most common intraocular malignancy of childhood
- Incidence 2/3rd before 2 years of age
- No racial predisposition
- Higher incidence in males
- One in 20,000 live births
- Unilateral tumor presents within one year
- Bilateral: Between 2 years and 3 years.

Genetics

- 30–40% bilateral
- Unilateral: Somatic mutation
- Bilateral: Genetically determined by tumor suppressor gene
- Associated with deletion of q14 band of chromosome 13
- 2/3rd: Sporadic
- 1/3rd: Heritable
- Bilateral with affected parents: 45%
- Chance of siblings being affected without affected parents—5% chance of siblings being affected
- Unilateral with normal parents is < 1% chance in siblings.

Origin

- Tumor arises from premature cells of photoreceptors
- Usually multicentric origin.

Histopathology

There are two types:
 i. Differentiated
 ii. Undifferentiated.

Differentiated Retinoblastoma

- *Polygonal cells with darkly staining nuclei*
- *Scanty cytoplasm*
- Flexner-Wintersteiner rosettes:
  - Cells arranged in circular manner around empty space
- Homer-Wright rosettes:
  - Cells arranged in circles. Central space contains filaments
  - Lumen filled with eosinophilic material
  - Also seen in neuroblastoma or cerebellar medulloblastoma.
- Fleurettes:
  - Composed of rod and cone inner segments and represent retinal differentiation.

Undifferentiated Retinoblastoma

- Consists of anaplastic cells. Arranged in sheets.
- Around lumen of blood vessels—*Pseudorosette*
- Mitotic figures are numerous. Cells necrosis is widespread.

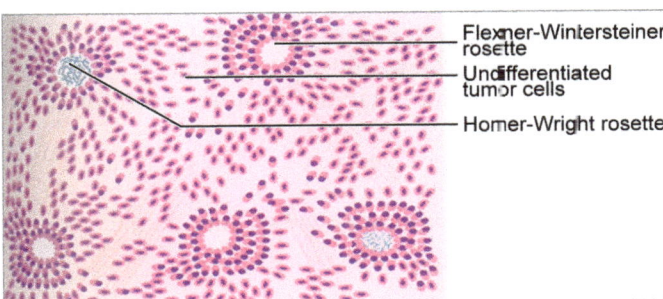

Fig. 14.1: Calcification made out in X-ray and ultrasonography.

Clinical Picture

There are four stages:
 I. Quiescent stage
 II. Glaucomatous stage
 III. Extraocular extension
 IV. Distant metastasis.

Stage I: Quiescent stage
- 6 months to 1 year
- Leukocoria: Amaurotic cat's eye
- Squint: Usually convergent
- Defective vision
- Rarely, child is old enough, he/she may complain.

Ophthalmoscopic Features
- Endophytum:
  - Grows into retina. Well circumscribed polypoid mass
  - Blood vessels and hemorrhage over the mass.
- Exophytum:
  - Grows outwards. Separates retina from choroid
  - Resembles exudative detachment
  - With ultrasonography, it can be differentiated from exudative detachment.

Stage II: Glaucomatous stage
- Quiescent stage left untreated
- Pain, redness, watery.

Signs:
- Eyeball enlarged, proptosis
- Intraocular pressure (IOP) raised, cornea hazy
- Resembles acute uveitis
- Pseudohypopyon/hyphema.

Stage III: Extraocular extension
- Tumor comes out of eyeball by bursting sclera
- Extraocular tissues involved. Rapid fungation
- Marked proptosis.

Stage IV: Distant metastasis
- Lymphatic spread:
  - Preauricular lymph nodes and neighboring lymph nodes.
- Direct extension:
  - Optic nerve: Brain.
- Bloodstream:
  - Cranial bones: Other bones
  - Other organs: Liver, lungs, etc.

International Classification
(Based on tumor size, location, and seeding)
- Group A—up to 3 mm in size
- Group B—> 3 mm, macular location subretinal fluid surrounding it
- Group C—with localized seeds
- Group D—with diffused seeds
- Group E—massive tumor needing enucleation.

Differential Diagnosis

Leukocoria

Leukocoria means whitish reflex in the pupillary area. It is also referred to as 'pseudoglioma' (see Miscellaneous chapter).

	Retinoblastoma	Pseudoglioma
IOP	Raised	Decreased or normal
Eyeball size	Increased or normal	Decreased
X-ray findings	Enlarged optic foramen Calcification	Normal optic foramen No calcification
Progression	Progressive	Usually nonprogressive

Causes of leukocoria
- Retinopathy of prematurity (retrolental fibroplasia)
- Persistent hyperplastic primary vitreous
- Cyclitic membrane
- Endophthalmitis
- Exudative retinopathy of coats
- Coloboma of choroid
- Congenital cataract.

Retinopathy of prematurity
It is a bilateral proliferative retinopathy of premature (<32 weeks of gestation) baby with low birth weight (<1,500 g) with history of prolonged exposure to oxygen.

Stages		
Stage 1	Flat demarcation line separating vascular and avascular retina	No treatment required. Only observation
Stage 2	Ridged demarcation line	No treatment required. Only observation
Stage 3	Fibrovascular proliferation	Laser photocoagulation or cryotherapy
Stage 4	Subtotal retinal detachment	Surgery
Stage 5	Total retinal detachment	Surgery

Persistent hyperplastic primary vitreous (See Q. 6, Page 99 of Chapter 12)
- It is a development disorder of the vitreous
- Usually unilateral
- Associated with microphthalmos.

Cyclitic membrane
- Fibrosis of plastic exudates behind the lens
- Seen in acute plastic iridocyclitis
- Coagulation of exudates on ciliary processes destroys its function
- Usually due to toxocariasis.

Endophthalmitis
Inflammation of internal structure of the eye, viz. choroid, retina and vitreous.

Exudative retinopathy of coats
This is an anomaly of retinal and optic nerve vasculature resulting in peripheral retinal aneurysm and massive subretinal exudation.

Coloboma of choroid
- It is a congenital anomaly due to incomplete closure of embryonic fissure
- Usually located inferonasally.

Congenital cataract
- Unilateral or bilateral opacity in the lens.

Diagnosis
- Examination under anesthesia
  - Fundus examination
  - Corneal diameter
  - IOP.
- Plain X-ray
  - Calcification: 75% of cases.

- Lactic dehydrogenase enzyme
  - Level is increased in aqueous humor.
- Ultrasonography
  - B-scan.
- CT scan
  - Optic nerve extension
  - Orbit spread
  - Central nervous system (CNS) spread.

Treatment
- Focal therapy
  - Argon laser photocoagulation for tumors < 3 mm.
    » Cryotherapy for anterior tumors.
  - Transpupillary thermotherapy-large spot diode laser-normal tissue spared.
- Local therapy
  - Radiation
    Plaque brachytherapy:
    » Too large for focal therapy
    » Away from disc or macula
    External beam radiotherapy:
    » Extensive vitreous seeding.
  - Enucleation:
    » Large unilateral tumor occupying more than half of globe
    » 10-15 mm optic nerve to be cut to test intracranial spread.
- Systemic chemotherapy
  - For bilateral tumor: Etoposide, vincristine and carboplatin
  - In unilateral tumor: To reduce size of tumor and later treated with focal therapy.

If optic nerve is involved
- After enucleation:
  - Radiotherapy—5,000 rads—applied to orbital apex
  - And periodical review to look for any recurrence.
- Palliative therapy
  - Is to be given for:
    » Retinablastoma with orbital extension,
    » Intracranial extension, distant metastasis.
  - Palliative therapy is a combination of:
    » Chemotherapy
    » Debulking of orbit or orbital exenteration
    » External beam radiotherapy (EBRT).

3. Discuss the types, pathology, clinical features, differential diagnosis, and treatment of malignant melanoma of the choroid.

Introduction
Incidence: 85% among uveal melanomas.
Age: 40–60 years.
Sex: Both sexes equally.
Race: Common in whites.
Site: Temporal half of choroid.

Types
- Circumscribe type
- Diffuse type.

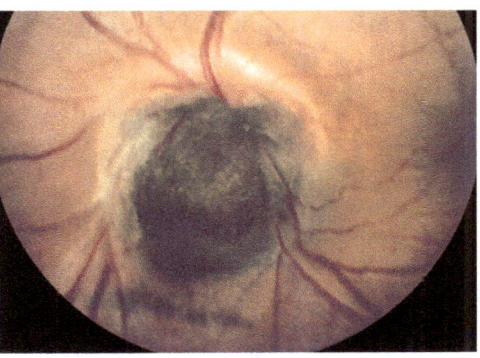

Fig. 14.2: Slaty-gray pigmentation in the retina.

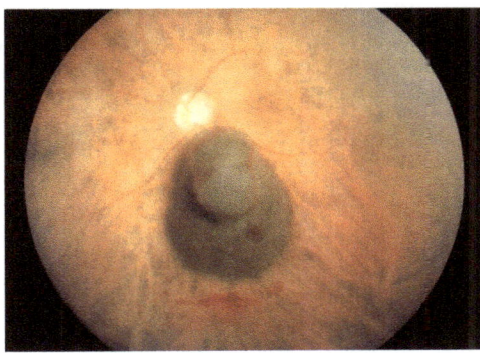

Fig. 14.3: Circumscribed malignant melanoma of choroid.

Circumscribe Type
- Always primary
- Single, unilateral—pigmented
- But metastasis from melanotic growth—unpigmented.

Diffuse Type
- Slaty-gray pigmentation in the retina
- Circumscribed malignant melanoma of choroid.

Pathology
Callender's classification (histological classification)
- Spindle cell melanoma
- Epithelioid cell melanoma
- Mixed cell melanoma
- Necrotic melanoma.

Clinical Features
- Mostly symptom free onset
- Visual impairment appears with involvement of macula/ with extension of retina detachment.

Stages of Tumor
- Quiescent
- Glaucomatous
- Stage of extraocular extension
- Stage of metastasis.

Quiescent Stage
- Tumor arises from outer layer of choroid
- Lens shaped mass pushing the retina over it
- Orange patches appear in RPE due to lipofuscin accumulation

- Becomes collar button/mushroom shaped when membrane of Bruch is ruptured
- Causes retinal detachment around tumor masses, even though the retina remains in contact with it.

Glaucomatous Stage

- Severe pain, visual deterioration due to increased IOP
- Secondary glaucoma due to:
  - Compression of vortex veins
  - Blockage of drainage channel
  - Direct invasion of anterior chamber
  - Obstruction of angle of AC by melanin pigment following tumor necrosis.

Stage of Extraocular Extension

- Spread through scleral emissary channel to involve bulbar surface of orbit
- Direct invasion of sclera/retina.

Stage of metastasis

- Hematogenous spread
- Other distant organs involved
- Mainly liver.

Differential Diagnosis

- Benign melanoma
- Hemangioma of choroid
- Rhegmatogenous detachment of retina
- Choroidal detachment
- Parasitic cyst of choroid
- Old choroidal hemorrhage.

Diagnosis

- Indirect ophthalmoscopy
- Slit lamp biomicroscopy with fundus contact lens
- Transillumination test
- Fluorescein angiography
- Radioactive phosphate (32p) uptake
- B-scan USG used when media is hazy and to exclude rhegmatogenous retinal detachment.

Prognosis

- **Good prognosis:** Spindle cell melanoma (81%, 10 years survival)
- **Poor prognosis:** Epithelial cell, mixed cell necrotic and diffuse types (<40% 10 years survival).

Treatment

- **Conservative:** For small melanomas.
- **Enucleation:** For large tumor with visual impairment.
- **Photocoagulation:** Tumors < 10 mm width, < 3 mm elevation

Tumors not located near foveola/subretinal fluid.

- **Irradiation:** Radioactive plaques—cobalt-60/ruthenium-106
- **Local resection:** For peripherally located tumors.
- **Cryotherapy (−60°C):** Done as primary procedure/secondary to photocoagulation.
- **Palliative:** Chemotherapy and radiotherapy for systemic metastasis.

4. Write short notes on exenteration.

This is a surgical procedure in which total excision of the orbital contents (including eyeball, extraocular muscles, fat, and periorbita) and the eyelids is done to remove a malignant growth that has advanced so much that it cannot be treated by irradiation or conservative surgical procedures.

Indications for Exenteration

- Extraocular extension of retinoblastoma, malignant melanoma.
- Squamous cell carcinoma of the eyelids involving bony orbit.

CHAPTER 15

Lids

1. What are the layers of eyelids?

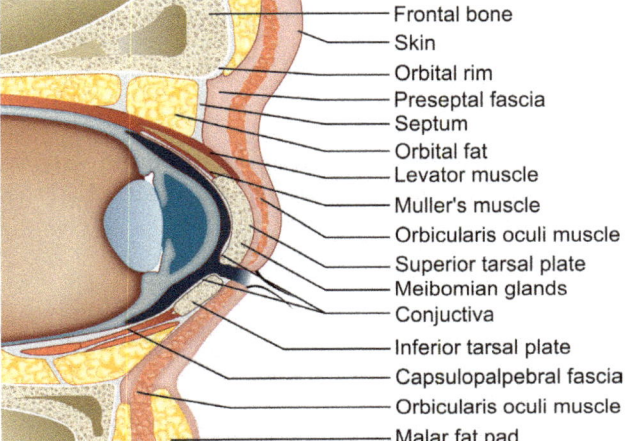

Fig. 15.1: Cross section of lids: From the front to back.

- Cutaneous layer (skin)
- Areolar layer (loose areolar tissue)
- Muscular layer (orbicularis oculi)
- Submuscular areolar tissue
- Fibrous layer (tarsal plate)
- Layer of smooth muscle (Muller's muscle)
- Conjunctival layer (mucous layer)
  - Gray line separates the fibrous layer from the muscular layer.

2. Write short notes on blepharitis.

Chronic inflammation of lid margin.

Types
- Squamous
- Ulcerative
- Posterior blepharitis or meibomitis
- Parasitic blepharitis—due to *Demodex folliculorum* and phthiriasis palpebrarum.

Squamous Blepharitis
- Due to seborrheic dermatitis
- Usually associated with dandruff of the scalp
- White colored scales accumulate among lashes
- Eyelashes fall out but are replaced without distortion
- On removal of scales, the underlying surface is red.

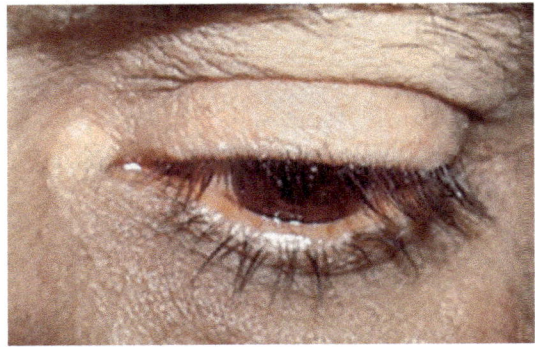

Fig. 15.2: Squamous blepharitis.

Ulcerative Blepharitis
- Yellow scales glue the lashes together
- Hyperemia, telangiectasia and scaling
- On removing of the crusts, small ulcers are seen around the base of the lashes. These ulcers bleed. Lashes fall and replaced by misdirected ones
- Caused by *Staphylococcus aureus* and *epidermidis*
- Secondary changes caused by hypersensitivity to *Staphylococcus* exotoxins are:
  - Mild papillary conjunctivitis
  - Marginal keratitis.

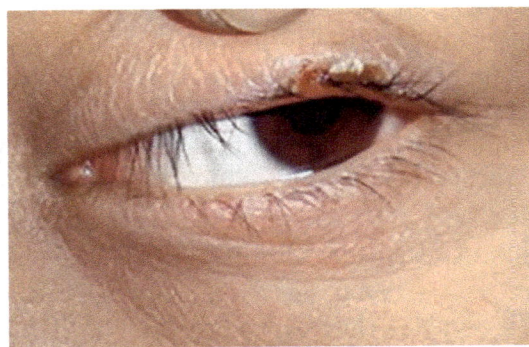

Fig. 15.3: Ulcerative blepharitis.

Symptoms
- Itching
- Redness
- Soreness
- Lacrimation

- Mild photophobia
- Lid crusting.

Sequela
- Trichiasis
- Tylosis (thickening of lid margin)
- Madarosis (loss of eyelashes)
- Poliosis (whitening of eyelashes)
- Ectropion
- Stye
  - Usually secondary to poor ocular hygiene, frequent rubbing of eyes, exposure to smoke and pollutants and asthenopia.

Differences between squamous and ulcerative blepharitis.		
Features	Squamous	Ulcerative
Etiology	Seborrhea	*Staphylococcus*
Deposits on eyelashes	Shiny waxy	Brittle scales/ulcers
Removal of deposits leaves	Hyperemic zone	Bleeding ulcers
Hair follicles	Not destroyed	Destroyed
Meibomian secretion	Vicarious	Normal
Eyelashes	Normal	Trichiasis, madarosis and poliosis
Lid margin may present	Chalazion	Stye
Conjunctiva	Mild conjunctivitis	Severe conjunctivitis
Dryness	Absent	Present
Corneal complications Punctate epithelial erosions Marginal ulcers	May be seen/absent	Commonly seen/present

Treatment

Local
- Removal of scales, crusts and diseased lashes
- Cleaning lid margin with 3% $NaHCO_3$, betadine, or baby shampoo and artificial tears.

Specific: Antibiotic eye ointment, betadine lotion applied for 2–3 weeks.
General: Improvement of general health and personal hygiene.
Dandruff of scalp: Selenium sulfide 2.5% shampoo twice weekly.

Posterior Blepharitis

Systemic tetracycline or doxycycline or erythromycin and antibiotic steroid eye ointment at the lid margin.
- Parasitic blepharitis—removal of nits by forceps and antibiotic ointment to the lid margin.
- Delousing of patient and family members.

3. Write short notes on hordeolum externum (stye).

Acute suppurative inflammation of Zeis or Moll's glands.

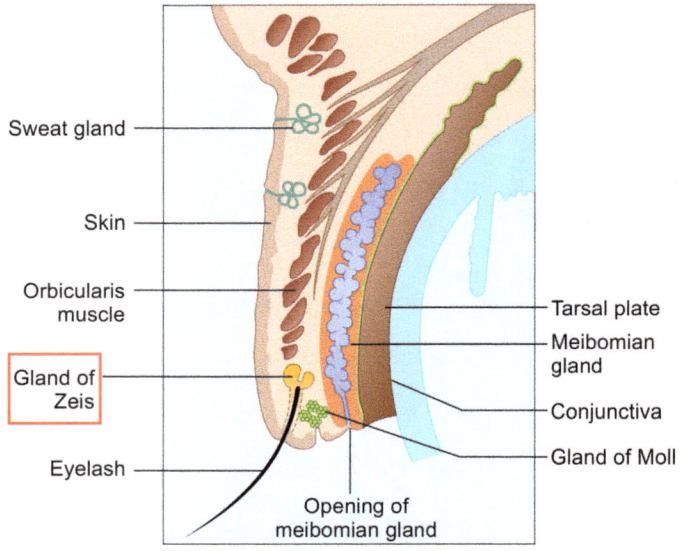

Fig. 15.4: Zeis gland.

Etiology

Due to staphylococcal infection associated with boils, acne, common in children and young adults. Also seen in immunocompromised person.

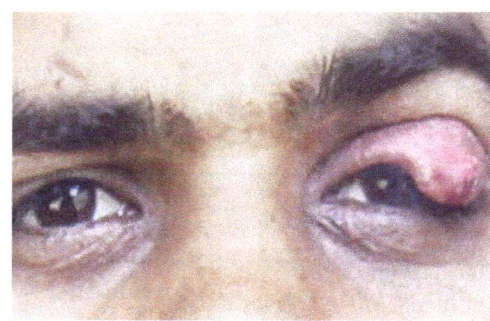

Fig. 15.5: Stye.

Symptoms

Acute pain along the lid margin.

Signs

Tender, hard swelling seen near lid margin. An abscess may form pointing near the base of lashes. The pain subsides if it gets ruptured. There are two stages:
- Stage of cellulitis
- Stage of abscess.

Treatment

Hot fomentation in early stage:
- Systemic—broad spectrum antibiotic
- Analgesics and anti-inflammatory drugs
- Removal of pus by pulling or epilating the involved lash or incision and drainage
- In the case of recurrent stye, diabetes and refractive errors have to be ruled out.

4. Write short notes on chalazion.

Chronic granulomatous inflammation of the meibomian gland.

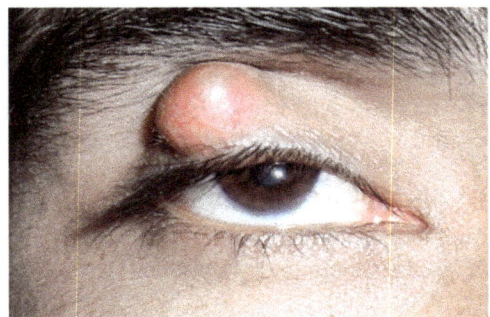

Fig. 15.6: Chalazion (tarsal or meibomian cyst).

Etiology

Due to chronic irritation caused by an organism of low virulence:
- Small, nontender, hard swelling in the lid, slightly away from the lid margin
- Cosmetic problem
- May cause astigmatism against rule due to pressure on the cornea.

Sequela

- Spontaneous resolution
- Contents may extrude through conjunctiva to resemble fungating mass
- Calcification
- Meibomian cell carcinoma
- May get a secondary infection and form hordeolum internum
- A marginal chalazion occurs in ducts of the meibomian gland. The granulation tissue projects as a reddish gray nodule on the intermarginal strip.

Differential Diagnosis

Features	Hordeolum externum	Hordeolum internum	Chalazion
Affected gland	Zeiss gland	Meibomian gland	Meibomian gland
Pathology	Suppurative inflammation	Suppurative inflammation	Granulomatous inflammation
Pain	Present	Severe pain	Painless
Signs	Localized tender swelling near lid margin, pus pointing on the base of an eyelash	Yellowish point seen on the palpebral conjunctiva on everting the lid	Nontender swelling, away from lid margin, purplish discoloration seen on palpebral conjunctiva corresponding to swelling
Treatment	Hot fomentation, systemic, local antibiotic eye ointment and analgesics, removal of affected eyelash, incision and drainage of abscess through horizontal incision at the lid margin	Systemic and local antibiotic eye ointment, analgesics, vertical incision and curettage through palpebral conjunctiva	If small intralesional injection of triamcinolone. Vertical incision and curettage through palpebral conjunctiva

Treatment

- Incision and curettage: The lid is everted and a vertical incision is made with 11 blade and mucoid material scooped out and the cavity curetted. A vertical incision is made to avoid damage to adjacent meibomian glands.
- Intralesional injection of triamcinolone may help in smaller chalazion.

5. Write short notes on hordeolum internum.

Acute suppurative inflammation of the meibomian gland
- Occurs due to secondary infection of chalazion
- Symptoms are more than in stye because the gland is larger and is embedded deeply in dense fibrous tissue.

Treatment

Broad-spectrum antibiotics and anti-inflammatory drugs to control pain. Latter incision and curettage as for chalazion.

6. What is molluscum contagiosum?

It is a viral infection of the lids, commonly affecting children. It is caused by a poxvirus.

Clinical Features

They are multiple, pale, waxy, umbilicated swellings around the lid margin.

Complications

Chronic follicular conjunctivitis and superficial keratitis.

Treatment

They should be incised and expressed and the interior touched with 5% povidone-iodine or pure carbolic acid.

7. Write short notes on trichiasis.

Etiology

- Stage IV trachoma
- Spastic entropion in an elderly person
- Tight bandaging
- Ulcerative blepharitis
- Scars of lid.

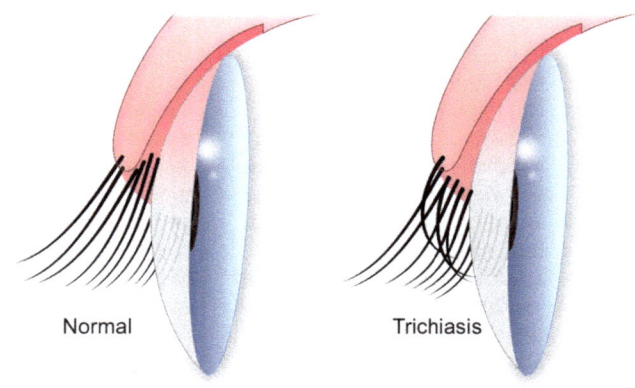

Fig. 15.7: Eyelashes are misdirected backwards and rub against the cornea.

Symptoms
- Foreign body sensation and photophobia
- Redness of conjunctiva and lacrimation.

Signs
- Misdirected cilia touching the cornea
- Blepharospasm and photophobia if the cornea is involved
- Superficial corneal opacities.

Complications
- Chronic conjunctivitis
- Recurrent corneal abrasions
- Non-healing corneal ulcer.

Treatment
- If single or few cilia are involved, epilation or electrolysis at the root of a hair follicle
- When many cilia are misdirected, surgical correction similar to cicatricial entropion is advised.

8. Write short notes on entropion.

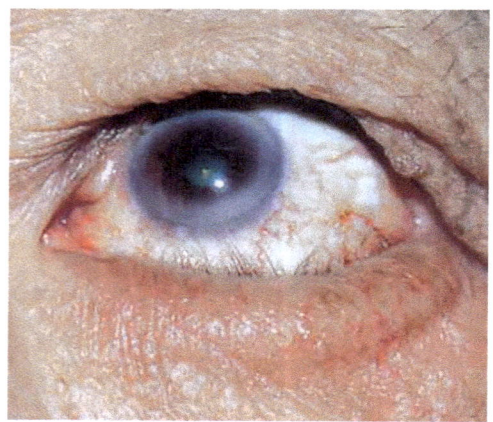

Fig. 15.8: Entropion (lid margin rolls inwards).

Types
- Senile or involutional: Affects only lower lid
- Spastic: Due to spasm of orbicularis oculi of the lower lid due to tight bandaging. Occurs in the lower lid of old people
- Cicatricial: Due to the contraction of palpebral conjunctiva involves both lids. It occurs in trachoma stage IV, ulcerative blepharitis, burns, Stevens-Johnson syndrome, diphtheritic membranous conjunctivitis and pemphigus (pemphigoid)
- Congenital entropion is rare due to deformity of the tarsal plate. It involves lower lid only.
- Mechanical: Due to lack of support provided by eyeball—seen in phthisis bulbi or enucleated or eviscerated eyes.

Symptoms and Signs

Same as for trichiasis and those of disturbances of stability of tear film. They are foreign body sensation, irritation, abrasion and corneal ulcer.

Three grades
i. *Mild:* Posterior border of lid inturned.
ii. *Moderate:* Intermarginal strip rotates inwards.
iii. *Severe:* Entire lid margin rolls inwards.

Senile Entropion
- Seen in old age.
- Usually above 60 years.

Etiology
- Overriding of preseptal part of orbicularis over the pretarsal part with atrophy of subcutaneous tissue with ageing
- Inturning of lower lid tarsus due to weak lower lid retractors and laxity of medial and lateral ligaments
- Loss of posterior support in enophthalmos due to atrophy of orbital fat.

Treatment

Aim of surgery: To restore vertical and horizontal tautness of lid:
- Reattach retractors to the tarsal plate
- Shortening of the horizontal width of the tarsal plate
- Forming a cicatrix between pretarsal and preseptal parts of orbicularis:
  - *Short term relief:* By sticking an adhesive tape to pull lower lid outwards.
  - *Everting sutures:* 5-0 vicryl chromic catgut from the conjunctiva to skin of lid adjacent to the inferior border of tarsus creates cicatricial barrier that maintains eyelid in an everted position.
  - *Modified wheeler operation:* Skin incision—parallel to lower lid. Orbicularis is dissected and 3 mm strip of muscle is double-breasted and stitched together with excision of the base-down triangle of tarsus. Redundant (excess) skin is excised.
  - *Quickert's procedure:* Transverse lid split + everting sutures + horizontal lid shortening.
  - *Modified Jones procedure:* Inferior lid retractors are plicated or attached to the tarsus.

Spastic Entropion

Due to spasm of orbicularis oculi:
- Evert the lid by pulling it with adhesive plaster
- Botulinum toxin injected into pretarsal orbicularis to prevent it from overriding.

Cicatricial Entropion

Treatment: Mild to moderate cases with thickened tarsus is treated with wedge resection of tarsus. If tarsus is not thickened, modified Burrow's operation or tarsal fracture is done. Very extensive scarring may necessitate the replacement of conjunctiva by a mucous membrane graft and a distorted tarsal plate by cartilage graft.

Congenital Entropion

The abnormal tarsal plate is resected. Abnormal skin fold is excised.

9. Write short notes on ectropion.

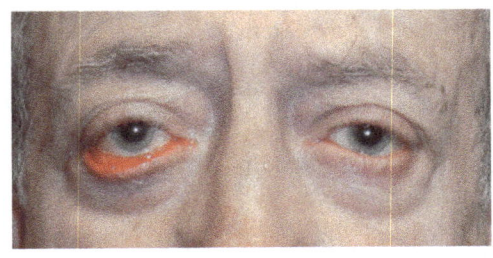

Fig. 15.9: Ectropion (outward turning of eyelid margin).

Types
- Senile or involutional
- Spastic
- Cicatricial
- Mechanical
- Paralytic
- Congenital
- *Senile* ectropion occurs only in lower lid due to horizontal laxity of the eyelid, medial canthal or lateral canthal laxity
- *Spastic:* Due to blepharospasm when lids are well supported by the globe. Occurs in children and young adults
- *Cicatricial:* Due to scarring of the skin by chronic conjunctivitis, blepharitis, injuries, burns, ulcers, etc.
- *Mechanical:* Due to the dragging of lid tumor with its weight
- *Paralytic:* Paralysis in orbicularis as in facial palsy—affecting lower lid
- *Congenital:* Due to deficient eyelid skin—skin grafting to be done.

Symptoms

Epiphora and constant watering of the eyes.

Signs
- Conjunctiva becomes dry and thickened
- Chronic conjunctivitis due to exposure, exposure keratitis.

Three grades
i. *Mild:* The only punctum is everted
ii. *Moderate:* Palpebral conjunctiva is visible
iii. *Severe:* Lower fornix is exposed.

Treatment
- *Spastic:* Underlying cause of blepharospasm is treated
- *Cicatricial:* Free lid margin from scar tissue and restore lid to normal position.

Mild cases

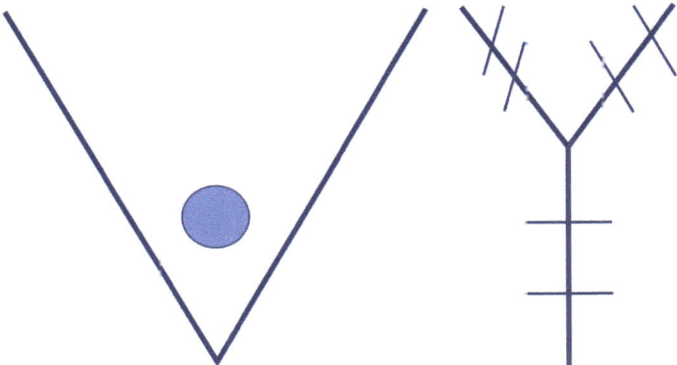

Fig. 15.10: V-Y operation.

V-shaped incision is made in the skin of the lower lid that includes the scar. Skin is excised and the wound is sutured in **Y**-shaped pattern thus correcting ectropion.

Extensive scarring: Excision of scar tissue and application of skin graft. Split skin graft or full-thickness grafts are taken from the upper lid, behind the ear, inner side of upper arm or thigh.

Senile Ectropion

Depending on the severity the following operations are done:
- Mild to moderate cases, a horizontal spindle-shaped piece of conjunctiva subconjunctival tissue is removed 5 mm from the punctum and margins are sutured
- For severe cases in mid portion of the lower lid, full-thickness shortening of the lid is done

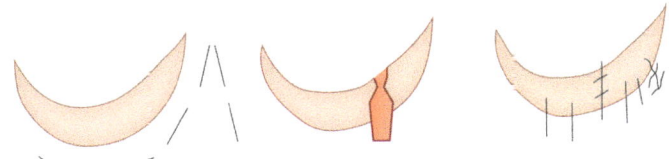

Fig. 15.11: Bryon Smith modification of Kuhnt Szymancwski's procedure.

Full thickness inverted house (pentagon) shaped excision at least 5 mm away from punctum is done and margins are sutured.
- Bryon Smith modification of Kuhnt Szymanowski's procedure: For severe ectropion which is more marked in the lateral half of the lid. A base up pentagonal full thickness excision from the lateral third of lid is combined with triangular excision of skin from the area just lateral to lateral canthus to elevate the lid
- Medial ectropion is corrected by modified lazy T operation in which medial vertical pentagon of full thickness lid is excised 4 mm lateral to lower punctum.

Paralytic Ectropion

It occurs due to paralysis of facial nerve, in Bell's palsy, parotid surgeries, trauma and tumors such as an acoustic neuroma.

Treatment

Initially lubricants and taping of the lid is done. For a permanent solution, lateral tarsorrhaphy is indicated. In this operation, the palpebral aperture is shortened by uniting the lids at lateral canthus. The edges of the upper and lower lids are freshened for requisite distance and then sutured.

10. Write short notes on symblepharon.

Etiology

Due to formation of the raw surface on two opposing surfaces. Causing adhesions during healing of:
- Burns, ulcer, diphtheria, operative scar
- Ocular pemphigus
- Steven Johnson's syndrome

Types
- Anterior—lid margin is involved
- Posterior—fornix is involved
- Total—both lids get completely adherent to the globe.

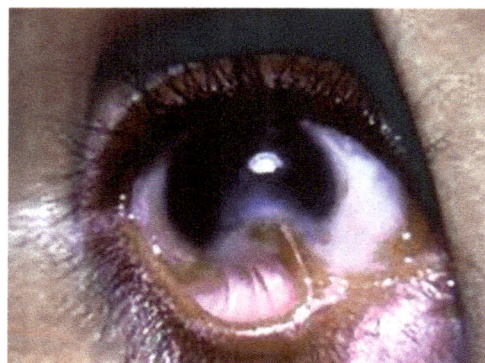

Fig. 15.12: Symblepharon (Adhesion of palpebral and bulbar conjunctiva).

Symptoms
- Cosmetic disfigurement
- Difficulty in lid movements
- Diplopia due to restricted mobility of the eye
- Lagophthalmos—inability to close lids properly.

Signs

Bands of fibrous tissue stretching between lid and globe are seen.

Treatment
- *Prophylaxis:* Applying eye ointment and moving a glass rod in the fornices several times a day
- Bandage contact lens
- Bands once formed need excision and the raw surfaces to be covered by conjunctival or buccal or amniotic membrane graft.

11. Discuss the types, evaluation, and treatment of ptosis.

Ptosis

Drooping of lids is called ptosis.
It is due to the weakness of levator palpebrae superioris or Muller's muscle.

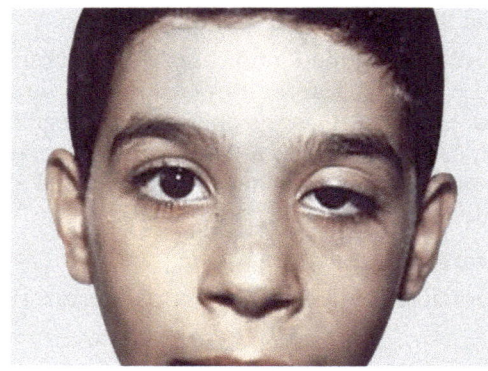

Fig. 15.13: Ptosis (dropping of left upper lid below its normal position which is 2 mm below upper limbus).

Pseudoptosis
- Lack of support—phthisis bulbi
- Contralateral lid retraction—thyrotoxicosis
- Ipsilateral hypotropia
- Brow ptosis (blepharochalasis)
- Dermatochalasis (excessive eyelid skin).

Classification
- Congenital
- Acquired
  - Neurogenic (oculomotor nerve palsy)
  - Myogenic (myopathy or myasthenic)
  - Traumatic
  - Mechanical—lid tumor
  - Aponeurotic—senile, postoperative
  - **Evaluation:**
    » Marginal reflex distance
    » Upper lid excursion—elevator action
    » Vertical fissure height
    » Upper lid crease
    » Bell's phenomenon
    » Associated features.

Marginal reflex distance
- Distance between upper lid margin and light reflex
- Mild ptosis—2 mm of droop
- Moderate—3 mm
- Severe—4 mm or more.

Upper lid excursion or levator action
- Normal—15 mm or more
- Good—12 mm or more
- Fair—5-11 mm
- Poor—4 mm or less.

Vertical fissure height
- Distance between upper and lower lid margin. Comparison determines unilateral ptosis.

Upper lid crease
- Distance between lid margin and lid crease in downgaze
- Female—10 mm (normal)
- Male—8 mm (normal)
- Absent in congenital ptosis
- High lid crease suggests aponeurotic ptosis.

Bell's phenomenon
(Upward rotation of eyeball on attempted lid closure)
- If it is poor—risk of postoperative corneal exposure
- Presence indicates intact superior rectus function.

Ocular movements
- Weakness of superior rectus
- Weakness of superior rectus and inferior oblique of one eye—double elevator palsy.

Marcus Gunn Jaw-winking Phenomenon
- Changes in lid position on attempted masticatory movements or side to side movement of jaws
- Indicate congenital synkinetic phenomenon.

Corneal sensation
Tensilon or neostigmine test: To exclude myasthenia gravis
10% phenylephrine test: To differentiate Horner's syndrome.
Schirmer's test: For corneal dryness (see chapter: Lacrimal Apparatus).

Management

Mild ptosis: Fasanella-Servant operation
Tarsus-conjunctival excision along with Muller muscle.

Moderate-to-severe ptosis
- Frontalis sling operation—if poor levator action
- Levator resection—if levator action is good
    - Everbusch operation—skin approach
    - Blaskowics operation—conjunctival approach.

12. Write short notes on lagophthalmos.

Lagophthalmos is a Greek word meaning incomplete closure of eyelids.

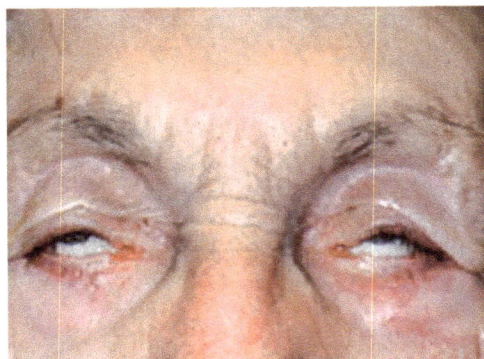

Fig. 15.14: Lagophthalmos of both eyes in a comatosed patient.

Causes
- Bell's palsy
- Postsurgical—following ptosis correction, eyelid reconstruction, inferior rectus recession
- Thyroid ophthalmopathy
- Lower lid ectropion
- Proptosis
- Extremely ill or comatosed patients.

Clinical Features
- Exposure keratopathy—burning sensation, increased lacrimation, tear film instability, decreased break uptime
- Inferior corneal ulcer.

Differential Diagnosis
- Neurotrophic keratopathy
- Dry eye syndrome.

Treatment
- Tear supplements and lubricating eye ointment
- Temporary corneal protection—bandage contact lens.

Surgical
- Lower lid ectropion—surgery
- Orbital decompression for thyroid ophthalmopathy
- **Lateral tarsorrhaphy:** Operation to create adhesions between the lateral part of upper and lower lid margins to narrow the palpebral aperture. Permanent tarsorrhaphy is done by splitting upper and lower lid margins after de-epithelializing the lid margins and then suturing them by lamellae
- Treat the cause.

13. What is Bell's palsy?

It is paralysis of one side of face due to facial nerve dysfunction.

Causes
- Exposure keratitis
- Viral infections
- Idiopathic.

Clinical Features
- Weakness of upper and lower facial musculature.
- Flat nasolabial fold
- Drooping of angle of mouth on the side of paralysis
- Lagophthalmos.

Treatment—Treat the Underlying Cause
- Artificial tears
- Temporary tarsorrhaphy
- Facial massage or electrical stimulation of affected facial musculature
- Oral steroids—Prednisolone 1 mg/kg/day for 4 days, then tapering over 10 days.

14. What are the indications and methods of Tarsorrhaphy?

Indications
- Lagophthalmos
- Bell's palsy
- Neurotrophic keratitis
- Exposure keratitis from proptosis due to thyroid orbitopathy.

Methods

Two types

i. In central tarsorrhaphy apposing area of intermarginal strips are freshened and two double armed sutures are used to suture the lids after excising the lashes. This is usually permanent.
ii. In lateral tarsorrhaphy, the palpebral aperture is shortened by uniting the lids at lateral canthus after freshening the intermarginal strip at that area. This is usually temporary.

15. Write short notes on lid tumors.

Benign

- Xanthelasma or xanthoma
- Cysts—Moll's gland
- Nevus
- Hemangioma
    - Capillary
    - Cavernous
- Lymphangioma
- Neurofibromatosis.

Malignant

- Squamous cell carcinoma (Epithelioma)
- Basal cell carcinoma
- Other: Lymphoma, lymphosarcoma, malignant melanoma, metastatic tumor, leukemia.

Treatment: Excision with radiation.

Xanthoma

- Yellowish round plaque. Usually seen in upper lid close to the medial canthus
- May be symmetrical
- Elderly, obese female who have diabetic or hyperlipoproteinemia.

Treatment: Excision or treated with trichloroacetic acid.

Cysts

- Retention cyst of Moll's gland
- Small, clear or whitish cysts—seen among the base of cilia in old people.

Treatment: Incision.

Nevus

Pigmentation seen on the lid margin.

Treatment: Excision.

Hemangioma

- *Capillary:* Red or port-wine stain. Dilated capillaries.
- *Cavernous:* Bluish in color. Dilated large venous spaces located deeper, localized and encapsulated. May increase in size on lowering the head, crying or coughing
    - Part of Sturge-Weber syndrome
    - May be associated with choroidal or leptomeningeal hemangioma.

Treatment

- Spontaneous regression
- Injection of a sclerosing agent
- Intralesional triamcinolone
- Cryosurgery
- Surgical excision.

Lymphangioma: Rarely Involves Lid.

Neurofibromatosis (Plexiform neuroma)

- Von Recklinghausen disease
- Phakomatosis involves lids and orbit
- Lids are swollen
- Skin: Shows multiple thickened nerves like knots, cords or bag of worms and
- Glioma of the optic nerve.

Malignant Tumors

Squamous Cell Carcinoma:

- Usually seen at edges of skin in elderly people
- Preauricular and submandibular lymph nodes are enlarged.

Basal Cell Carcinoma—(Rodent Ulcer)

- Occur near medial canthus and is more common
- Starting as pimple, ulceration or induration
- Grows deeper and all around
- Locally malignant
- Lymph gland not involved
- Basal cell carcinoma is radiosensitive.

Chapter 16: Lacrimal Apparatus

1. Describe briefly the anatomy of lacrimal apparatus.
- Lacrimal gland
- Lacrimal passage.

Lacrimal Gland—Two Parts
i. Orbital lobe—orbital roof.
ii. Palpebral part—superior fornix.

Lacrimal Passage
- Lacrimal puncta
  - 6 mm from the medial canthus
  - On the posterior border of the lid margin

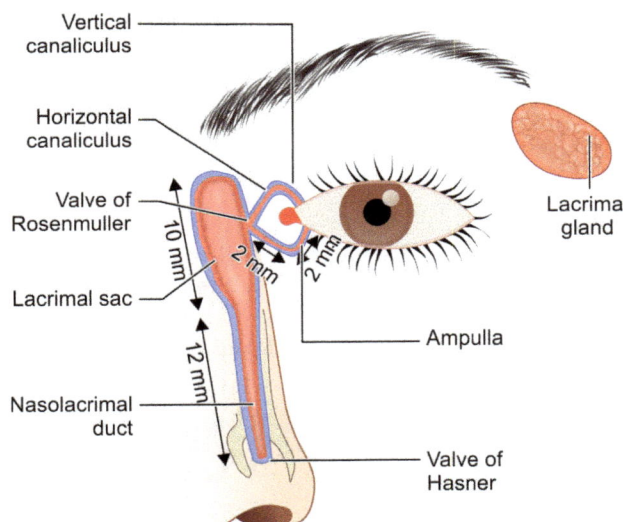

Fig. 16.1: Lacrimal apparatus.

- Lacrimal sac
  - Lies in lacrimal fossa
    » formed by lacrimal bone and
    » frontal process of the maxilla
    » 10 mm in length
  - Opens into the nasolacrimal duct
- Nasolacrimal duct
  - 12 mm in length
  - Opens into the inferior meatus of the nose
  - Directed downwards, slightly outwards and backwards.

Lacrimal Apparatus

Dacryocystitis
Inflammation of the lacrimal sac.

Classification
- Congenital
- Acquired
  - Acute
  - Chronic.

2. Describe the etiology, clinical features, differential diagnosis, and treatment of congenital dacryocystitis.
Dacryocystitis in the newborn.

Etiology
- Failure in the canalization of nasolacrimal duct (NLD)
- Lumen blocked by epithelial debris
- Commonly at the inferior end.

Symptoms
- Epiphora
  - Normally tears are secreted only 3–4 weeks after birth
- Purulent discharge or conjunctivitis.

Signs
- Sticky mucopurulent discharge
- Persistent epiphora
- Regurgitation on pressure over the sac area.

Differential Diagnosis
- Ophthalmia neonatorum
- Congenital glaucoma.

Complications
- Recurrent conjunctivitis
- Lacrimal abscess
- Fistula formation.

Treatment
- **Conservative**
  - Massage over lacrimal sac area and clear the discharge several times by downward pressing from sac area towards ala of the nose
  - Increase in hydrostatic pressure helps to open up membranous occlusion, followed by instillation of antibiotic drops 3-4 times daily
- **Surgical**
  - Probing of the nasolacrimal duct through upper punctum after 3 months of age
  - Dilate the punctum and pass probe vertically downwards, then inwards until the lacrimal bone is reached; 9–12 months of age is the ideal time for probing
  - The probe is then rotated towards the midline and pushed down the nasolacrimal duct
  - Lacrimal duct syringing
  - Intubation with silicon tube after 2 years of age
  - To be kept for 6 months
  - Dacryocystorhinostomy (DCR) after 4 years.

3. Describe the etiology, clinical features, complications, and treatment of acute dacryocystitis.

Acute suppurative inflammation of the lacrimal sac.

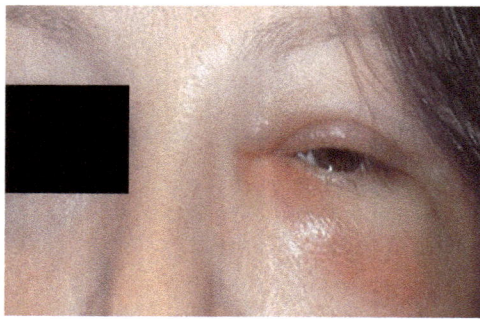

Fig. 16.2: Acute dacryocystitis.

Two Forms:
i. Acute suppurative dacryocystitis
ii. Acute suppurative pericystitis

Acute Suppurative Dacryocystitis
- Acute exacerbation of chronic dacryocystitis
- May start spontaneously.

Etiology
Pneumococcus, *Staphylococcus*, and Streptococci are usual pathogens.

Symptoms and Signs
- Marked swelling, redness, and tenderness of the skin over the sac area
- Conjunctival congestion
- Submaxillary lymph nodes enlargement
- Lacrimal fistula—if the abscess bursts repeatedly.

Clinical Picture
Three stages:
i. Stage of cellulitis
ii. Stage of lacrimal abscess
iii. Stage of fistula formation.

Stage of Cellulitis
- Painful swelling in lacrimal sac region
- Epiphora
- Fever and malaise
- Redness and edema
  - May spread to lids and cheek

Stage of Lacrimal Abscess
- Occlusion of canaliculi due to edema
  - Sac filled with pus distends
  - Anterior wall ruptures
  - Forms pericystic swelling—lacrimal abscess
  - Points below and outer side of the sac.

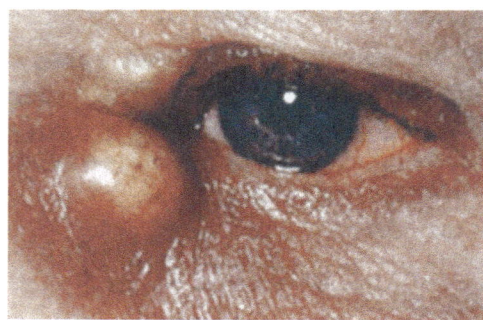

Fig. 16.3: Lacrimal abscess.

Stage of Fistula
- Lacrimal abscess discharges
- Leaving external fistula below the medial palpebral ligament
- May open internally into nose forming an internal fistula.

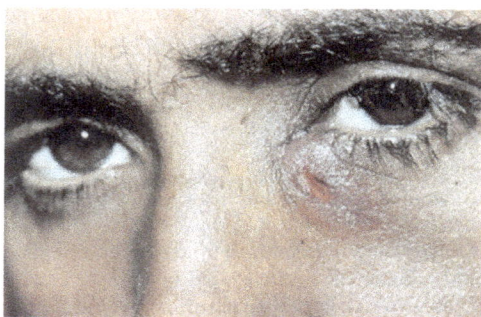

Fig. 16.4: Stage of external lacrimal fistula—left eye.

Complications
- Orbital cellulitis and thrombophlebitis
- Cavernous sinus thrombosis
- Ulcer with minor trauma to the cornea.

Differential Diagnosis
- Inflamed sebaceous cyst
- Furuncle
- Acute sinusitis
- Dental abscess
- Acute mucocele of frontal or anterior ethmoidal sinuses.

Treatment
- Systemic antibiotics
- Analgesics and anti-inflammatory drugs
- In lacrimal abscess: Vertical incision and drain the pus
- In lacrimal fistula: Excision of the fistulous tract and removal of the sac.

Acute Suppurative Pericystitis
- Infection of perilacrimal tissue
- Symptoms are similar to acute dacryocystitis
- May burst to form a fistula
- Treatment: Same as for acute dacryocystitis.

4. Describe the etiology, clinical features, complications, and management of chronic dacryocystitis.

Common suppurative inflammation of the lacrimal sac that usually results from obstruction of the nasolacrimal duct.

Etiology
- Stasis of tear fluid in the lacrimal sac.
- It occurs due to inflammation of the mucosa of the nasolacrimal duct.
- Mucosa becomes swollen and congested causing block favoring stasis.
  - Source of infection—from neighboring structures—nose, sinuses, conjunctiva and pericystic tissue.

Factors responsible for stasis and inflammation:
- Anatomical factors
  - Narrow bony canal—Male:Female = 1:3
  - Hypertrophied inferior turbinate
  - Deviated nasal septum
  - Polyps in the nose.
- General infection: Influenza, mumps, chicken-pox
- Lacrimation: Excess secretion-retention
  - Atony of the sac—chronic inflammation—Block foreign bodies in canaliculi or sac.

Clinical Features
Depending on the type:
- Catarrhal—commonest
- Encysted
- Suppurative.

Catarrhal Form
- Swelling in the lacrimal sac region below the level of the inner canthus
- Swelling: Not freely mobile
- Skin over the swelling is normal
- No tenderness
- Regurgitated material is mucoid
- Syringing: Nonpatency with regurgitation of fluid from upper punctum.

Encysted Mucocele
- Obstruction at the upper part of NL duct and sac canalicular junction
- In a closed sac: Encysted mucocele forms
- No regurgitation
- Syringing: Fluid comes back from the same punctum.

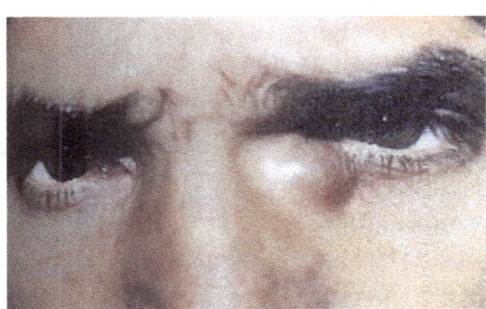

Fig. 16.5: Lacrimal mucocele.

Suppurative Form
- Erythema of the skin over sac
- Conjunctival congestion
- Epiphora
- Syringing: Discharge of pus.

Complications
- Unilateral conjunctivitis
- It can be a source of infection
- Hypopyon ulcer with minor trauma to cornea
- Eczema of lower lid
- Ectropion due to repeated wiping of tears.

Differential Diagnosis
- Lacrimal sac tumor
  - Bloodstained discharge
- Cold abscess
- Dermoid cyst
- Sebaceous cyst
- Mucocele of the anterior ethmoidal sinus or frontal sinus.

Investigations
- Nasal examination
  - To exclude deviation of septum, growth and atrophic rhinitis
- Radiological examination
  - Dacryocystography
    » Lipiodol, urografin, or iodized oil outlines the lacrimal excretory passage. X-ray is taken immediately and after 15 minutes to find out the size of the sac and site of obstruction
  - Substraction macrodacryocystography
    » Done with canalicular catheterization
  - Gamma scanning
    » Radioactive tracer (technetium) instilled into the conjunctival sac. Its excretion is visualized by a gamma camera.

Treatment

- **In recent cases**
  - Repeated syringing of the nasolacrimal duct with frequent instillation of antibiotic drops—reduces swelling of inflamed mucosa and restore the patency by clearing epithelial debris
- **In recurrent cases**
  - Dacryocystectomy (DCT)
  - Dacryocystorhinostomy
- **Insertion of tube**
  - Lester Jones tube
  - Pawar's implant—inserted into the lacrimal sac
  - Facilitates drainage of tears into nasal cavity.

Dacryocystectomy

- Complete excision of the lacrimal sac
- Advantage: Operation is easy and takes less time
- Disadvantage: Watering persists.

Dacryocystorhinostomy

- Conventional
  - From skin approach: Nasal drainage operation
  - Advantage: No postoperative epiphora
  - Early steps are as same as excision of the sac. Nasal mucosa in middle meatus is anastamosed with medial wall of sac
- Endonasal DCR
  - Approach from the nose
  - No skin incision
  - Success: 80%

Features	Endoscopic DCR	External DCR
External scar	Absent	Present
Blood loss during surgery	Less	More
Operating time	Less (15–30 min)	More (45–60 min)
Cost	Expensive	Cheap
Success rate	Less (70–80%)	More (90–95%)
Surgical technique	Needs skill in endoscopy	Endoscopy not required

- Endolaser DCR
  - Diode laser—approach from canaliculi
  - Takes less time
  - Success: 70%.

Contraindications for DCR

- Atrophic rhinitis
- Tumors of lacrimal sac
- Rhinosporidiosis
- Tuberculosis of lacrimal bone
- Bleeding diseases
- Extremes of age.

5. Write short notes on tear film.

Tears form a thin (7.6–8 μ) layer over the cornea and conjunctiva which is known as tear film. It consists of 3 layers:
  i. Inner mucin layer (0.2 μ)
   - Produced by the goblet cells. It consists of glycoproteins
  ii. Aqueous layer (6.5–7.5 μ)
   - Lacrimal gland and accessory glands of Krause and Wolfring—constitute 90% of the tear film
   - Content—water with dissolved salts, glucose, lysozymes, lactoferrin, immunoglobulin A and lactoferrin
  iii. Outer lipid layer (0.1 μ) produced by the Meibomian glands. It consists of cholesterol esters.

Functions

- Mucous layer: Converts corneal epithelium to the hydrophilic surface
- Aqueous layer: Aids oxygenation, removes debris and antimicrobial
  - Barrier to ocular infection
  - Optical clarity
- Lipid layer: Reduces evaporation and aids lubrication
  - Prevents lid margin overflow.

6. Describe the etiology, investigations, and treatment of dry eye.

Dry eye is a clinical condition of ocular discomfort caused by deficient tear production and/or excessive tear evaporation.
- Mucin deficiency
- Aqueous tear deficiency
- Lipid deficiency
- Impaired eyelid function
- Corneal epitheliopathies.

Punctate epithelial erosion filaments and plaques.

Mucin Deficiency: Dry Eye

- Hypovitaminosis A
- Severe conjunctival scarring
- Trachoma, Steven-Johnson syndrome, chemical burns, radiation and ocular phemphigus
- Goblet cell dysfunction.

Aqueous Deficiency: Dry Eye

- Pure keratoconjunctival sicca (KCS)—only lacrimal glands are damaged by mononuclear cells
- Primary Sjögren's syndrome (Sicca complex), KCS and dry mouth
- Secondary Sjögren's syndrome—sicca complex and conjunctival tissue disease (usually rheumatoid arthritis)
- Riley day syndrome (familial dysautonomia)
- Idiopathic hyposecretion.

Lipid Deficiency: Dry Eye

- Congenital absence of meibomian glands
- Chronic blepharitis and meibomitis
- Neurological lesion of non-Sjögren KCS.

Impaired Eyelid Function: Dry Eye

- Bell's palsy
- Dellen
- Symblepharon
- Lagophthalmos
- Ectropion.

Miscellaneous Causes
- Computer vision syndrome
- After LASIK surgery
- After keratoplasty.

Tests for Dry Eye
- Tear film break up time (BUT)
- Schirmer's test
- Rose Bengal staining
- Tear lysozyme
- Tear lactoferrin
- Tear film osmolarity.

Tear Film Break Up Time
The interval between a complete blink and appearance of first randomly distributed dry spots on the cornea.
- Normal: 15–30 seconds
- Deficiency: < 10 seconds
- Indicates mucin deficiency.

Schirmer's Test
- Measures total tear secretion
- 5 mm × 35 mm strip of Whatman 41 filter paper is used
- Normal: > 15 mm in 5 minutes
- Mild to moderate: 5–10 mm
- Severe dry eye: < 5 mm
- Aqueous deficiency dry eye (KCS).

Rose Bengal Staining
- Stains devitalized cells
- Propracaine used for less irritation
  - Three staining patterns are seen
  i. C pattern: Fine punctate stain in the interpalpebral area—suggests mild dry eye
  ii. B pattern: Extreme staining
     » Moderate dry eye
  iii. A pattern: Confluent staining of cornea and conjunctiva
     » Severe dry eye.

Treatment
- Tear substitutes
- Topical mucolytics for excessive mucosa
- Tear conservatives
- Immunosuppressants
- Cholinergic agents
- Omega 3 fatty acid.

Tear Substitutes
- 0.3% Hyper mellose, 0.25 to 0.7% methyl cellulose (HPMC)
- 1.4% polyvinyl alcohol and povidone
- 0.1% sodium hyaluronate
- 0.5 or 1% carboxymethyl cellulose
- Preservative free drops, gels, and ointments.

Topical Mucolytics
5% acetylcysteine

Tear Conservatives
- Measures to decrease evaporation
  - Air humidification
  - Protective spectacles
  - Lateral tarsorrhaphy
- Measures to decrease the drainage
  - Temporary punctal occlusion by
    » Collagen implants
    » Cyanoacrylate adhesive
  - Permanent occlusion by
    » Electrocauterization, or
    » Argon laser.

Immunosuppressants
In refractory cases, cyclosporin 0.05% or 0.1% twice daily reduces cell mediated inflammation of the lacrimal tissue.

Cholinergic Agents
Oral cholinergic agents such as pilocarpine.

7. Describe how tears are secreted and drained.
Tears are mainly secreted by lacrimal glands situated in the upper and lateral part of orbit. Accessory lacrimal glands (in the fornix) also secrete tears.

Secretion of Tears
- Afferent: Lacrimal branch of the ophthalmic division of 5th nerve
- Efferent: Parasympathetic secretomotor fibers from the superior salivary nucleus.

Accessory Lacrimal Glands
- Krause and Wolfring
  - Krause: 42 in upper fornix, 6–8 in the lower fornix
  - Wolfring: Near the upper border of superior tarsus and lower border of inferior tarsus.

Elimination of Tears
- Tears flow down and medially via the lacus lacrimalis in the inner canthus
- Drained by lacrimal passage into the nasal cavity
- Done by lacrimal pump mechanism by fibers of orbicularis inserted on the lacrimal sac
- When the eyelids close, contraction of these fibers distends the fundus of the sac and creates negative pressure and siphons the tear into the lacrimal sac
- When eyelids open, Horner's muscle (fibers of orbicularis) relaxes causing collapse of the lacrimal sac and positive pressure is created which forces the tears travel down the nasolacrimal duct into the nose.

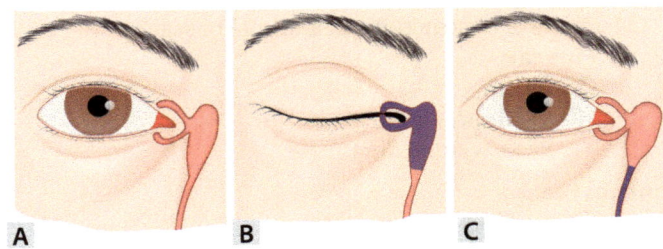

Figs. 16.6A to C: Lacrimal pump mechanism.

8. Describe the causes and investigations of watering eyes.

Etiology
- Hyperlacrimation: Increased secretion of tears
- Epiphora: Obstruction to drainage of tears.

Causes of Hyperlacrimation
- Primary
- Reflex
- Central.

Primary Hyperlacrimation
- Direct stimulation of the lacrimal gland
- Early stages of lacrimal gland tumors and cysts
- Parasympathomimitic drugs.

Reflex Hyperlacrimation
- Stimulation of sensory branches of fifth nerve due to irritation of cornea or conjunctiva
  - Affections of lids:
    » Stye, hordeolum internum, trichiasis, concretions and ectropion
  - Affections of conjunctiva: All types of conjunctivitis
  - Affections of the cornea: Corneal abrasions, corneal ulcers and nonulcerative keratitis
  - Affections of Sclera: Episcleritis and scleritis
  - Affections of the uveal tissue: Iritis and iridocyclitis
  - Acute glaucoma
  - Endophtalmitis and panophthalmitis
  - Orbital cellulitis.

Central Hyperlacrimation
Due to emotional states.

Causes of Epiphora
- Inadequate drainage of tears:
  - Lacrimal pump failure due to lower lid laxity or weakness of orbicularis

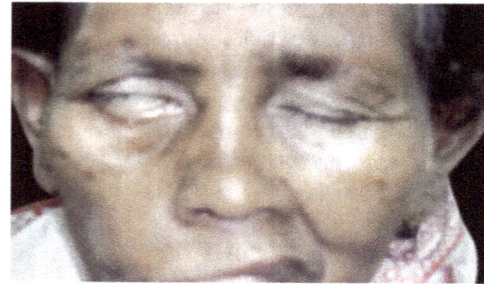

Fig. 16.7: Bell's palsy (right side).

- Mechanical obstructions in lacrimal passage:
  - Punctal
  - Canaliculi
  - Lacrimal sac
    » Nasolacrimal duct

Punctal Causes
- Eversion of lower punctum:
  - Old age, chronic blepharitis and ectropion
- Punctal obstruction:
  - Congenital obstruction of puncta
  - Cicatricial closure
  - Injuries and infections
  - Small foreign bodies, cilia
  - Prolonged use of drugs like IDU, pilocarpine.

Causes in Canaliculi
- Foreign body
- Trauma
- Stricture
- Canaliculitis—Actinomyces.

Causes in Lacrimal Sac
- Congenital mucous membrane folds
- Traumatic stricture
- Dacryocystitis
- Dacryolithiasis
- Specific infections—Tuberculosis, syphilis
- Tumors
- Atony of sac.

Causes in Nasolacrimal Duct
- Congenital—noncanalization
  - Partial canalization
  - Imperforated membranous valve
- Acquired stricture: Traumatic or inflammatory tumors and diseases of surrounding bones.

Clinical Evaluation
- Examination with diffuse illumination using magnification
- Causes of reflex hypersecretion and punctal causes of epiphora
  - Swelling in sac area.

Regurgitation Test
- Reflux of mucopurulent discharge
- Chronic dacryocystitis

Fluorescein Dye Disappearance Test
- 2 drops of dye instilled in both conjunctival sac
- After 2 minutes
  - No dye in conjunctival sac: Normal
  - Prolonged retention of dye: Inadequate drainage like atony of sac or mechanical obstruction.

Lacrimal Syringing Test
- Saline passes with pressure on syringing.

Partial Obstruction
- No fluid passes
- Reflux through same punctum
  - Obstruction in same canaliculi or common canaliculi
- Reflux through upper punctum
  - Obstruction in lower sac or nasolacrimal duct.

Probing and Irrigation
- Blunt tipped lacrimal cannula on a 2 mL saline-filled syringe
- Advanced through canaliculus to enter lacrimal sac
- The cannula comes to hard stop or soft stop.

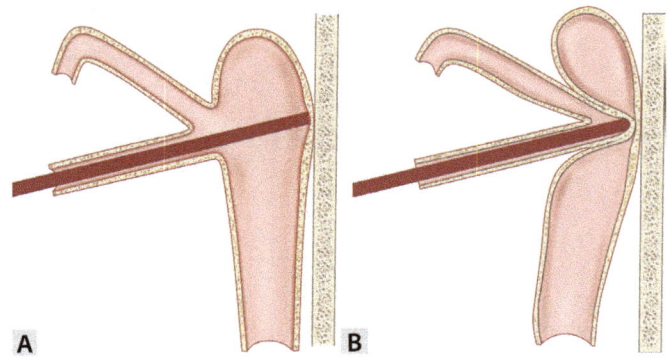

Figs. 16.8A and B: Hard and soft stop.

Nasolacrimal Duct Block
Hard Stop
- Cannula enters lacrimal sac
- Comes to a stop at medial wall of sac
- Rigid lacrimal bone is felt
  - Canaliculi are patent
- If saline passes into nose on irrigation
  - Stenosis or subtle lacrimal pump failure
- If it does not and sac distends—reflux through upper punctum NLD obstruction.

Canalicular Block
Soft Stop
- Cannula stops at the junction of common canaliculus and sac—at lateral wall of sac
- Sac is not entered—spongy feeling is felt
- On irrigation,
  - Reflux through lower punctum—denotes lower canalicular obstruction
  - Reflux through upper punctum—denotes obstruction of common canaliculus.

Jones Dye Tests
- **Jones primary test** (Test 1):
  - To differentiate partial obstruction of lacrimal passages from hypersecretion
- Method:
  - 2 drops of 2% fluorescein dye is instilled in the conjunctival sac
    » Cotton bud dipped in xylocaine is placed in inferior meatus
  - After 5 minutes:
    » Stained cotton bud indicates adequate drainage and cause is hypersecretion— test is positive
  - Unstained cotton bud—test is negative
    » Indicates partial obstruction or failure of lacrimal pump (negative test)

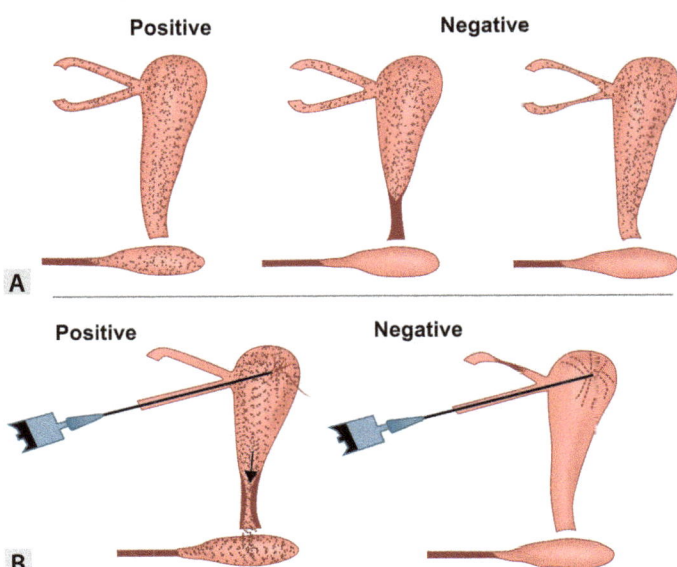

Figs. 16.9A and B: Jones dye testing.

- **Jones secondary test** (Test 2):
  - When test 1 is negative, lacrimal syringing is done with cotton bud in inferior meatus
  - Staining (positive test) of cotton bud suggest partial obstruction
  - No staining (negative test) indicates pump failure.

Dacryocystography
- Exact site, nature and extent of block can be inferred
- Lipiodol is pushed in the sac with a lacrimal cannula
- X-ray is taken at 5 and 30 minutes
- Entire passage can be visualized, fistulae, diverticular stone or tumor in sac can be seen
- Subtraction macrodacryocystography gives better visualization.

Radionuclide Dacryocystography
- Lacrimal scintillography
- Noninvasive technique
- Radioactive traces (technetium) is instilled into the conjunctival sac
- The passage is visualized with gamma camera
- To assess functional efficiency of lacrimal drainage apparatus.

9. Write short notes on regurgitation test.
Regurgitation on pressure over lacrimal sac area (ROPLAS) is a simple test to perform. A firm pressure is applied over the sac area and noted for regurgitation. If there is regurgitation, the test is positive. When positive the type of regurgitation is noted—watery, mucoid, mucopurulent or blood stained. Clear watery fluid is seen in atonic sac. Mucoid or mucopurulent discharge is indicative of nasolacrimal obstruction. Blood stained fluid is seen in malignancy or stone in the sac.

CHAPTER 17

Injuries to the Eye

1. Classify injuries to the eye. Describe the presentation and treatment of chemical injuries.

Classification
- Chemical
- Thermal
- Radiational
- Mechanical.
- **Chemical injuries**
  - Alkaline injuries
  - Acidic injuries.

Alkaline Injuries
- Lime from fresh mortar
- Lime during white washing
- Laboratory alkalies
  - For example: *Ammonia, sodium hydroxide, etc.*
    » *Household detergents, drain cleaners*
    » *Lime powder packets*
    » *Color powders in Holi.*

Pathogenesis
- Presents as dull cornea with corneal ulcer
- Causes necrosis of the surface epithelium and occlusion of the limbal vasculature
- Dry eye at later stages.

Ocular Chemical Injury Severity

Grade	Signs and symptoms	Prognosis
1	Cornea clear and limbal ischemia absent	Excellent
2	Cornea hazy, iris details absent, limbal ischemia < 1/3	Good
3	Total loss of corneal epithelium, stromal haze obscures iris, ischemia 1/3–1/2 limbus	Poor
4	Cornea opaque, ischemia > 1/2 limbus	Dismal

Acidic Injuries
- Caused by hydrochloric acid and sulphuric acid during toilet cleaning or tiles cleaning
- Laboratories, car battery, and refrigeration workshops, vegetable preservatives
- Less severe than alkaline injuries
- Coagulates surface layer
- Does not penetrate the eye.

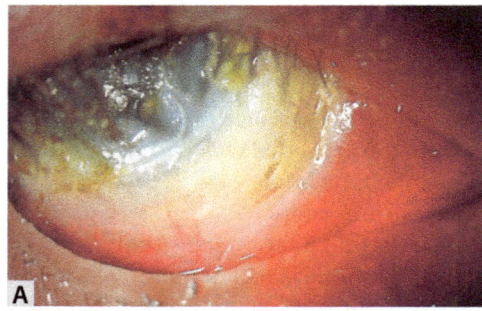
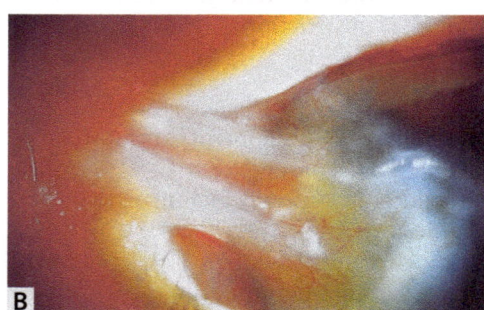

Figs. 17.1A and B: A. Grade 4 chemical injury with totally opaque cornea; B. Conjunctival adhesions following chemical injury.

Treatment
- Removal of irritant material
- Copious irrigation
- Fornices are washed with saline till pH returns to normal or for 30 minutes continuously
- Cycloplegics—cyclopentolate
- Antibiotic ointment
- Oral doxycycline 100 mg bd
- Judicious use of steroids
- Prevention of symblepharon by glass rodding.

2. Describe management of thermal injuries.

- Thermal energy or due to infrared rays
- Commonly due to cigarette, hot metals, oils, welding arc or exposure to fire and electrical short circuits.

Treatment

- Removal of foreign material in burns
- Debride necrotic epithelium
- 1% cyclopentolate eye drops
- Antibiotic ointment.

3. Describe the causes, clinical features and treatment of injuries due to radiation.

- Commonly due to ultraviolet rays
- Exposure during sunbathing, snow or water skiing
- Highly reflective surface like snow and water increase the risk of injury
- Long exposure to X-rays and UV rays can cause cataract
- Infrared rays cause photoretinitis
  Solar macular burn.

Pathogenesis

- Produces local cell death
- Causes inflammation and sloughing of the affected tissues.

Clinical Features

- Burning pain
- Photophobia
- Lacrimation
- Foreign body sensation
- Loss of epithelium and stromal edema.

Treatment

- Cold compresses
- Apply cooled clothes or pad to affected eye
- Cyclopentolate 1%
- Analgesics.

4. Write short notes on photophthalmia.

This refers to multiple epithelial erosions of cornea which occur due to the effect of ultraviolet rays in the range from 311 mm to 290 nm.

Causes

- Exposure to welding arc
- Bright light of short circuit
- Snow blindness: Due to reflection of UV rays from snow surfaces in mountains.

Clinical Features

There is a latent period of 4 to 5 hours between the exposure and onset of symptoms. Patient presents with severe burning pain, lacrimation, photophobia and blepharospasm. Conjunctiva is congested and the cornea shows multiple spots on fluorescein staining.

Pathogenesis

There is desquamation of corneal epithelium causing multiple epithelial erosions.

Prophylaxis

Wearing of protective glass crooks B1 or B2.

Treatment

- Cold compresses
- Patching with antibiotic eye ointment for 24 hours since epithelium regenerates in 24 hours
- Lubricating eye drops
- Analgesics and tranquilizers
- Cycloplegics if there is severe corneal involvement.

5. Classify mechanical injuries to the eye and describe the clinical features of blunt injuries to the eye.

- Closed globe injury
- Open globe injury.

Closed Globe Eye Injuries

Without full thickness defect of corneoscleral coat: Usually due to blunt trauma.

- Contusion or concussion
- Lamellar laceration
- Superficial foreign bodies.

Open Globe Eye Injuries

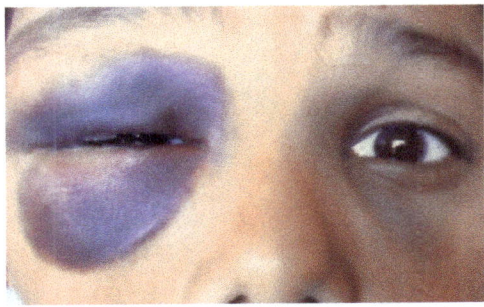

Fig. 17.2: Ecchymosis of lids.

- Lacerations (outside to inside break)
  - Penetrating injuries (has entry wound)
  - Perforating injuries (has entry and exit wound)
  - Lamellar lacerations—partial thickness injury of coats of eyeball
  - Intraocular foreign body (IOFB).
- Ruptures (inside to outside break).

Blunt Injuries

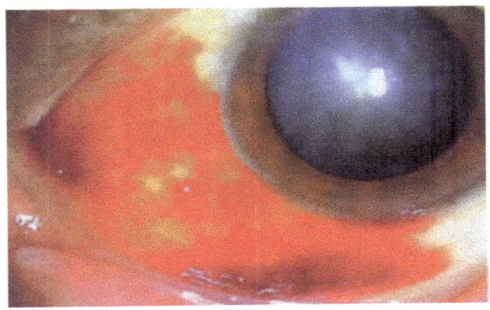

Fig. 17.3: Subconjunctival hemorrhage.

Injuries to the Eye

- Due to concussion or contusion
- Coup or direct—corneal abrasion
- Counter coup—damage due to pressure waves.

Conjunctiva: Subconjunctival Hemorrhage

- Bright red sharply delineated area
- Rupture of small blood vessels in the conjunctiva.

Due to local injury	Due to injury to skull
Appears immediately	Appears after few hours to 24 hours
Moves with movement of conjunctiva	Does not move
Bright red color	Bluish purple
Posterior limit seen	Not seen as it is coming from back

Treatment
- Assurance
- It gets absorbed in 2 weeks.

Cornea

- Abrasion to cornea
- Corneal opacity due to edema of stroma and folds in DM
- Blood staining of cornea will occur in cases of recurrent hyphema, long-standing large hyphema associated with increased IOP and decompensated endothelium.

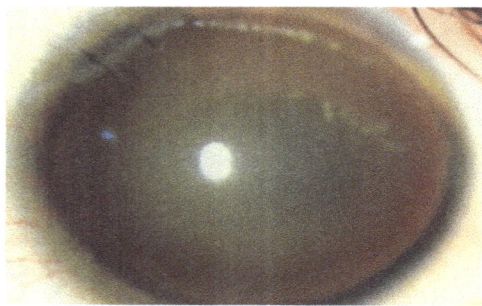

Fig. 17.4: Blood staining of cornea.

Sclera

- Rupture of globe with prolapse of uveal tissue
- Superonasal rupture is common as inferotemporal area is vulnerable to injury.

Anterior Chamber: Traumatic Hyphema

- Primary and secondary hemorrhage
- Reduce IOP.

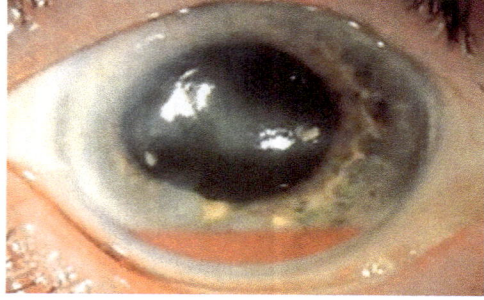

Fig. 17.5: Hyphema.

Treatment

Topical Steroids
- IOP > 35 mm Hg for 5 days or > 50 mm Hg for 3 days:
  - Do paracentesis and let out the blood clot
  - Saline irrigation of anterior chamber
  - Antifibrinolytic—aminocaproic acid.

Iris and Ciliary Body

- Traumatic miosis
- Traumatic mydriasis

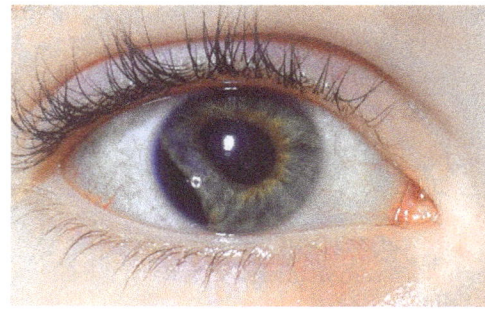

Fig. 17.6: Iridodialysis.

- Radial tears of iris
- Iridodialysis.
  - Iris is torn from ciliary attachment
  - D-shaped pupil
  - Dark biconvex area near limbus
  - Uniocular diplopia and glare
- Anti-flexion of iris
- Pigmented portion of iris faces forward
- Retroflexion of iris
- Total inversion of iris
- Aniridia or irideremia
  - Iris is completely torn from ciliary attachment
  - It contracts and forms a little ball which sinks to the bottom of anterior chamber
- Cyclodialysis
  - Ciliary body gets detached from sclera.

Lens

- Vossius ring: Circular ring of brown pigment seen on the anterior capsule of the lens

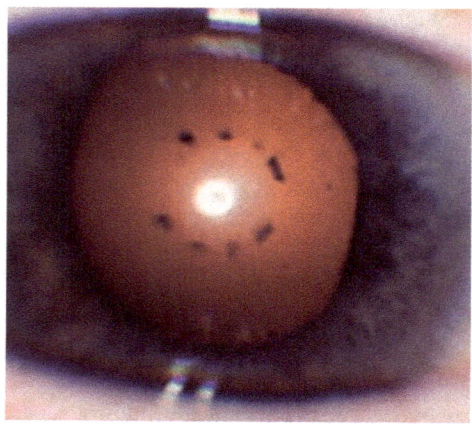

Fig. 17.7: Vossius ring.

- Imprint of pupil
- Rosette shaped cataract.
  - Feathery opacity can occur early or after one year of injury in the posterior cortex

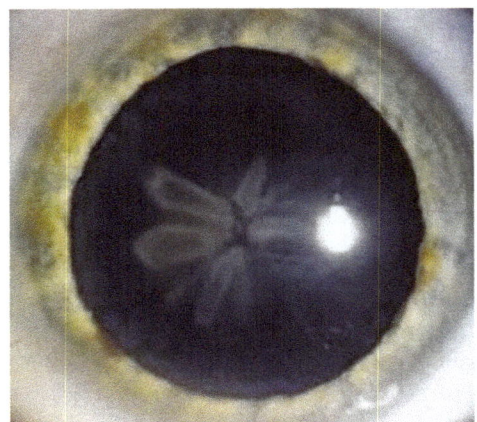

Fig. 17.8: Rosette shaped cataract.

- Subluxation or dislocation of lens
- Tear of lens capsule with absorption of lens
- Total lens opacification.

Vitreous

- Posterior vitreous detachment
- Vitreous hemorrhage
- Pigmented opacities in fluid vitreous
- Vitreous herniation into anterior chamber
- Vitreous loss in case of globe rupture.

Choroid

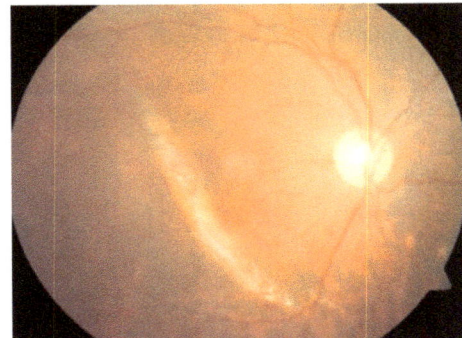

Fig. 17.9: Choroidal rupture.

- **Choroidal rupture**
  - Single or multiple, temporal to macula
  - Crescent shaped and concentric
  - Exposing white sclera.
    » Direct rupture at the point of injury
    » Occur anteriorly parallel to ora serrata
    » Indirect rupture occurs opposite to point of injury countercoup.
- **Choroidal hemorrhage**

Retina

- Cloudy swelling of sensory retina at macula—Berlin's edema

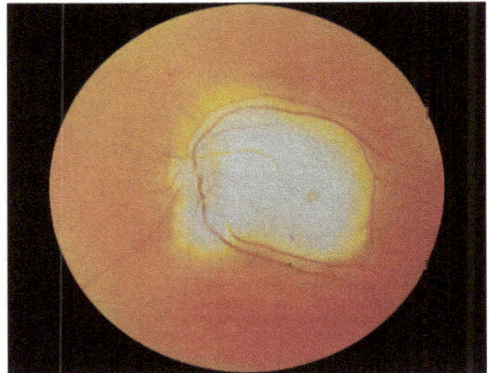

Fig. 17.10: Fundus picture: Berlin's edema.

- Gives gray appearance
- Cherry red spot at macula
- Spontaneous resolution is possible in 6 weeks
- Severe case associated with pigmentary degeneration and macular hole.

Retinal Break

- Retinal dialysis, equatorial tears and macular hole all predispose to retinal detachment
- Retinal detachment common in the upper nasal quadrant in injuries.

Optic Nerves

- Optic neuropathy
- Compression of nerves and its blood supply due to post-traumatic inflammation
- Optic nerve avulsion
  - Due to sudden extreme rotation or anterior displacement of the globe.

6. Describe the clinical features, and treatment of perforating injuries to the eye.

Perforating Injury

- Causes severe damage to eye due to immediate trauma and infection
- It is an ocular emergency
- Signs of perforation of eyeball
  - Decreased visual acuity
  - Low intraocular pressure
  - Shallow anterior chamber or hyphema
  - Alteration in pupil size or shape
  - Hole in iris
  - Wound traction in cornea, lens or vitreous.

Ruptured Globe

- Full thickness wound
- Signs of open-globe injury:
  - Severe subconjunctival hemorrhage and edema
  - Choroidal pigment visible through sclera
  - Lacerated cornea
  - Shallow anterior chamber
  - Vitreous hemorrhage
  - Reduced IOP.

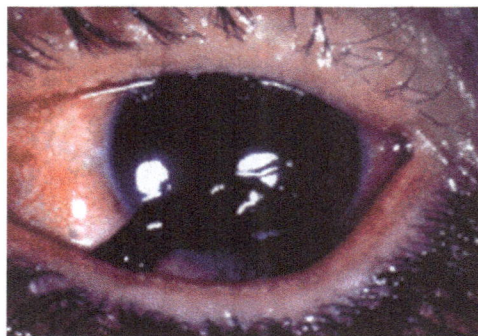

Fig. 17.11: Ruptured globe.

Corneal Perforation: Iris Prolapse

Aim of Treatment
- To save the vision
- To prevent sympathetic ophthalmia.

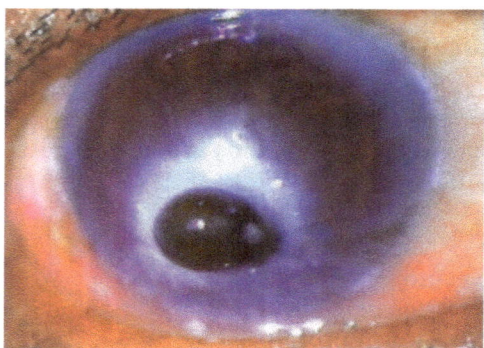

Fig. 17.12: Corneal perforation—iris prolapse.

Principles of Treatment
- Proper suturing
- Free uveal tissue from cornea or corneoscleral wound
- Control and prevention of infection
- Close follow-up with topical antibiotics atropine and steroids.

7. Write short notes on intraocular foreign body (IOFB).

- Effects of retained foreign body:
  - Mechanical effect
  - Infection
  - Specific chemical action of the metal
  - Degenerative changes:
    » Inert metals glass, platinum, porcelain, gold, silver, etc.
    » Little reaction with encapsulation—lead in shot gun pellets
    » Local suppuration: Aluminium, nickel, mercury, pure copper and zinc
    » Iron and copper alloy (< 85% copper) undergo electrolytic dissociation and gets deposited throughout the eye.

8. Write short notes on siderosis bulbi.

- A piece of steel is the commonest IOFB, ferrous foreign body undergoes dissociation.
- Deposition of iron on lens epithelium and retina exerts toxic effects on cellular enzyme systems.

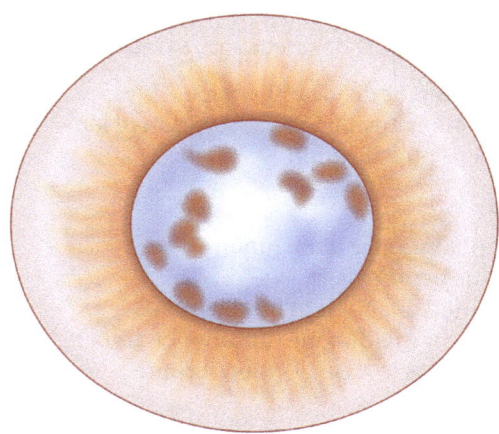

Fig. 17.14: Siderosis bulbi due to iron deposits. Iron deposits occur within 6 months to 2 years of injury.

- Radial iron deposits on anterior lens capsule
- Reddish brown staining of iris
- Secondary glaucoma due to trabecular damage
- Pigmentary retinopathy
- ERG—attenuation of b wave.

9. Write short notes on chalcosis.

- Pure copper-violent endophthalmitis
- Alloy with less than 85% copper- chalacosis
- Gets deposited in membrane structures

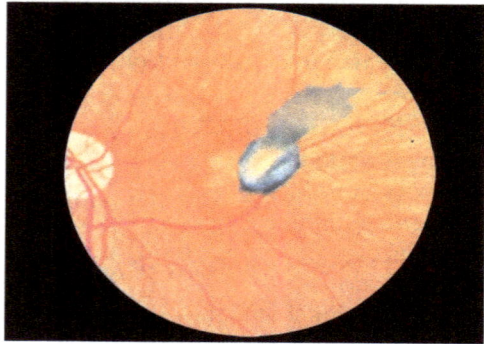

Fig. 17.13: Degenerative changes due to IOFB.

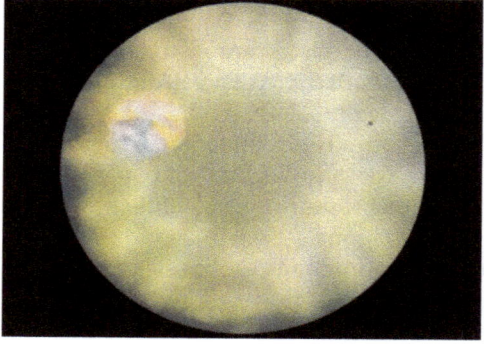

Fig. 17.15: Sunflower cataract.

- Kayser-Fleischer (KF) ring-golden brown ring deposition of copper on descemet's membrane—similar to Wilson's disease
- Sunflower cataract—deposition under posterior capsule of lens. Brilliant golden green
- Golden plaque deposited on the posterior pole:
    » Copper less retinotoxic than iron
    » Visual function may be preserved
    » Reflect the light with a metallic sheen.

10. What is the reaction of organic material injury to the eye?

- Wood splinter, other vegetable matter, eyelash or caterpillar hair
- Produces proliferative reaction with formation of giant cells
- May carry infection.

CHAPTER 18

Orbit

1. Describe the anatomy of orbit.

- Pyramidal shaped
- Above—anterior cranial fossa
- Below—maxillary sinus
- Apex—optic foramen
- Base—orbital margins
- Volume—30 cc.

Orbital Walls

- Formed by seven bones—sphenoid, ethmoid, lacrimal, frontal, maxillary, palatine, and zygoma. [SELF MPZ]
- Medial wall—maxilla, ethmoid, lacrimal, and sphenoid (MELS)
- Lateral wall—Zygoma, sphenoid (ZS)
- Roof—frontal, sphenoid (FS)
- Floor—maxilla, palatine, and zygoma (MPZ).

Orbital Apertures

- Superior orbital fissure
- Inferior orbital fissure
- Optic foramen and canal.

Superior Orbital Fissure

- Lies between lesser and greater wings of sphenoid
- Communicates with middle cranial fossa
- Common tendinous ring divides it into 3 parts:
    i. The part above the tendinous ring transmits:
        » Lacrimal nerve
        » Frontal nerve
        » Trochlear nerve
        » Superior ophthalmic vein
        » Recurrent lacrimal artery.
    ii. The part within the tendinous ring transmits:
        » Superior division of 3rd nerve
        » Nasociliary nerve
        » Inferior division of 3rd nerve
        » Abducent nerve
    iii. The part below the tendinous ring transmits inferior ophthalmic vein.

Inferior Orbital Fissure

- It separates inferior and lateral walls of the orbit.
- Lies between maxilla and greater wing of sphenoid.
- Connects orbit with infratemporal and pterygopalatine fossa.

Optic Canal

- Lies between lesser wing and body of sphenoid.
- Optic nerve, ophthalmic artery, and sympathetic nerve plexus.

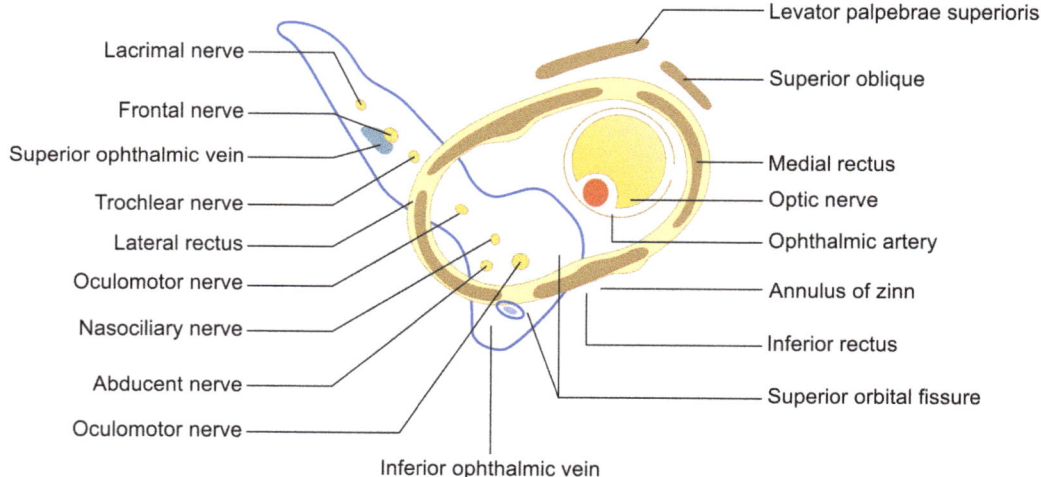

Fig. 18.1: Superior orbital fissure.

Surgical Spaces of Orbit

Four surgical spaces:
i. **Subperiosteal space:** Space between periorbita and bones of orbit.
ii. **Central space:** Lies between four recti
   - Cone shaped space: Contain vital structures
   - Space occupying lesion produces axial proptosis.
iii. **Peripheral space:** Space between muscle cone and periosteum of orbit
   - Space occupying lesion produces eccentric proptosis.
iv. **Subtenon's space:** Space between Tenon's capsule and globe
   - Tendonitis produces mild proptosis.

2. Write short notes on cavernous sinus thrombosis.

Cavernous sinus thrombosis can occur due to extension of thrombosis from various sources which communicates with the cavernous sinus.

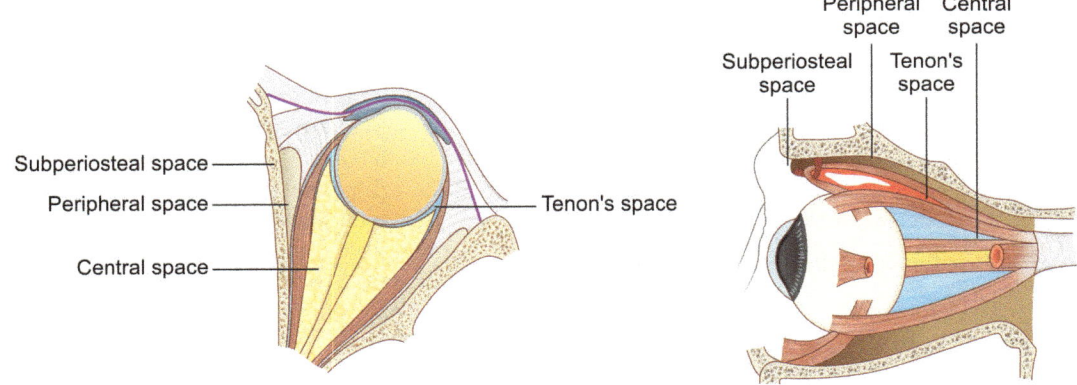

Fig. 18.2: Surgical spaces of orbit.

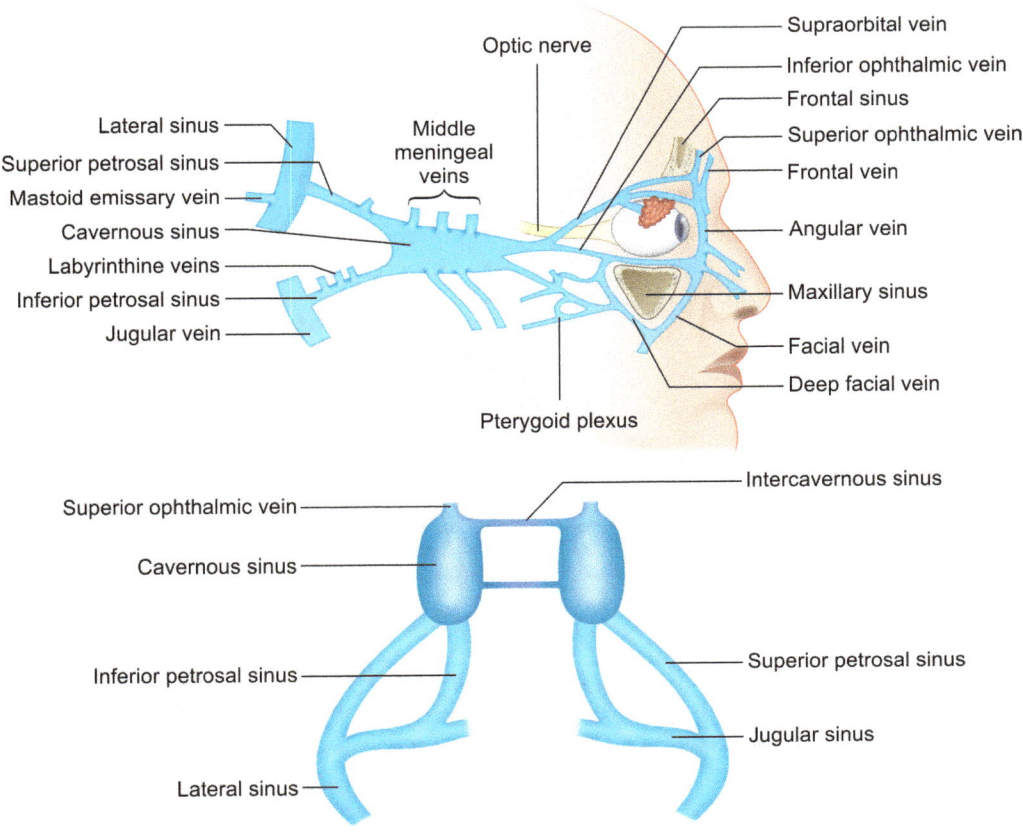

Fig. 18.3: Cavernous sinus.

Communications of Cavernous Sinus

- Superior and inferior ophthalmic veins enter the sinus anteriorly
- Superior and inferior petrosal sinuses leave the sinus posteriorly
- Intercavernous sinuses (transverse sinuses) communicate with the other side.

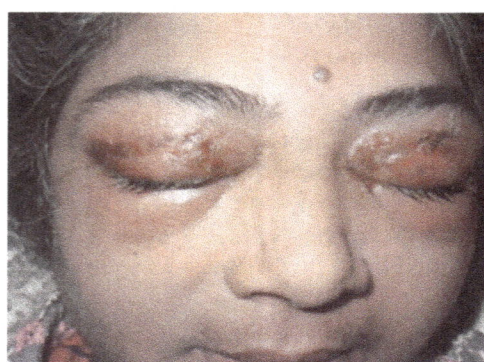

Fig. 18.4: Cavernous sinus thrombosis.

Etiology

- Spread of infection from orbital cellulitis
- Otitis, facial furuncles and erysipelas
- *Staphylococcus aureus*
- *Streptococcus pneumonia*
- *Aspergillus*.

Symptoms

- Same as for orbital cellulitis
- Severe supraorbital pain due to ophthalmic division of trigeminal nerve involvement
- High grade fever, rigor, and vomiting.

Signs

- Edema over mastoid process of affected side
- Paralysis of 6th nerve of other eye denotes bilateral involvement.

Complications

- Meningitis
- Cerebral abscess.

Treatment

- Antibiotics—intravenous broad spectrum
- Analgesics and anti-inflammatory drugs
- Anticoagulant therapy may be helpful in dissolving the thrombus.

3. Write short notes on Graves' ophthalmopathy.

This term is used to denote typical ocular changes which include lid retraction, lid lag and proptosis. Other terms used are endocrine exophthalmos, malignant exophthalmos, dysthyroid ophthalmopathy, ocular Graves' disease, and thyroid eye disease.

Etiology

- Exact cause is obscure
- Maybe present in hyper, hypo or euthyroid states. Maybe associated with:
    - Disturbance of endocrine system
    - Increased secretion in thyrotrophic hormone
    - Increased secretion of exophthalmic producing substances and long acting thyroid stimulators.

Pathogenesis

Delayed hypersensitivity or autoimmune reaction to thyroglobulin leading to edema; infiltration, deposition of fat, mucopolysaccharides, and fibrosis.

Common Signs of Graves' Disease

- Lid retraction
- Lid lag (upper and lower)
- Infrequent blinking
- Exophthalmos
- Diplopia
- Lid edema and chemosis
- Conjunctival injection over insertion of recti
- Increased IOP on elevation
- Superior limbic keratopathy.

Classification of American Thyroid Association: [Mnemonic: NO SPECS]

- Class 0: No signs and symptoms
- Class 1: Only signs, no symptoms
- Class 2: Soft tissue involvement with signs

Differential diagnosis.			
Features	CS thrombosis	Orbital cellulitis	Panophthalmitis
Laterality	Initially unilateral soon becomes bilateral	Unilateral	Unilateral
Degree of proptosis	Moderate	Marked	Minimal
Vision	Not affected in early stages	Not affected in early stages	Loss of vision from the beginning
Cornea and AC	Clear in early stages	Clear in early stages	Hazy due to corneal edema. Hypopyon is present.
Ocular movement	Marked limitation	Marked limitation	Painful and limited
Edema in mastoid	Present	Absent	Absent
General symptoms	Marked	Mild	Mild

- Class 3: Proptosis
- Class 4: Extraocular muscle involvement
- Class 5: Corneal involvement—exposure to keratitis
- Class 6: Sight loss due to optic nerve involvement.

Clinical Types
- Thyrotoxic exophthalmos
  - Seen in hyperthyroid patients
  - Exophthalmos in mild to moderate
  - Weakness of convergence only.
- Thyrotropic exophthalmos
  - Seen in euthyroid patients
  - Exophthalmos is severe
  - External ophthalmoplegia may occur.

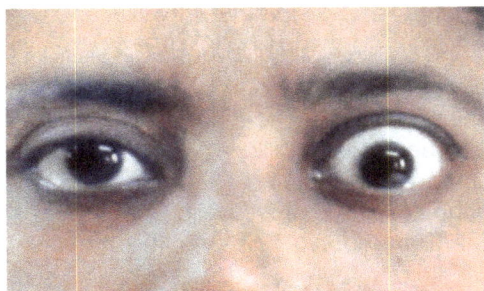

Fig. 18.5: Thyrotoxic exophthalmos.

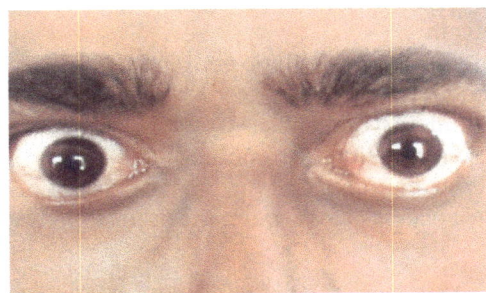

Fig. 18.6: Thyrotropic exophthalmos.

Eye signs in Graves' disease.		
Feature	Signs	Causes
Retraction of upper eyelid	Dalrymple's	Overactive Muller's muscle
Upper lid lag when patient looks down	Von Graefe's	Overactive Muller's muscle
Eversion of upper lid is difficult	Gifford	Lid edema
Infrequent blinking and incomplete closure	Stellwag	Lid edema and staring looks
On looking up, the upper lid tends to move faster than the globe	Kocher's	Overactive Muller's muscle
Trembling of eyelids	Rosenbach	Sympathetic overaction
Fullness of eyelid	Enroth	Edema of lids

Management
- Topical artificial tear drops
- Guanethidine 5% eye drops to decrease lid retraction
- Systemic steroids
- Lateral tarsorrhaphy
- Extraocular muscle surgery to correct diplopia in primary gaze
- Orbital decompression.

Investigations
- Thyroid function tests: T3, T4, TSH and radioactive iodine uptake
- Positional tonometry: An increase in IOP in upgaze, helps in subclinical cases
- Ultrasonography: To note extraocular muscle thickness and accumulation of retro orbital fat
- CT scanning: To confirm ultrasound findings.

4. Classify orbital inflammations.

Acute Orbital Inflammations
- Preseptal cellulitis
- Orbital cellulitis
- Orbital osteoperiostitis
- Tendonitis
- Cavernous sinus thrombosis.

Chronic Orbital Inflammations
Specific Inflammations
- Tuberculosis
- Syphilis
- Actinomycosis
- Mycotic infections—mucormycosis
- Parasitic infestations.

Chronic Nonspecific Inflammations
- Idiopathic (inflammatory pseudotumor)
- Tolosa Hunt syndrome
- Chronic orbital periostitis.

5. Write short notes on preseptal cellulitis.
Infection of subcutaneous tissues anterior to orbital septum.

Causes
- *Staphylococcus aureus*
- *Streptococcus pyogenes.*

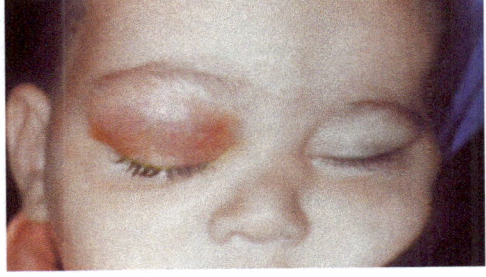

Fig. 18.7: Preseptal cellulitis.

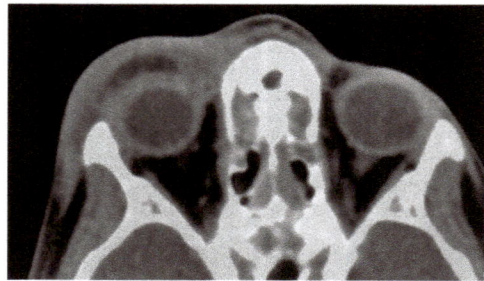

Fig. 18.8: CT scan of right eye.

Mode of Infection

- Exogenous
  - Skin laceration
- Contiguous
  - Acute hordeolum or dacryocystitis
- Endogenous
  - Middle ear and upper respiratory tract infections.

Clinical Feature

Inflammatory edema of eyelids and periorbital skin.

Complication

Spreads posteriorly to become orbital cellulitis.

Differential diagnosis.		
Features	Preseptal cellulitis	Orbital cellulitis
Age of onset	< 5 years	>5 years
Lid edema	Marked	Present
Proptosis	Absent or mild	Present
Chemosis (conjunctival edema)	Absent or mild	Marked
Ocular movements	Painless and full	Painful and restricted
Visual acuity	Normal	Reduced

Treatment

Oral antibiotics and anti-inflammatory drugs.

6. Write short notes on orbital cellulitis.

Acute infection of soft tissue of orbit behind the orbital septum.

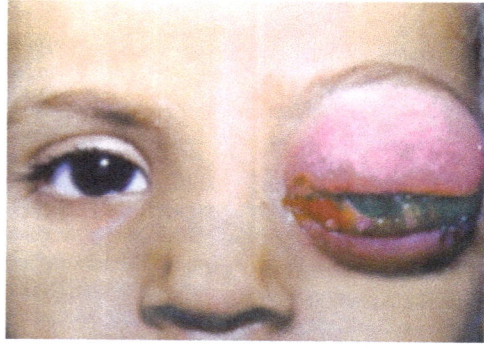

Fig. 18.9: Orbital cellulitis of left eye.

Causative Agents

- *Staphylococcus aureus, Streptococcus pyogenes*
- *Streptococcus pneumoniae, Haemophilus influenzae.*

Mode of Infection

- Exogenous—trachoma
- Contiguous—from adjacent structures
- Endogenous—blood spread
- Postsurgical—due to orbital surgery or paranasal sinus surgery.

Clinical Feature

- Symptoms—swelling and severe pain increased by ocular movement
  - Fever, prostration and defective vision.

Signs

- Lid edema
- Marked chemosis
- Axial proptosis
- Restriction of ocular movement
- Fundus: Congestion of veins and disc edema.

Complications

- Ocular
  - Exposure keratitis, occlusion of central retinal artery or vein
  - Endophthalmitis, optic neuropathy.
- Intracranial
  - Meningitis, brain abscess
  - Cavernous sinus thrombosis.
- Subperiosteal abscess along medial orbital wall.
- Orbital abscess—post-traumatic or postoperative.

Treatment

- Intravenous broad spectrum antibiotics:
  - Ceftazidime 1 g tds and Metronidazole 500 mg tds
  - Vancomycin to be given if there is penicillin allergy.
- Analgesics and anti-inflammatory drugs
- Surgical intervention: In case of orbital or subperiosteal abscess.

7. Classify the proptosis. Enumerate the causes, investigations and treatment of proptosis.

The protrusion of the eyeball is known as proptosis. It is a condition where there is forward displacement of the eyeball beyond orbital margin with the patient looking straight head.

Classification

It can be classified on the basis of onset, location, laterality and etiology.
- Onset
  - Sudden or gradual
- Location
  - Axial and eccentric

- Laterality
  - Unilateral and bilateral
- Based on etiology.

Unilateral Proptosis
- **Congenital**
  - Dermoid
  - Congenital cystic eye ball
  - Orbital teratoma.
- **Inflammatory**
  - Orbital cellulitis.
- **Vascular**
  - Retrobulbar hemorrhage
  - Orbital varices
  - Hemangioma.
- **Cysts of orbit**
  - Parasitic cysts
  - Hydatid and cysticercosis.
- **Tumors of orbit**
  - Primary
  - Secondary
  - Metastatic.
- **Mucocele of paranasal sinuses**
  - Frontal
  - Ethmoidal
  - Maxillary.

Bilateral Proptosis
- **Developmental anomalies of skull**
  - Craniofacial dysostosis, e.g., oxycephaly, and Crouzon's syndrome
- **Osteopathies**
  - Osteitis deformans
  - Rickets
  - Acromegaly.
- **Inflammatory**
  - Cavernous sinus thrombosis.
- **Endocrine exophthalmos**
  - Thyrotoxic or thyrotropic.
- **Tumors**
  - Lymphoma or lymphosarcoma
  - Secondaries from neuroblastoma
  - Leukemic infiltrates.
- **Systemic diseases**
  - Amyloidosis
  - Wegener's granulomatosis.

Causes of Acute Proptosis
- Orbital emphysema
- Fracture of medial orbital wall
- Orbital hemorrhage
- Rupture of ethmoidal mucocele.

Causes of Intermittent Proptosis
- Orbital varices
- Periodic orbital edema
- Recurrent orbital hemorrhage
- Highly vascular tumors.

Causes of Pulsating Proptosis
- Pulsating vascular lesions
- Caroticocavernous fistula
- Saccular aneurysm of ophthalmic artery
- Intermittent cerebral pulsation due to deficient orbital roof
- Meningoencephalocele
- Neurofibromatosis.

Investigations
- Clinical evaluation
- Laboratory investigations
- Imaging techniques
  - Noninvasive
  - Invasive
- Histopathological studies.

Clinical Evaluation
- History
- Local examination
- Systemic examination.

History
- Age of onset
- Duration
- Progression
- Associated symptoms.

Local Examination
- Inspection
- Palpation—compressibility
- Auscultation—bruit
- Transillumination
- Visual acuity
- Pupil reaction
- Fundus
- Ocular motility
- Exophthalmometry.

Systemic Examination
- To look for—thyrotoxicosis
  - Tumors elsewhere.

Histopathological Studies
- Fine needle aspiration biopsy
- Incisional biopsy
- Excisional biopsy.

Management
- Artificial tear drops
- Guanethidine 5% eye drops for lid retraction
- Systemic steroids
- Lateral tarsorraphy
- Squint surgery or orbital decompression.

8. What are the differences between proptosis and exophthalmos?

Proptosis	Exophthalmos
'Pro' means forward "Ptosis" means falling	"Exo" means outward "Ophthalmos" means eye
Mostly unilateral	Mostly bilateral
Can occur at any age	Affects adults between 20–40 years of age
Either sex affected	Affects females 4:1
Etiology is varied	Mostly endocrine
Passive protrusion due to space occupying lesion	Dynamic process due to active changes taking place in muscles and tissues of the orbit

9. Mention the investigations for diagnosing orbital tumors and the indications for referral.

Examination: Visual acuity, pupillary reaction, ocular motility, palpation and exophthalmometry
Imaging techniques: X ray of orbit, CT scan, B scan ultrasonography, MRI

To study the vasculature, orbital venography, carotid angiography or MR angiography can be performed.

Inflammatory lesions usually resolve with antibiotics and anti-inflammatory agents. If they do not resolve, it is better to get ENT and neurological opinion.

10. Write short notes on orbital tumors.

Orbital tumors are rare. They can be classified as benign and malignant or primary, secondary, and metastatic.

Common orbital tumors.		
Origin	Children	Adult
Congenital	Dermoid cyst, teratoma	–
Vascular	Capillary hemangioma, lymphangioma	Cavernous hemangioma Hemangiopericytoma, orbital varices
Neural	Optic nerve glioma, plexiform neurofibroma	Optic nerve meningioma Schwannoma, neurofibroma
Mesenchymal	Rhabdomyosarcoma	Fibrous histiocytosis
Hemopoietic	Acute myeloid leukemia, histiocytosis	Lymphomas
Metastatic	Neuroblastoma, Ewing's sarcoma, Wilms' tumor	Breast, lungs and prostatic carcinoma

Treatment: Surgical Removal by Orbitotomy

- Anterior orbitotomy: This is best suited for tumors that are present anteriorly without extending deep into orbit or into the cranium. The approach is through upper or lower lids.
- Lateral orbitotomy: (Kronlein-Berke approach) is used for deeper tumors. This involves cutting the lateral wall.
- Transfrontal orbitotomy (Naffziger approach): This is done through the orbital roof and is best suited when the optic foramen is enlarged or for deeper tumors in posterior third of orbit.
- Temporofrontal orbitotomy—access to orbit through roof, anterior and middle cranial fossa simultaneously.

11. Write short notes on blowout fractures of orbit.

Blow out fractures are fractures which occur when the orbital walls are pressed indirectly. It is due to sudden rise in orbital pressure by a striking object greater than 5 cm in diameter. Blowout fracture is nature's way of protecting the globe from injury.

Clinical Features

- Periocular ecchymosis, subconjunctival hemorrhage and epistaxis
- Diplopia
- Enophthalmos
- Infraorbital anesthesia involving lower lid, cheek, upper lip and teeth.

Investigations

- Plain X-ray orbit (Water's view): Hanging drop sign in maxillary sinus due to herniation of orbital fat
- CT scan
- Forced duction test.

Management

- Avoid nose blowing, systemic antibiotics, analgesic and anti-inflammatory drugs and cold compresses.
- Surgical repair to restore continuity of orbital floor with or without orbital implant.
The optimum time for surgery is 10–14 days after injury.

Chapter 19: Neuro-ophthalmology

1. What are pupillary reflexes and list their pathways?

Pupillary Reflex
- Light reflex
- Near reflex
  - Convergence reflex
  - Accommodation reflex
- Psychosensory reflex.

Light Reflex
- Light shown to one eye
- Both pupils constrict
- Constriction of same pupil—direct light reflex
- Constriction of other pupil—indirect light reflex.

Afferent Pathway
- Impulses from retina
- Optic nerve
- Optic tract
- Pretectal nucleus in the midbrain
- Internuncial fibers connecting the pretectal nucleus with Edinger-Westphal nucleus of both sides
- This connection forms the basis of consensual light reflex
- Damage to internuncial fibers results in the light near dissociation.

Efferent Pathway
- From Edinger-Westphal nucleus in midbrain to 3rd nerve
- Inferior division of 3rd nerve
- Nerve to inferior oblique
- Ciliary ganglion
- Short ciliary nerve
- Sphincter pupillae
  - Convergence reflex
  - Accommodation reflex

Near Reflex
- Contraction of pupil on seeing near object
- Impulses from medial rectus
- Oculomotor nerve
- Mesencephalic root of fifth nerve
- Nucleus of Perlia
- Edinger-Westphal nucleus of both sides
- Motor fibers of the third nerve
- Accessory ciliary ganglion
- Sphincter pupillae.

Accommodation Reflex
- Impulses from retina
- Optic nerve
- Optic tract
- Lateral geniculate body
- Optic radiation
- Striate cortex of occipital lobe
- Occipito-mesencephalic tract
- Nucleus of perlia
- Edinger-Westphal nucleus of both sides
- Oculomotor nerve
- Accessory ciliary ganglion
- Sphincter pupillae and ciliary muscle.

Psychosensory Reflex
Dilatation of pupil in response to psychic and sensory stimuli.

2. Describe abnormal pupillary reactions.
- Afferent pupillary defect
  - Total afferent pupillary defect (TAPD)
  - Relative afferent pupillary defect (RAPD)
- Efferent pupillary defect
  - Direct and consensual reflex absent on the affected side.

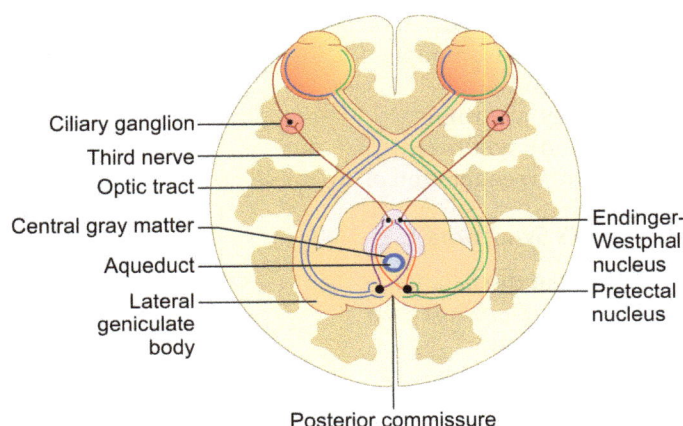

Fig. 19.1: Light reflex pathway.

Causes
- Parasympatholytic drugs
  - Atropine, homatropine, cyclopentolate
- Sympatholytic drugs
- Internal ophthalmoplegia
- Third nerve palsy.

Total Afferent Pupillary Defect
- Amaurotic pupil
  - Due to complete optic nerve lesion
  - No light perception
  - Afferent eye stimulated—both pupils do not react
  - Normal eye stimulated—both pupils react.

Relative Afferent Pupillary Defect (RAPD)
Marcus Gunn pupil

Causes
- Incomplete optic nerve lesion
- Severe retinal disease
- Swinging flash light test
- Each pupil stimulated in rapid succession
  - When abnormal pupil stimulated
  - Ill sustained contraction
- Usually seen in unilateral optic neuritis.

Other Causes of Abnormal Pupil
- Argyll Robertson pupil
- Adie's tonic pupil
- Wernicke's hemianopic pupil.

3. What is Argyll Robertson pupil?
- Accommodative reflex present
- Light reflex is lost
- Usually bilaterally miotic
- Light near dissociation
- Dilates well to atropine
- Seen in neurosyphilis
- Lesion at pretectal nucleus
- Damage to internuncial neuron
- Pupil—small and irregular due to focal iris atrophy.

4. What is Adie's pupil?
Adie's Tonic Pupil
- Unilateral (80%), dilated
- Usually in women (70%)
- 20–50 years of age
- Segmental contraction of pupil
- Due to selective activation of small segments of sphincter margin
- Light near dissociation
- Light reflex absent
- Slow tonic contraction of iris in near response
- Bright light accentuates parasympathetic palsy—larger pupil is abnormal.

Causes
- Parasympathetic denervation
- Super sensitivity: Ciliary ganglion affected due to herpes simplex virus (HSV)-1, measles, chickenpox
- Adie's syndrome: Loss of deep tendon reflexes secondary to degeneration of dorsal root ganglion cells
- Loss of neuron in ciliary ganglion.

5. What is Wernicke Hemianopic pupil?
- Site of lesion-optic tract
- Incongruous homonymous hemianopia
- Pupil response to light is normal in intact field absent in hemianopic field
- Contralateral hemianopic pupillary reaction.

6. What is Horner syndrome?
- Ipsilateral interruption of sympathetic outflow to the head and neck
- Unilateral triad of miosis, ptosis and anhidrosis and the mild enophthalmos
- Miosis: Dilator muscle paralysis
- Ptosis: Muller muscle paralysis
- Enophthalmos: Muller muscle paralysis
- Anhidrosis (absence of sweating): Sympathetic denervation
- Heterochromia iridis present in congenital Horner's syndrome
- Dim illumination accentuates sympathetic palsy: Smaller pupil is abnormal.

7. What is Hutchinson's pupil?
Unilateral dilated poorly reactive pupil in comatosed patients due to ipsilateral supratentorial mass causing uncal herniation entrapping 3rd nerve.

8. Write short notes on light near dissociation.
- Light reflex absent
- Near response intact.

Etiology
Damage to internuncial neuron which connects pretectal and Edinger-Westphal nucleus seen in:
- Argyll Robertson pupil
- Adie's pupil
- Riley day syndrome
- Parinaud's syndrome
- Aberrant regeneration of 3rd nerve.

Parinaud's Syndrome
- Light near dissociation
- Paralysis of upward gaze
- Lid retraction
- Dorsal midbrain lesion.

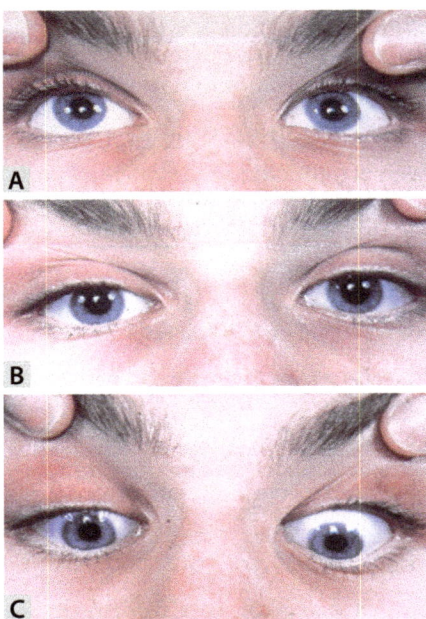

Figs. 19.2A to C: Parinaud's dorsal midbrain syndrome: A. Defective upgaze; B. Straight eye in primary position; C. Normal downgaze.

9. What is anisocoria?
Difference in size of pupils.

Causes
- 3rd nerve palsy
- Pharmacological
- Adie's pupil
- Iris damage
- Greater in bright light: The large pupil is abnormal
  - Defect in parasympathetic innervation - as in Adie's pupil
- Greater in dim light: Smaller pupil in abnormal
  - Defect in sympathetic innervation—as in Horner's syndrome
- Difference is same in both: Physiological.

10. Mention causes of dilated and constricted pupil.

Dilated pupil	Constricted pupil
3rd cranial nerve palsy	Horner's syndrome
Adie's tonic pupil	Argyll Robertson's pupil
Pharmacological mydriasis	Pharmacological miosis
Iris abnormalities	Iris abnormalities
Trauma	Pontine hemorrhage

11. Describe etiology, clinical features, differential diagnosis, and management of optic neuritis.

Inflammation of Optic Nerve
- Acute
  - Papillitis
  - Retrobulbar neuritis
  - Neuroretinitis
- Chronic
  - Toxic amblyopia.

Etiology
- Idiopathic
- Hereditary (Leber's disease)
- Demyelinating disorder
- Inflammation (from surrounding structures)
- Endogenous.

Demyelinating Diseases
- Multiple sclerosis
- Neuromyelitis optica (Devic's)
- Schilder's disease.

Endogenous Causes
- Acute infections—influenza, mumps, measles, and herpes zoster
- Septic foci—teeth, tonsil, and throat
- Metabolic—diabetes.

Papillitis
Acute inflammation of the optic nerve head with rapid loss of vision.

Pathogenesis
- Inflammation of a nerve or its sheath
- Loss of myelin sheath
- Degenerative changes and gliosis.

Symptoms
- Profound loss of vision
- Usually unilateral
- Sudden onset and rapid deterioration.

Signs
- Direct light reflex-sluggish
- Marcus Gunn pupil-(RAPD)
- Ill sustained contraction
- Fundus
  - Vitreous is cloudy
  - Blurred disc margin
  - Soft exudates near disk
  - Cup–Obliterates
  - Vein–Dilated, perivascular sheathing
- Field defect: Central or centrocecal scotoma
- Pulfrich phenomenon—altered perception of moving objects
- Uhthoff's sign—worsening of symptoms with exercise or increased body temperature.

Differential diagnosis

Features	Papilledema	Papillitis	Pseudoneuritis
Laterality	Usually bilateral	Usually unilateral	Usually bilateral
Vision	Transient attack of blurred vision	Sudden marked loss	Depends on degree of refractive error
Pain	Absent	May be present with ocular movements	Absent
Media	Clear	Haze	Clear
Disc swelling	2–6 D	< 3 D	Varies as per refractive error
Peripapillary edema	Present	Present	Absent
Venous engorgement	More marked	Less marked	Absent
Retinal exudates	More marked	Less marked	Absent
Macula—shape of exudates	Star	Fan	Absent
Fields	Enlarged blind spot	Central scotoma	No defect
Fundus fluorescent angiogram	Leakage of dye	Minimal	Absent

Treatment
- Injection methylprednisolone 1 g IV daily for 3 days followed by oral prednisolone 1 mg/kg for 11 days
- Injection methylcobalamin 500 mcg daily for 10 days
- Treatment of cause
- Intramuscular injection—interferon β1A.

12. Write short notes on retrobulbar neuritis.

Acute inflammation of optic nerve behind eyeball.

Symptoms
- Sudden loss of vision in acute cases
- Pain on ocular movements: Superiorly and medially.

Signs
- Pupil—ill sustained contraction
- Color vision—affected
- Fundus:
  - No visible sign
  - Temporal pallor may be present.

Differential Diagnosis of Retrobulbar Neuritis
- Malingering
- Hysterical
- Cortical
- Anterior ischemic optic neuropathy
  - Malingering: Pretending loss of vision
  - Hysterical: Psychiatric illness: To get attention

- Cortical blindness:
  - Occlusion of posterior cerebral artery
  - Hemorrhage or tumor in posterior cortical region.

Clinical Features of Cortical Blindness
- Formed visual hallucination involving hemianopic field
- Anton's sign—denial of blindness
- Riddoch's phenomenon—ability to perceive kinetic but not static targets.

Treatment of Retrobulbar Neuritis
- Retrobulbar injection of dexamethasone
- Systemic steroids
- Vasodilator
- Injection methylcobalamin 500 mcg daily for 10 days.

Neuroretinitis

Inflammation of disc and neighboring retina involving macula:
- Macular exudates in star pattern
- Often follows viral infection
- Not due to demyelination.

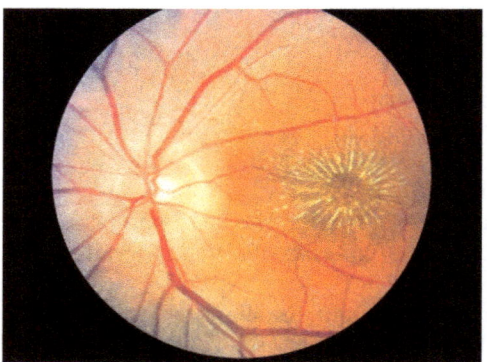

Fig. 19.3: Neuroretinitis.

Treatment
- As per optic neuritis
- Often self-limiting.

13. Describe anterior ischemic optic neuropathy (AION).

Segmental or generalized infarction of anterior part of optic nerve occlusion of posterior ciliary arteries.

Types
- Arteritic
- Nonarteritic—seen in hypertension or arteriosclerotic persons.

Arteritic Type
- Also called giant cell arteritis
- Predilection for large and medium sized arteries
- Especially superficial temporal, ophthalmic and posterior ciliary arteries

- Affects elastic tissue in walls of arteries
- Age group > 65 years.

Clinical Features
- Sudden profound unilateral loss of vision
- Periocular pain
- Preceded by transient visual obscuration
- Scalp tenderness
- Severe headache and neck pain
- Tender inflamed nodule in arteries
- Fundus: Disk—pale and swollen
  - Splinter hemorrhage on disc margin
  - Disc becomes atrophic in 2 months.

Differential diagnosis.

Features	Arteritic AION	Non-arteritic AION
Age	> 60 years	40–60 years
Etiology	Giant cell arteritis	Seen in hypertensives, arteriosclerotic patients
Symptoms	Scalp tenderness, headache, vision <6/60	Painless, vision >6/60
Laterality	Bilateral in 90%	Bilateral in <30%
Optic disc	Swollen, pale	Hyperemic
ESR	>40 mm/hour	<40 mm/hour
Treatment	Intravenous steroids followed by oral steroids	Control of hypertension and diabetes, levodopa - carbidopa for 2 months

Investigations
- ESR > 60 mm Hg
- Raised C-reactive protein
- Temporal artery biopsy
- Fields—inferior altitudinal defect.

Treatment
- IV Methyl prednisolone 1 g daily for 3 days followed by oral prednisolone 80 mg for 3 days, 60 mg for 3 days, 40 mg for 3 days.
- Reduce weekly gradually and continue 10 mg daily for 1 to 2 years.

Non-arteritic Type

Mono-ocular sudden painless loss of vision. Disk and fields are same as in arteritic type.

Investigations
- Abnormal lipid profile
- Increased viscosity of blood

Treatment
- Underlying disease
- Stop smoking
- Low dose aspirin to prevent affection of other eye
- Levodopa, Carbidopa combination for 3 weeks. Double the dose for the next one month.

14. Describe etiology, clinical features, differential diagnosis, and management of papilledema.

Definition

Non-inflammatory edema of optic disc, usually secondary to raised intracranial pressure (ICP).

Disc swelling not associated with raised ICP is called "Disk edema".

Etiology
- Raised ICP
- Orbital space occupying lesions
- Ocular causes.

Raised ICP
- Intracranial space occupying lesions:
  - Brain tumors, abscess, tuberculoma, etc.
  - Space occupying lesions of cerebellum, mid brain, parieto-occipital region produce papilledema more rapidly
- Meningitis, encephalitis
- Subarachnoid hemorrhage
- Pseudotumor cerebri
- Systemic conditions
  - Malignant hypertension
  - Toxemia of pregnancy
  - Leukemia and polycythemia.

Orbital Space Occupying Lesion

Tumors, abscess, cellulitis, pseudotumors, endocrine exophthalmos.

Ocular Causes

Central retinal vein occlusion, increased IOP, ocular hypotony.

Pathogenesis of Papilledema

Stasis of axoplasmic transport in prelaminar region of optic disc due to alteration in the pressure gradient across the lamina cribrosa.

Foster Kennedy Syndrome
- Pressure atrophy of optic nerve on the side of lesion due to direct pressure
- Papilledema on the other side due to raised intracranial pressure.

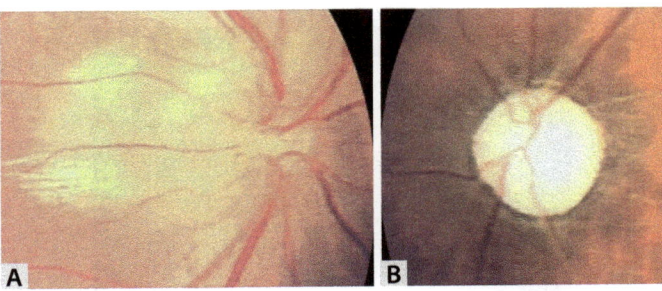

Figs. 19.4A and B: Foster-Kennedy syndrome. A. Papilledema due to generalized raised intracranial pressure; B. Optic atrophy due to mass lesion in optic nerve.

Causes

Tumor of frontal lobe, pituitary or olfactory groove meningioma.

Clinical Features of Papilledema

Symptoms
- Recurrent attacks of transient blurred vision
- Vision remains normal till last stage
- General symptoms: Headache, projectile vomiting.

Signs
Fundus examination.

Stages
- Early—established
- Late or chronic—atrophic

Early Papilledema
- Disk
  - Color: Hyperemic and mild elevation
- Margins Blurred: Nasal margins first followed by superior, inferior, and temporal margin
- Absence of spontaneous venous pulsation (absent in 20% of normals)

Established Papilledema
- Disc: Marked hyperemia
- Margin: Indistinct
- Cup: Obliterated
- Disc edema: 3-6 D
- Veins: Dilated and tortuous
- Hemorrhage: Peripapillary

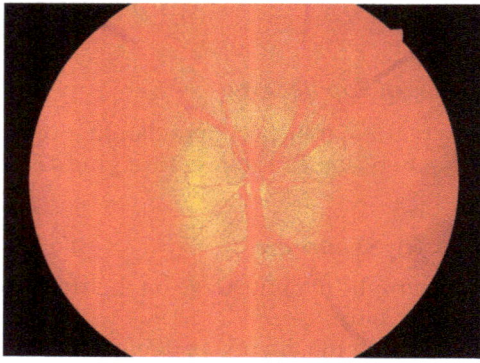

Fig. 19.5: Early papilledema.

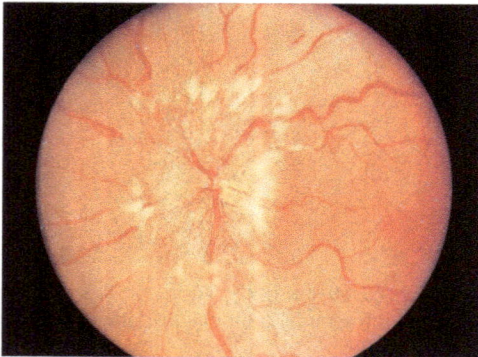

Fig. 19.6: Established papilledema.

- Exudate: Cotton wood spots
- Macula: Macular star
- Paton's line (due to retinal folds)
- Fundus fluorescein angiography (FFA): Dilated disc capillaries.

Late or Chronic
- Later increasing hyperfluorescence beyond disc margin in FFA
- Disc markedly elevated
- Champagne cork appearance.

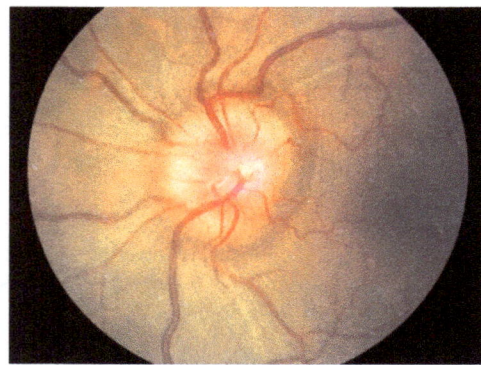

Fig. 19.7: Late or chronic papilledema.

Atrophic or End Stage
- Postpapilledemic optic atrophy
- Disc greyish white
- Pale disc with indistinct margin
- Vessels attenuation and sheathing
- Fields—enlarged blind spot and later progressive contraction of visual fields.

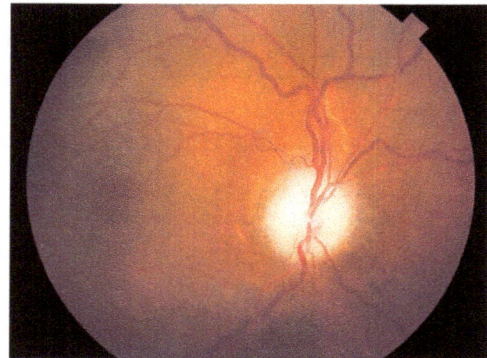

Fig. 19.8: Atrophic or end stage papilledema.

Differential Diagnosis
- Papillitis
- Pseudoneuritis
- Malignant hypertension
- Central retinal vein occlusion (CRVO)
- Toxemia of pregnancy
- Bilateral anterior ischemic optic neuropathy (AION)
- Drusen of optic nerve head.

Treatment
- Treat the underlying cause
- Surgical decompression before visual field changes occur

- Immediate medical treatment—diuretics, oral acetazolamide and intravenous mannitol
- Papilledema takes 4–6 weeks to appear and resolves in same duration when treated.

15. Describe etiology, clinical features, differential diagnosis, and management of optic atrophy.

Degeneration of optic nerve resulting from damage to axons from retinal ganglion cells to lateral geniculate body.

Types
- Ascending type
  - Toward brain—takes 1 week
- Descending type
  - From optic tract towards disc—takes 1 month.

Pathology
- Degenerative and excessive gliosis
  - Consecutive and post-neuritic optic atrophy
- Degenerative and orderly gliosis
  - Primary optic atrophy
- Degenerative and negligible gliosis
  - Cavernous, glaucomatous and ischemic optic atrophy.

Clinical Types
- Primary optic atrophy
- Consecutive optic atrophy
- Postneuritic optic atrophy
- Glaucomatous
- Ischemic or vascular.

Primary Optic Atrophy
- Lesion is behind optic disc
- No sign of inflammation
- Usually seen in lesions of CNS disease.

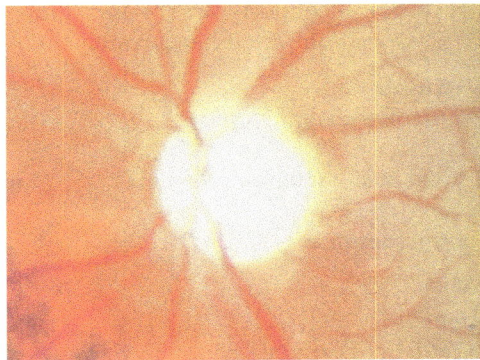

Fig. 19.9: Primary optic atrophy.

Etiology
- Multiple sclerosis
- Idiopathic retrobulbar neuritis
- Pituitary tumor
- Toxic amblyopia
- Tabes dorsalis
- Leber's hereditary optic atrophy
- Trauma to optic nerve.

Fundus of Primary Optic Atrophy
- Disk: Grayish white or white
- Margin: Defined
- Lamina cribrosa: Visible
- Retinal vessels and surrounding retina normal.

Consecutive Optic Atrophy
Secondary to degeneration of inflammation of choroid and retina.

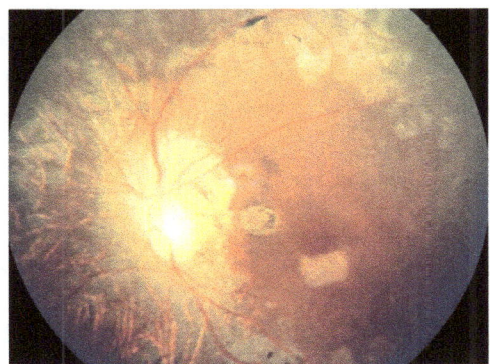

Fig. 19.10: Consecutive optic atrophy.

Causes
- Retinitis pigmentosa
- Diffuse chorioretinitis
- Pathological myopia.

Fundus
- Disc: Yellowish waxy color
- Margins: Ill defined
- Vessels: Attenuated
- Retina: Usually abnormal.

Postneuritic Optic Atrophy (also called Secondary Optic Atrophy)
Due to longstanding papilledema or papillitis.

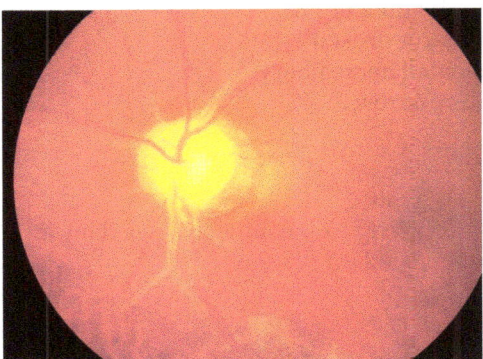

Fig. 19.11: Postneuritic optic atrophy (also called secondary optic atrophy).

Fundus
- Disc: Dirty white
- Margins: Blurred
- Cup: Filled
- Lamina cribrosa: Not seen

- Vessels
  - May be attenuated
  - Perivascular sheathing
- Macula
  - Stippling may be seen.

Features	Primary	Secondary
Clinical appearance	Chalky white	Grayish in color
Margins	Sharply defined	Blurred
Cup	Deep	Obliterated
Laminar dots	Seen	Not seen
Glial proliferation	Absent	Marked
Sheathing of vessels	Not present	Present
Previous optic disc edema	Absent	Present

Difference between primary and secondary optic atrophy.

Glaucomatous Optic Atrophy

Cause: Raised IOP.

Fundus
- Disc: Deep and wide cupping
- Margins: Well defined
- Vessels: Bayonetting sign
- Vessels appear broken at the margin and nasal shifting
- Neuroretinal rim: Pale.

Vascular (Ischemic) Optic Atrophy

Due to ischemia other than glaucoma.
- Central retinal artery occlusion (CRAO): Giant cell arteritis
- Severe hemorrhage and anemia
- Quinine poisoning.

Fundus:
- Pale disc
- Vessels: Marked attenuation.

Differential Diagnosis of Optic Atrophy

- Optic nerve hypoplasia
- Disc coloboma or pit
- Optic nerve drusen
- Myelinated nerve fibers
- Tilted optic disc.

Treatment
- As per the cause
- Injection Methylcobalamin 500 mcg daily for 10 days
- To be repeated every week.

16. Describe etiology, types, clinical features, differential diagnosis, and management of toxic amblyopia.

Refers to chronic retrobulbar neuritis caused by poisons like tobacco, alcohol, etc.
- Frequently bilateral
- Permanent visual loss.

Etiological Types

- Tobacco
- Ethyl alcohol
- Methyl alcohol
- Lead
- Quinine
- Chloroquine
- Ethambutol
- Oral contraceptives.

Tobacco Amblyopia

It occurs in men who are smokers, heavy drinkers, and have a diet deficient in proteins, and vitamin B complex. It occurs after one year of exposure. The causative factor is cyanide in tobacco leaves.

Pathogenesis

Degeneration of ganglion cells in macula and papillomacular bundle.

Pathology
- Ascending degeneration of ganglion cells
- Failure of choline synthesis
- Choline is precursor of myelin.

Clinical Features
- Increasing fogginess of vision
- Vision reduced to 6/60
- Defective near vision
- Fundus:
  - Normal or slight temporal pallor
- Field
  - Centrocecal scotoma.

Treatment
- Abstinence from tobacco
- General nutrition to be improved
- Injection methylcoblamin 500 mcg daily for 1 week
- Vasodilators.

Ethyl Alcohol Amblyopia

- Seen in chronic alcoholism with malnutrition
- Occur in association with tobacco amblyopia.

Clinical Features
- Similar to tobacco amblyopia
- Fundus
  - Normal or slight temporal pallor
- Field
  - Central scotoma.

Treatment
- Abstinence
- Improvement of general health
- Vitamin B complex
- Vasodilators.

Methyl Alcohol Amblyopia

Intake of methylated spirit in adulterated beverages.

Pathogenesis
- Methyl alcohol is oxidized to formic acid and formaldehyde
- They cause edema followed by degeneration of ganglion cells and retina
- Results in blindness due to optic atrophy.

Clinical Features
- 4–5 mL—visual loss
- 30 mL—death
- Headache, dizziness, vomiting, abdominal pain, delirium, stupor, and death
- Acidosis due to imperfect oxidation of methyl alcohol
- Formation of formaldehyde and formic acid in blood and tissue
- Fundus
  - Edema of disk and surrounding retina
  - Postneuritic optic atrophy
- Field
  - Central scotoma
  - Peripheral contraction.

Diagnosis
- Occurs in group
- Abdominal pain, vomiting, and dizziness
- Characteristic odor due to formic acid in breath and sweat.

Treatment
- Gastric lavage
- 3% sodium bicarbonate 200 cc IV
- 100 cc every 6 hours
- Oral 5 g powder
- Ethyl alcohol substitution in early stages—90 cc every 3 hours for 3 days
- Injection methylcobalamin 1 g IM daily for 6 days
- Injection furosemide 20 mg 6th hourly.

Lead Amblyopia
- Used in pottery industry
- Optic neuritis, optic atrophy, retinopathy.

Quinine Amblyopia
- More than 60 mg daily in susceptible individuals
- Pupil dilated and fixed
- Deafness and tinnitus
- Fundus:
  - Pallor of disc and attenuation of vessels
  - Retinal edema
- Field
  - Tubular vision.

Chloroquine Amblyopia
- Toxicity: Retinopathy, myopathy
- Fundus:
  - Bull's eye lesion in macula
  - Pigmentary retinopathy
  - Attenuated vessels.

Ethambutol Amblyopia
- Upper limit 15 mg/kg
- Toxicity occurs 2 months after therapy
- Fundus
  - Optic neuritis
  - Swollen disc with splinter hemorrhages
  - Color vision is affected
- Field
  - Central scotoma
  - Reversible when stopped.

Oral Contraceptives
- Increased risk of vascular occlusion
- Infarction of optic nerve head
- Hypertension, migraine, and vascular disorder.

CHAPTER 20

Squint

1. Define squint.
Ocular misalignment either with abnormalities in binocular vision or anomalies of neuromuscular control. It literally means to look obliquely.

2. What is the incidence of squint?
- Incidence: 2%
- By 1 year 50% become evident
- By 4 year 80% become evident.

3. What is orthophoria, heterophoria, and heterotropia?
- Orthophoria: Perfect ocular balance
- Heterophoria: Ocular deviation kept latent by the fusional mechanism—latent squint
- Heterotropia: Ocular deviation that is manifest and not kept under control by the fusional mechanism—manifest squint.

4. Classify squint.
- Pseudostrabismus
  - Pseudoesotropia: Broad epicanthal fold
  - Hypertelorism (wide inter pupillary distance): Pseudoexotropia
- Heterophoria (latent)
  - Esophoria: Exophoria
  - Hyperphoria: Hypophoria
- Heterotropia (manifest).

Comitant Squint
Although the eyes are misaligned, they retain their abnormal relation to each other in all directions of gaze. Here the afferent pathway or the central mechanism mediating fixation and fusional reflexes are abnormal.

There is no symptom. No diplopia or limitation of ocular movement. The primary deviation is equal to the secondary deviation. There will be cosmetic disfigurement. No binocular vision.

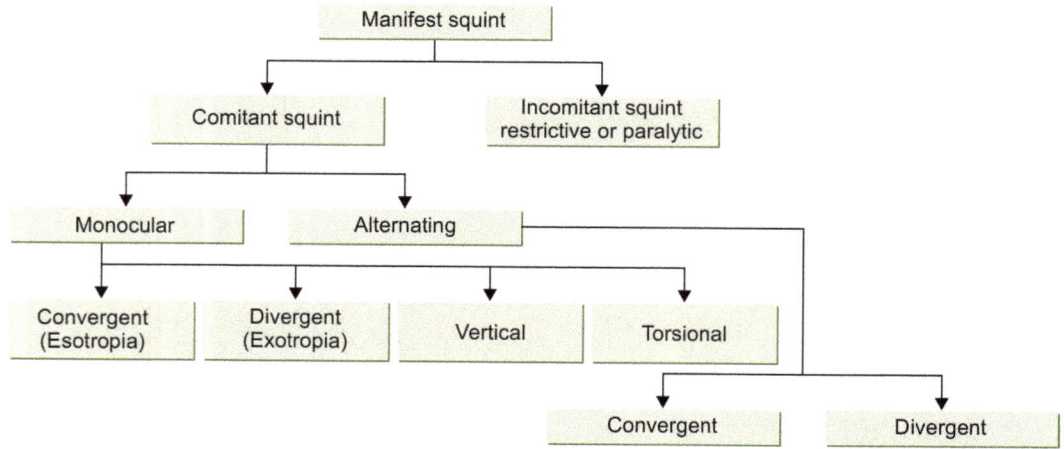

Tests for concomitant squint are:
i. Hirschberg test
ii. Cover test
iii. Synoptophore test

Management is given in question no 18 of the same chapter.

Incomitant Squint

Eyes are misaligned but it is not the same in all directions of gaze. Efferent pathway is abnormal.
- Incomitant squint may be paralytic or restrictive
- In paralytic squint the afferent pathways and centers are intact but the efferent mechanism breaks down
- In restrictive squint, there is a mechanical factor such as tight or fibrosed muscle which leads to a limitation of movements. The ocular deviation in the primary position is much smaller in proportion to the limitation of ocular movement. Common types of restrictive squint are:
    - Duane's retraction syndrome
    - Brown's superior oblique sheath syndrome
    - Dysthyroid ophthalmopathy
    - Strabismus fixus
    - Orbital trauma like blowout fracture.

5. What is primary and secondary deviation?

Primary Deviation

It is the deviation measured with normal eye fixing and paretic eye deviating.
- Normal eye fixation
- Other eye deviation.

Secondary Deviation

It is the deviation measured with the paretic eye fixing and the normal eye deviating.
- Deviated eye fixation
- Normal eye deviation.

6. What are the differences between comitant and incomitant squint?

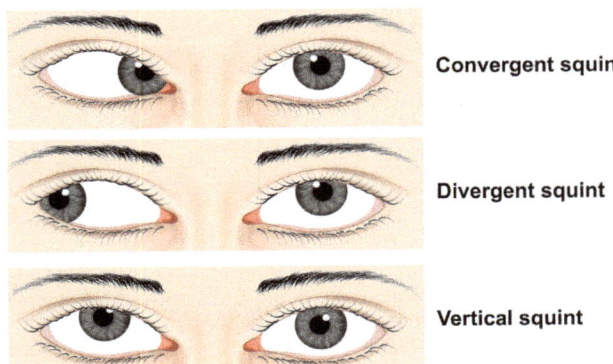

Fig. 20.1: Types of squint.

Features	Comitant squint	Incomitant squint
Degree of squint	Same in all direction	Varies with eye position
Diplopia	Absent	Present
Ocular movements	Full	Restricted
False projection	Absent	Present
Abnormal head posture	Absent	Usually present
Secondary deviation	Same as primary	More than primary

7. What is esotropia and exotropia?

Esotropia (Convergent Squint)

The eye is rotated so that cornea deviates nasally and the fovea is rotated temporally and visual axes converge.

Exotropia (Divergent Squint)

The eye deviates temporally and the fovea is rotated nasally and visual axes diverge.

8. What is vertical squint?

Vertical strabismus can be hyper or hypo.

In Hyper Type

- Cornea deviated superiorly
- Fovea rotated inferiorly.

In Hypo Type

- Cornea deviated inferiorly
- Fovea is rotated superiorly.

9. List different gaze positions.

- **Uniocular movements:** Duction
- **Binocular movements:** Version
- **Primary position:** Patient fixes eyes on an object in a straight ahead posture
- **Secondary position of gaze:** 4

From primary position moving the eye to right, left, up or down.

Tertiary Positions—4

i. Dextroelevation—up and right
ii. Levoelevation—up and left
iii. Dextrodepression—down and right
iv. Levodepression—down and left

Cardinal Positions—6

i. Dextroversion
ii. Levoversion
iii. Dextroelevation
iv. Levoelevation
v. Dextrodepression
vi. Levodepression

10. What is the origin, insertion, and action of extraocular muscles?

Extraocular Muscles

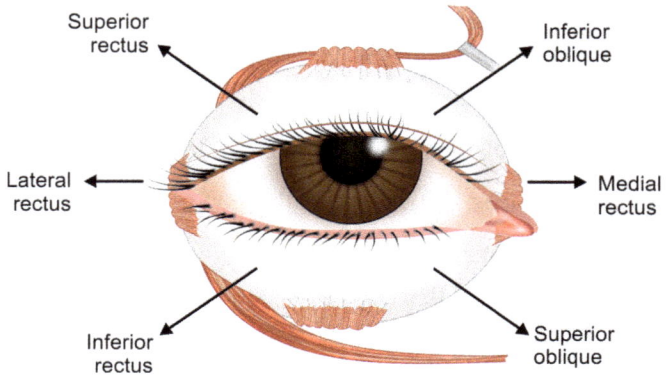

Fig. 20.2: Field of action of extraocular muscles.

Origin

All except inferior oblique arises from annular tendon of Zinn – Present around optic foramen at apex of orbit.

Inferior Oblique

Arises from medial wall and floor of orbit.

Insertion of Muscle

- Medial rectus: 5.5 mm from limbus
- Inferior rectus: 6.6 mm from limbus
- Lateral rectus: 7 mm from limbus
- Superior rectus: 7.7 mm from limbus
- Superior oblique: Above and lateral to posterior pole
- Inferior oblique: Below and lateral to posterior pole.

Actions of extraocular muscles.			
Muscle	Primary	Secondary	Tertiary
Medial rectus	Adduction	—	—
Lateral rectus	Abduction	—	—
Superior rectus	Elevation (best in abduction)	Intorsion	Adduction
Inferior rectus	Depression (best in abduction)	Extorsion	Adduction
Superior oblique	Intorsion (best in adduction)	Depression	Abduction
Inferior oblique	Extorsion (best in adduction)	Elevation	Abduction

Intorsion

Eye is rotated so that superior pole of vertical meridian is moved nasally and inferior pole rotated temporally.

Extorsion

Superior pole of vertical meridian moved temporally and inferior pole rotated nasally.

11. What are the laws of ocular motility?

- **Sherrington's law of reciprocal innervation**
  - Increased innervation accompanied by decreased innervation to its antagonist. For example, when medial rectus contracts, lateral rectus relaxes and vice versa.
- **Herring's law of equal innervation**
  - Equal and simultaneous innervation flows to the yoke muscle (contralateral synergist)
  - Basis of secondary deviation. For example right lateral rectus and left medial rectus contract simultaneously for dextroversion movements.

12. What are antagonists and synergists?

Synergists

Muscles having same primary action in same eye.
For example, superior rectus and inferior oblique of same eye act as elevators.

Antagonist

Antagonist having opposite action in same eye:
- Medial rectus and lateral rectus
- Superior rectus and inferior rectus
- Superior oblique and inferior oblique

Yoke Muscle—Pair of Muscles

- **Contralateral synergist:** One from each eye which contract simultaneously during version
  - *Dextroversion:* Right lateral rectus and left medial rectus; *Dextroelevation:* Right superior rectus and left inferior oblique; *Dextrodepression:* Right superior oblique and left inferior rectus
  - *Similarly to look left:* Levoversion, levoelevation and levodepression
- **Contralateral antagonist:** *Pair of muscles*
  - One from each eye having opposite action
  - Right lateral rectus and left lateral rectus
  - Right medial rectus and left medial rectus.

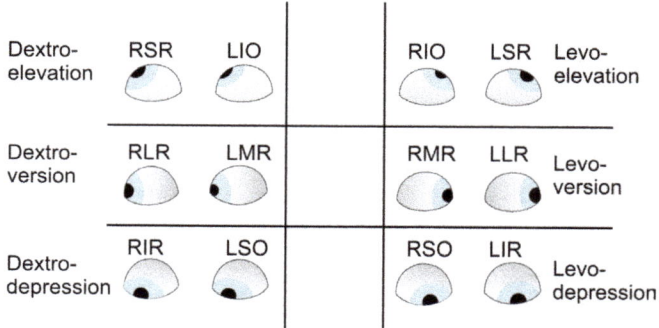

Fig. 20.3: Yoke muscles and their field of action.
(RSR: right superior rectus; LIO: left inferior oblique; LSR: left superior rectus; RIO: right inferior oblique; RLR: right lateral rectus; LMR: left medial rectus; LLR: left lateral rectus; RMR: right medial rectus; RIR: right inferior rectus; LSO: left superior oblique; LIR: left inferior rectus; RSO: right superior oblique)

13. What are the types of measuring angle of deviation in squint?

Useful for diagnosis and as a guide to treatment.

Corneal Reflection Tests
- Hirschberg's test
- Cover uncover test
- Alternate cover test
- Prism cover test
- Krimsky test.

Other Tests
- Using synoptophore
- Maddox rod
- Maddox wing.

Hirschberg Test
- Rough indication of angle of squint
- Degree of squint is assessed from the position of corneal reflex when light is thrown into the eye from a distance of 33 cm with ophthalmoscope or pen torch.

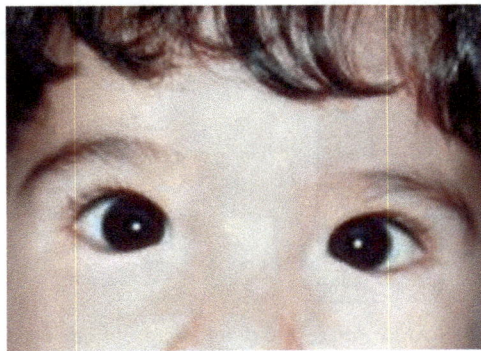

Fig. 20.4: Hirschberg's test showing left convergent squint.

Corneal Light Reflex – Hirschberg's Test
- 1 mm of deviation equals 7° of deviation
- 1° = 2 Prism diopter (2 PD)
- 7° = 15 PD
- Reflex of light at border of pupil—15° or 30 PD (prism diopters)
- Mid iris region (4 mm from center) 30° or 60 PD
- Limbus 45° or 90 PD.

Cover-uncover Test
To Detect Manifest Deviation
- Occlude each eye in turn and observe movement of uncovered eye
- Inward deviation reveals exotropia.

Uncover Test
To Detect Latent Deviation
- Occlude the first eye for a few seconds (less than 2 seconds)
- Look for movement of covered eye
- As the occluder is removed
- Repeat for other eye
- Inward movement of eye behind cover: Exophoria.

Alternate Cover Test
- Hold the occluder over one eye for 2 seconds to break fusion
  - Dissociates binocular fusion
- Rapidly move occluder to other eye
- Observe refixation shift of unoccluded eye
- Identifies full deviation (tropia + phoria)

- No shift = Orthophoria
- In cover test, movement of uncovered eye is observed. It is done to detect tropia or manifest squint
- In cover-uncover test, re-fixation movement of covered eye is observed. It is done to detect phoria or latent squint
- In alternate cover test, each eye is covered for 2 seconds alternatively. After the cover is removed, the examiner notes the re-fixation movement as it returns to pre-dissociated state.

Prism Cover Test
- Loose prisms or prism bar is placed in front of one eye with apex of prism pointing toward deviation and repeat the test till corrective movement of eye is neutralized
- The strength of prism which is needed for neutralization gives the objective angle of deviation.

All cover tests are performed for both distance and near. For near test, accommodative target is used.

Krimsky's Test
- In case one eye is blind, prisms are placed in front of seeing eye which fixates a light target
- Increasing strength of prism are applied till the corneal reflex is centered in the blind eye
- Prism reflection test
- Prism in front of fixing eye
- Spot light at 33 cm
- Measures manifest deviation.

Uses of Krimsky's Test
- Dense amblyopia in squinting eye
- In uncooperative patients
- Not useful in angle > 50 PD.

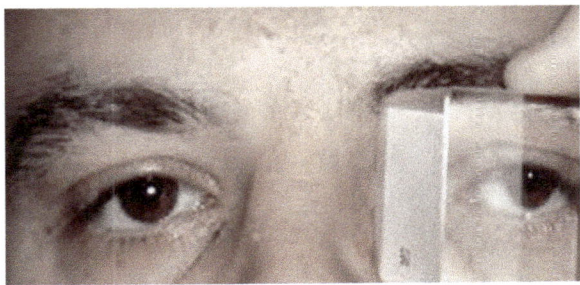

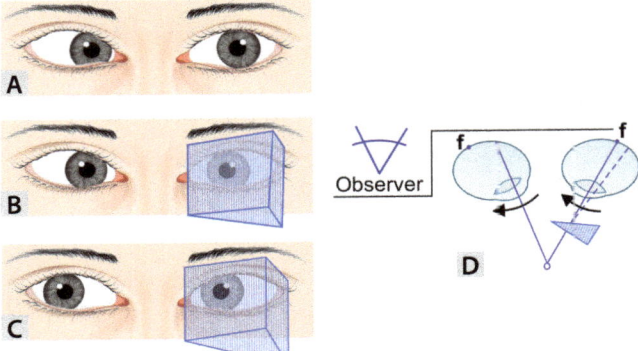

Figs. 20.5A to D: A. Right convergent squint; B. Prism over fixing eye; C. Squint neutralized by prism; D. Fixation movement of right eye.

Prism Cover Test

- More accurate
- Cooperation to maintain steady fixation
- Prism in front of squinting eye
- Apex of prism towards deviation
- Convergent squint—base out
- Alternate cover test is performed
- Prism negates movement
- Horizontal prism bar and loose vertical prism can be used.

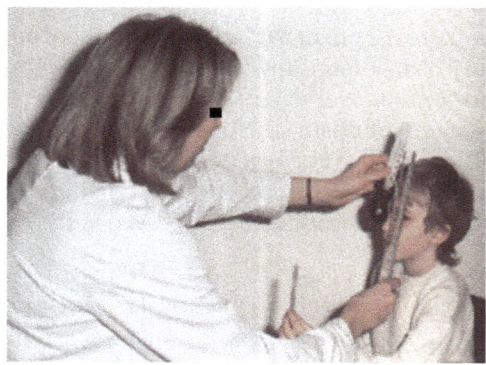

Fig. 20.6: Prism cover test.

Using Synoptophore

- Cover test principle
- Two picture slide in carriers
- Alternatively illuminated
- Movement of deviating eye
- Distance measurement
- More useful in:
  - Vertical and torsional deviation
  - To measure in 9 gaze positions.

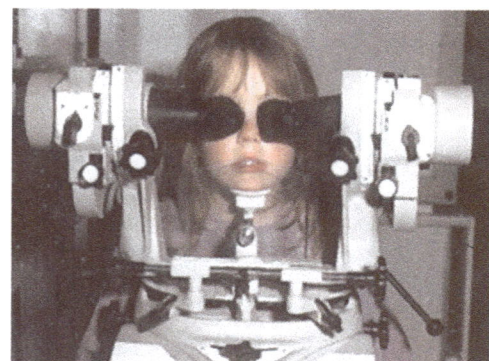

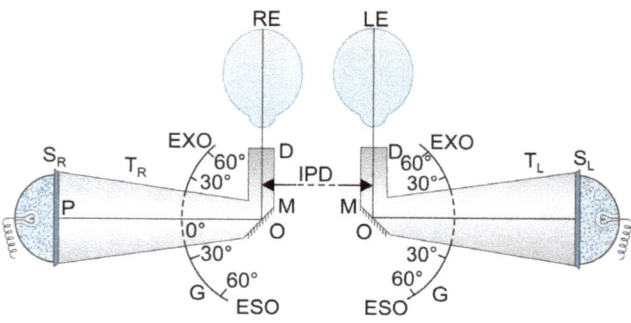

Fig. 20.7: Synoptophore.

14. How will you measure phoria for distant and near?

Maddox Rod Test

- To detect heterophoria for distance
- Fused cylindrical red glass rods in metallic disc is used (as in Maddox rod)
- Converts white spot of light to red streak
- Perpendicular to long-axis of rods. Due to dissimilar images of the two eyes, fusion is broken and heterophoria becomes obvious. The deviation can be measured by Maddox tangent scale or by prism placed in front of one eye with apex towards deviation.

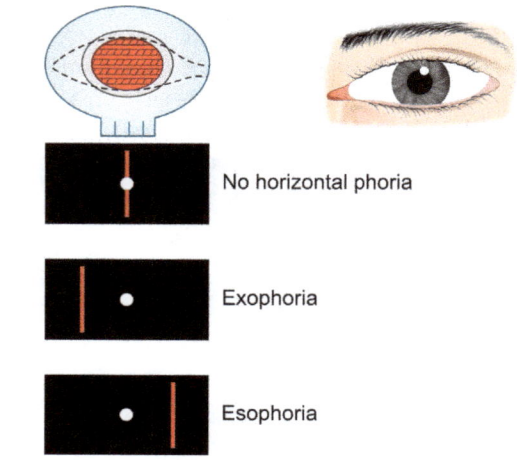

Fig. 20.8: Maddox rod test to detect heterophoria for distance.

Maddox Wing

Measures heterophoria for near:
- Red and white arrows seen by one eye
- Scale seen by other eye

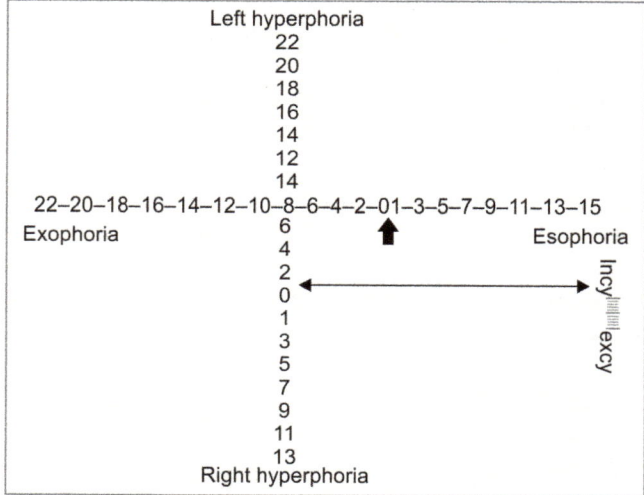

Fig. 20.9: Maddox wing test to detect heterophoria for near.

15. What are the binocular vision tests?

- Bagolini striated glasses
- Worth 4 dot test
- Synoptophore
- Tests for stereopsis

Bagolini Striated Glasses

Each lens is covered with fine striations which convert a point source of light into line similar to Maddox rod.
Two lenses are placed at 45° and 135° in front of each eye.

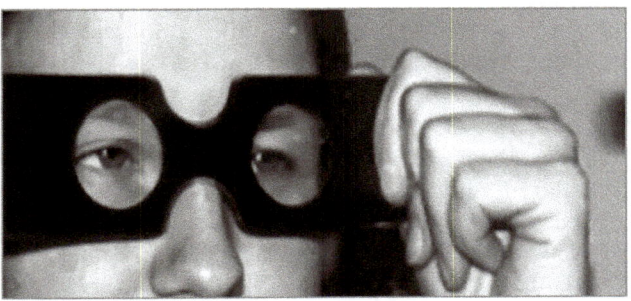

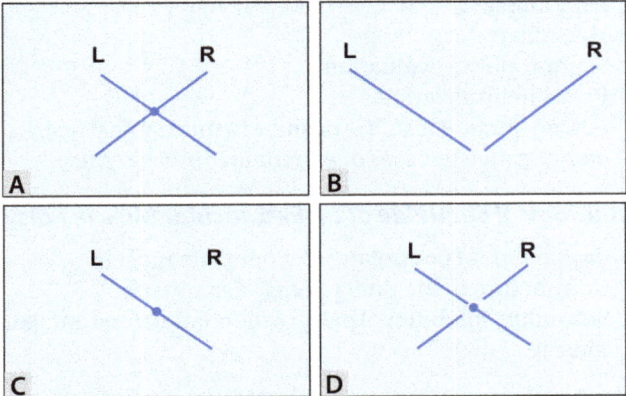

Figs. 20.10A to D: Possible results of the Bagolini striated lens test: A. Orthophoria; B. Diplopia; C. One eye suppression; D. Small gap denotes central suppression scotoma.

Synoptophore

It measures the angle of squint and state of binocular vision. It differentiates the three grades of binocular vision:
- Grade 1: Simultaneous macular perception
- Grade 2: Fusion
- Grade 3: Stereopsis.

Worth 4 Dot Test

- The patient wears the red lens in front of the right eye
- Green lens is placed on left eye
- The patients views the box with four lights (1 red, 2 green, 1 white)
- Usually incorporated in Snellen's test drum.

Tests For Stereopsis (same as Tests for Binocular Vision, Given in Physiology of Eye Chapter)

Frisby stereo test is commonly used. In this the patient is asked to identify the hidden circle in the squares with random shapes.

16. What are the types of esotropia?

Esotropia–Types

Comitant
- Accommodative:
  - Refractive (normal AC/A ratio)
  - Nonrefractive (high AC/A ratio)
  - Partially accommodative (mixed)
- Nonaccommodative:
  - Infantile
  - Acquired

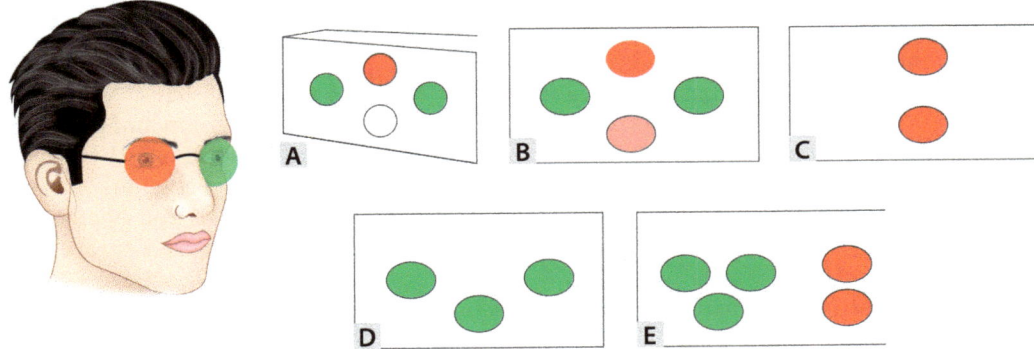

Figs. 20.11A to E: Worth 4 dot test: A. and B. Normal; C. Left eye suppression; D. Right eye suppression; E. Diplopia.

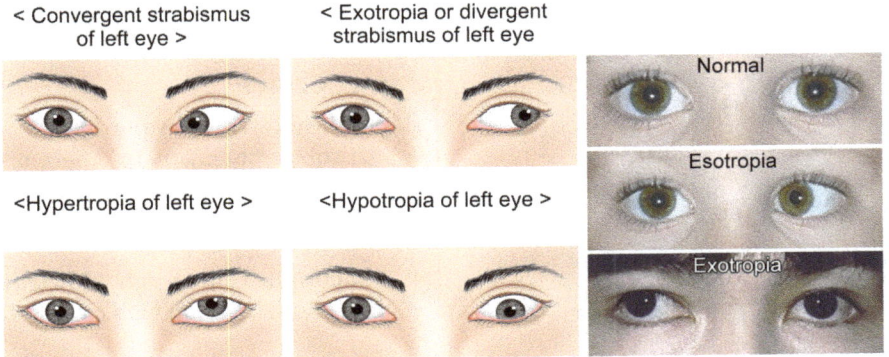

Fig. 20.12: Deviations in left eye.

Incomitant
- Paralytic
- Restrictive

17. What are the types of exotropia?

Types
- Convergence insufficiency: Exotropia at near > Distance fixation
- Divergence excess: Exotropia at distance > Near fixation
- Basic type: Exotropia at near = Distance fixation

18. What is the management of comitant squint?

Management of Heterophoria
- Correct refractive error
- Orthoptic exercises
- Prism
- Improvement of general condition

Management of Heterotropia
- *Concomitant squint management*
  - Nonsurgical
    - » Optical correction   - Prism
    - » Orthoptic exercises - Treatment of amblyopia
    - » Medical treatment   - Botulinum toxin
  - Surgical
- *Incomitant squint management*
  - Treat underlying cause
  - Surgical correction.

19. What are the principles of squint surgery?

- Muscle weakening procedures: Recession, marginal myotomy, and myectomy
- Muscle strengthening procedures: Resection, tucking, and advancement
- Procedures that change the direction of muscle action:
  - Vertical transposition of horizontal recti to correct A and V pattern
  - Posterior fixation suture (Faden procedure) to correct dissociated vertical deviation
  - Transplantation of insertion of muscle in paralytic squint.

20. Write short notes on paralytic squint.

Definition

It is ocular deviation due to paresis or paralysis of extraocular muscle.

Symptoms
- Diplopia
- Abnormal head posture
- History of injury
- Diabetes
- History of signs or raised intracranial pressure.

Signs
- Secondary deviation is > primary deviation
- Restriction of ocular movements (of paralyzed eye)
- Head is turned towards the direction of action of paralyzed muscle
- False projection or orientation due to increased innervational impulses to paralyzed muscle.

Diagnosis
- Cover test
- Ocular motility
- Weakness of paralyzed muscle
- Overaction of direct antagonist of paralyzed muscle
- Spread of comitance
- Diplopia test
- Hess chart
- Synoptophore evaluation
- Prism neutralization
- Forced duction test: It is positive in mechanical restriction and negative in cases of extraocular muscle palsy.

Pathological Sequelae of an Extraocular Muscle Palsy
- Overaction of contralateral synergistic muscle
- Contracture of the direct antagonist muscle
- Secondary inhibitional palsy of the contralateral antagonist muscle.

Management
- Acute phase: Medical
- Occlusion of paralytic eye to eliminate diplopia
- Prism
- Botulinum toxin to prevent contraction of antagonist.

Surgical
- Done after 6 months
- To restore binocular vision and cosmesis
- Strengthen paralyzed muscle by resection and weaken overacting muscle by recession
- Transplantation of insertion of adjacent muscles to the site of insertion of paralyzed muscle.

21. What is amblyopia?

Amblyopia means dull vision.

Definition

Partial or complete loss of vision in one or both eyes in the absence of ophthalmoscopic or other marked objective signs.

Types – Causes
- Strabismic: Due to squint
- Anisometropic: Due to difference in refractive power of more than 3 D between the eyes
- Form vision deprivation: Due to congenital cataract or any opacity in visual axis
- Ametropic: Due to high refractive power
- Meridional: Due to high astigmatism.

Treatment

- Correction of refractive error
- Occlusion: Full time or part time of good eye
- Penalization by cycloplegic—atropine is used to blur the normal eye
- Pleoptics—stimulating fovea of an amblyopic eye with prolonged sessions of dazzling light flashes to improve vision
- CAM stimulators—consists of viewing rotational high contrast stripes of different sizes
- Levadopa: Carbidopa.

22. What are the clinical features of third nerve palsy?

- Eye is divergent and depressed
- Ptosis due to paralysis of levator muscles
- Divergent squint with intorsion
- Limitations of movements in all direction except outwards
- Pupil is semidilated and fixed
- Loss of accommodation
- Diplopia on raising the upper lid.

23. What are the clinical features of fourth nerve palsy?

- Abnormal head posture, chin depression, head tilt and face turn to opposite side (normal side)
- Diplopia in downgaze—difficulty in walking downstairs
- Eyeball deviated upward and inward
- Restriction of ocular movement on downward and inward (common cause of isolated fourth nerve palsy is trauma).

24. What are the clinical features of sixth nerve palsy?

- Eyeball rotated inwards (convergent squint)
- Defective abduction of the eye
- Face turn towards the field of action of paralyzed muscle.

CHAPTER 21

Ocular Manifestations of Systemic Diseases

- Diabetes mellitus
- AIDS
- Tuberculosis
- Syphilis
- Leprosy
- Nutritional deficiency.

1. Enumerate the ocular manifestations in diabetes mellitus.

Ocular manifestations in diabetes mellitus.	
Lids	Chalazion, hordeolum internum/externum, blepharitis, ptosis (III nerve palsy), xanthelasma
Conjunctiva	Microcirculatory abnormalities, vasoconstriction of conjunctival vessels
Cornea	Decreased sensation, neurotrophic ulcers, increased thickness, persistent epithelial defects, infective keratitis, decreased endothelial cell count
Sclera	Episcleritis
Glaucoma	All types of glaucoma are common
Refraction	Index myopia, index hypermetropia and early presbyopia
Lens	Snow flake cataract, intumescent cataract
Vitreous	Asteroid hyalosis
Retina	Diabetic retinopathy, central retinal artery occlusion (CRAO), central retinal vein occlusion (CRVO), ocular ischemic syndrome
Optic nerve	Papillitis, anterior ischemic optic neuropathy, diabetic papillopathy
Cranial nerves	III, IV and VI nerve palsies
Orbit	Mucormycosis, orbital cellulitis

2. Describe the ocular manifestations in AIDS.

Etiology
- Caused by human immunodeficiency virus (HIV)
- RNA virus of human retrovirus family
- Immune complexes lead to small vessel disease
- Deficiency of T helper lymphocytes leading to inability to combat opportunistic infections.

Clinical Features
50–75% of adult AIDS patients manifest ocular lesions.
- Anterior segment lesions
- Posterior segment lesions
- Orbital infections
- Neuro-ophthalmic lesions.

Anterior Segment Lesions

Eyelids
- Herpes zoster ophthalmicus (HZO)
- Kaposi's sarcoma
- Molluscum contagiosum.

HZO
- Painful vesiculobullous dermatitis
- Involves ophthalmic branch of 5th Cranial nerve
- Caused by Varicella zoster virus
- Occurs when CD4 counts < 200/µL
- Treatment: Topical steroids, cycloplegics and intravenous drugs.

Kaposi's Sarcoma
- Seen in 25% of HIV patients
- Painless vascularized tumors affecting skin and mucous membranes
- Caused by Herpes virus type 8
- Multiple, small, blue-violet to black nodules affecting eyelid or conjunctiva. Rare in india.
- Treatment: Excision, radiotherapy or cryotherapy.

Molluscum Contagiosum
- Caused by DNA pox virus
- Multiple, pearly, papular umbilicated lesions affecting eyelid, skin and conjunctiva
- Treatment: Surgical excision, podophyllin or povidone iodine application.

Cornea
- Develop bacterial or fungal ulcer
- Herpes simplex keratitis.

Iris
Anterior uveitis with hypopyon.

Posterior Segment Lesions
- HIV retinopathy
- Cytomegalovirus retinitis

- Progressive outer retinal necrosis (PORN)
- Acute retinal necrosis (ARN)
- Toxoplasmic retinochoroiditis
- Mycobacterial infection.

HIV Retinopathy
- Seen in 50-75% of AIDS patients
- Cotton wool spots
- Retinal hemorrhages
- Microaneurysm
- Retinal ischemia.

Cytomegalovirus (CMV) Retinitis
- Retinal opportunistic infection
- Occur when CD4 < 50/µL
- Scattered yellowish white areas of necrotizing retinitis with hemorrhages and mild vitritis
- Cottage cheese or pizza pie appearance
- Progressive
- Incidence—30% before highly active antiretroviral therapy (HAART)
    - Now decreased.

Progressive Outer Retinal Necrosis
- Multifocal deep retinal lesion
- Retinal vessels—normal
- Dense white full thickness plaques
- Cracked mud appearance
- No vitreous inflammation
- Progressive and rapid.

Acute Retinal Necrosis
- Retinitis starts in extreme periphery
- Progressive circumferentially and rapid
- Lesions appear white with minimal hemorrhages
- Significant vitritis.

Treatment of viral retinitis
- Ganciclovir
- Foscarnet
- Cidofovir.

Toxoplasmic Retinochoroiditis
- Unifocal or multifocal
- Necrotising retinitis
- Similar to CMV retinitis.

Mycobacterial Infection
- Tuberculosis is common in HIV patients
- Present as choroiditis.

Orbital Infection
- Aspergillosis
- Mucormycosis.

Neuro-ophthalmic Infections
- Cranial nerve palsies
- Optic neuritis
- Pupillary abnormalities
- Brainstem ocular motility disorders.

3. Mention ocular manifestations in tuberculosis.

Ocular manifestations in tuberculosis.	
Lids	Ulceration of lid margin, ectropion
Conjunctiva	Purulent conjunctivitis, follicular conjunctivitis, pseudomembranous conjunctivitis, tuberculomas
Cornea	Phlyctenular keratoconjunctivitis, fascicular keratitis, interstitial keratitis
Uvea	Bilateral granulomatous anterior uveitis, conglomerate iris tubercles, choroidal granulomas, pars planitis, multifocal choroiditis
Retina	Eales's disease, retinal vasculitis
Sclera	Scleritis
Optic nerve	Optic neuritis, papilledema
Cranial nerves	Palsies
Orbit	Orbital cellulitis/abscess, periostitis, osteomyelitis, chronic dacryocystitis

4. Enumerate the ocular manifestations in syphilis.

Ocular manifestations in syphilis.	
Lids	Chalazion like induration, madarosis, symblepharon
Cornea	Interstitial keratitis
Iris	Acute plastic iritis
Pupil	Argyll Robertson pupil, internal ophthalmoplegia, paralysis of accommodation
Choroid, retina	Diffuse chorioretinitis, multifocal choroiditis, neuroretinitis
Optic nerve	Optic neuritis, papilledema, optic atrophy
Cranial nerves	III, IV and VI nerve palsies
Orbit	Periostitis, proptosis due to gumma in orbit

5. Mention the ocular manifestations in leprosy.

Ocular manifestations in leprosy.	
Lids	Madarosis, lagophthalmos, lower lid ectropion, trichiasis
Cornea	Exposure keratitis, neurotrophic keratitis, dry eye, pannus, interstitial keratitis
Lacrimal system	Acute dacryocystitis
Sclera	Episcleritis, scleritis, staphyloma
Uvea	Granulomatous uveitis, iris pearls, iris hole due to atrophy
Pupil	Miosis

6. Mention the ocular manifestations in nutritional deficiencies.

Ocular manifestations in nutritional deficiency.	
Vitamin A	Night blindness, xerosis, keratomalacia
Vitamin B1	Retrobulbar neuritis, Wernicke's encephalopathy
Vitamin B2	Corneal vascularization
Vitamin C	Hemorrhages in subconjunctiva, retina and orbit
Vitamin D	Zonular cataract in children

Ocular manifestations of vitamin A deficiency are given in Conjunctiva chapter.

CHAPTER 22

Community Ophthalmology

1. Define blindness.

World Health Organization (WHO) Definition of Blindness
- Vision < 3/60 in the better eye with the best correction
- Field restriction to 10 degrees.

National Programme for Control of Blindness (NPCB) Definition of Blindness
- Vision < 6/60 in the better eye with the best correction
- Field restricted to 20 degrees
  NPCB definition has been revised in 2017 as same as WHO definition, with the objective of generating data which can be compared with global estimate and achieve WHO goal of reducing the blindness prevalence of India to 0.3% of total population by the year 2020.

2. What is low vision? Mention the low vision aids.
(Refer question no. 13 for low vision aids)
- Vision 6/18 to 6/60 with the best correction in the better eye
- Restriction of the field as in anyone the following:
  - Reduction of field > 50 degrees
  - Hemianopia with macular involvement
  - Altitudinal defects.

Low Vision Aids
Types
Optical
- Contact lens
- Magnifying devices
- High plus reading glasses
- Microscopic lenses
- Telescopic lenses
- Projection devices.

Non-optical
- Large print books
- Large print typewriters
- Illumination devices to adjust the illumination.

3. Describe various types of blindness.

Economic Blindness
- Prevents from earning the wages
- Vision < 6/60
- Work vision.

Social Blindness
- Hampers social interaction
- Vision < 3/60
- Curtails movement
- Walk vision.

Manifest Blindness
- Vision < 1/60
- Daily living hampered.

Absolute Blindness
Inability to perceive light in any eye.

Legal Blindness
- Vision < 6/60
- Field restriction to 20 degrees
- Eligible for welfare measures.

Avoidable Blindness – 50%
- Includes preventable and curable blindness
- Preventable
  - Xerophthalmia
  - Trachoma
  - Glaucoma—early diagnosis
- Curable
  - Cataract
  - Refractive errors
  - Squint—early correction.

4. What is the prevalence of blindness in elderly age group?

Prevalence of blindness in elderly age group.	
Cataract	62.6%
Refractive error	19.7%
Glaucoma	5.8%
Posterior segment: Disorders	4.7%
Surgical complications	1.2%
Corneal opacities	0.9%
Miscellaneous	5.0%

5. What is the prevalence of blindness in children?

Prevalence of blindness in children.	
Whole eye anomalies	20%
Congenital cataract	11%
Corneal opacities	27%
Retinal affections	22%
Optic nerve and CNS affections	15%
Glaucoma	3%
Other causes	2%

Blindness statistics.		
	World	India
Blind	45 million	12 in millions
Low vision	135 million	36 in millions

Incidence of Blindness
- Every 5 seconds one adult goes blind
- Every 1 minute one child goes blind.

6. What is legal blindness?
Legal blindness is a level of vision loss that has been legally defined to determine eligibility for benefits. The clinical diagnosis refers to visual acuity of <6/60 or less in the better eye with best possible correction and/or visual field is 20° or less.

Legal Blindness - Categories of Visual Disability
Legal blindness is based on disability criteria and according to this, compensation is given to the individual.
- Better eye vision less than 3/60 or field less than 10°—100% impairment
- Better eye vision less than 6/60 or field less than 20°—75% impairment
- Better eye less than 6/18 or worse eye less than 6/60—40% impairment
- Better eye 6/6 and worse eye less than 1/60—one eyed—30% impairment.

7. What is childhood blindness and how will you control it?

Definition
Corrected vision < 6/60—below 15 years.

Prevalence
- Developing countries—0.8 per 1,000
- Developed countries—0.3 per 1,000

Anatomical Classification
- Whole globe—20%
- Cataract—11%
- Corneal opacity—27%
- Retina—22%
- Glaucoma—3%.

Etiological Classification
- Corneal scarring
- Congenital anomalies of whole eye
- Retinal dystrophies
- Cataract
- Optic atrophy.

Ocular Trauma
20-40% of one eyed blindness.

Avoidable Blindness
- 30%—preventable
- 20%—treatable.

Preventable Causes
- Vitamin A deficiency
- Malnutrition
- Ophthalmia neonatorum
- Congenital rubella
- Birth hypoxia
- Trachoma.

Vitamin A Deficiency
- Nutrition education
- Breastfeeding
- Food supplementation
- Food fortification.

Malnutrition
- Diarrhea
- Protein deficiency
- Eruptive fevers.

Ophthalmia Neonatorum
- Ocular prophylaxis of newborn
- Topical antibiotics after cleaning the eyelids.

Congenital Rubella
- MMR vaccine
- Immunization of girls before puberty or before marriage.

Birth Hypoxia
- Good antenatal care
- Care during delivery.

Treatable Causes
- Cataract
- Glaucoma
- Corneal scar
- Refractive error and early treatment of squint.

Congenital Cataract
- Prompt surgery
- Good refractive correction.

Glaucoma
- Early diagnosis
- Prompt surgery.

Corneal Scar
Keratoplasty.

Refractive Error
School eye screening.

Control of Blindness
- Primary level
- Secondary level
- Tertiary level.

Primary Level
- Health Education
- Vitamin A rich food
- Safe water and basic sanitation
- Maternal and child health care
- Immunization
- Early treatment of corneal injuries.

Secondary Level
- Management of corneal injuries and ulcers
- Refraction and prescription of glasses
- Cataract surgery.

Tertiary Level
- Retinopathy of prematurity: Screening and treatment
- Treatment of amblyopia and squint correction
- Genetic counselling and research.

Role of Vision 2020 Program
- Pediatric ophthalmology units
- Eye banking and corneal transplantation
- Training of personnel
- Strengthening school eye screening program.

8. What are the causes of corneal blindness?
a. Corneal ulcer
b. Corneal trauma
c. Keratomalacia due to Vitamin A deficiency
d. Corneal dystrophies
e. Trachoma

Corneal opacity due to trauma is the most common cause of childhood blindness.

9. Write short notes on district blindness control society (DBCS).

Aim of DBCS
To decentralize blindness control activities in the country.

Formation of DBCS
- Introduced in 1991 as pilot project in Salem for Tamil Nadu
- Extended to all districts in 1994.

Features of DBCS
- Autonomous society to implement NPCB
- Decentralized planning, management and monitoring
- Empowered to utilize and raise funds
- Forum for community participation.

Composition
- Government Sector
- NGO's
- Private practitioners
- Media
- Social service organizations
- Other bodies interested in eye care.

Organizational Set-up
- Chairman – District collector
- District program manager:
  - Member secretary and technical advisor
  - District ophthalmic surgeon or HOD (ophthalmology) of medical college.
  - Members – NGO's and private sector.

Functions of DBCS
- To plan, implement, and monitor all blindness control activities in the district
- To assess magnitude of blindness in the district
- To prepare annual plan of action
- Organization of school eye screening
- To organize training course for eye care personnel
- Collection, compilation and reporting of eye care activities to state blindness control society
- To conduct review meeting of paramedical ophthalmic assistants (PMOA's)
- Information education communication (IEC) activities in eye care in the district.

10. Discuss the objectives, organizational structure, and activities of national program for control of blindness (NPCB).
- Objectives
- Organizational structure
- Levels of eye care service delivery
- Main activities
- Highlights of revised pattern.

Objectives of NPCB
Goal-Reduction in prevalence of blindness
- To reduce backlog of blindness
- To develop comprehensive eye care services in every district
- To expand coverage of eye care services to underserved areas
- To provide high quality eye care services to the population
- Providing support for equipment, material and training.

Organizational Structure of NPCB
- *Central level*
  - Directorate General of Health Services
  - Ministry of Health and Family Welfare, New Delhi
- *State level*
  - State ophthalmic cell
  - State blindness control society
  - Directorate of health services

- State health societies
- (State health secretary is the chairman)
- *District level*
  - District Blindness Control Society (Collector is the chairman).

Levels of Eye Care Service Delivery

- Tertiary Level
- Secondary Level
- Primary Level

Tertiary Level

- Regional institutes of ophthalmology: Centers of excellence in eye care (NGOs and private sector)
  - Medical colleges.

Secondary Level

- District hospitals
- NGO eye hospitals.

Primary Level

- Taluk hospitals
- Upgraded PHC's
- Vision centers/PHCs.

Functions

Tertiary Level

- Centers of Excellence and Regional Institutes:
  - Overall leadership
  - Supervision and guidance to technical matters in planning and implementation of program
  - Sophisticated eye care
  - Specialized training program for medical personnel to arrange CME programs.

Secondary Level

- Treatment of common causes of blindness
- Mobile ophthalmic unit to conduct eye camps.

Primary Level

- Primary eye care
- Treatment of common eye diseases
- Correction of refractive error
- Vitamin A prophylaxis.

Main Activities of NPCB

- Cataract surgery with IOL implantation
- School eye screening
- Eye banking
- Eye care education
- Training of health personnel
- Teleophthalmology.

Five Steps to Control Blindness

i. Identify the blind and list them in village register
ii. Organize screening camps for detection of cataract, refractive errors, glaucoma, and diabetic retinopathy for referral
iii. Transport the patient to the base hospital for further management
iv. Free treatment at base hospital
v. Follow-up of operated cases, carrying out refraction and providing best corrective spectacles.

Eye Care Education

- Community participation in the control of blindness by training one link worker in each village
- Public awareness through various media channels.

Highlights of Revised Patterns of Assistance - From NPCB

- Development of facilities for all causes of blindness as per global initiative 'Vision 2020; the right to sight'
- To prevent and control of childhood blindness:
  - Strengthening school eye screening program
  - Increase in collection of donated eyes
  - Developing pediatric eye wards.

11. Write short notes on school eye screening program.

- Screen all children for refractive errors by teachers
- Train teachers
- Refer children with refractive errors to paramedical ophthalmic assistants (PMOA) for refraction and others district hospitals or NGO hospitals
- Prescription of spectacles and other advice
- Provide children from poor families with free glasses
- Screen on annual basis.

12. What is vision 2020? Discuss objectives and measures taken to prevent blindness in vision 2020.

- Vision 2020 was launched in 1999. It aims at elimination of avoidable blindness by the year 2020. It has unique partnership of World health organization (WHO), International agency for prevention of blindness (IAPB), International Nongovernmental organizations (INGOs)
  - Motto of vision 2020 is Right to Sight.

Goal of Vision 2020

- Comprehensive eye care
- Coverage of underserved areas
- Institutional support for equipment, material and training.

Main Objectives

- Reduction in the burden of blindness diseases
- Human resource development
- Development of eye care infrastructure.

Plan of Action

- Disease control
  - Cataract control
  - Refractive errors and low vision
  - Diabetic retinopathy
  - Glaucoma
  - Corneal blindness
  - Childhood blindness.

Reduction of Disease Burden

Cataract Control

Objective:
- To improve the quantity and quality of cataract surgery
- To eliminate curable blindness with vision <3/60 in the better eye
- As cost effective as immunization
  - The objective under cataract program is to improve the quantity and quality of cataract surgery
  - The target fixed by Government of India is as follows:
    » To increase the cataract surgical rate to
      - 500/100,000 by 2010
      - 550 by 2015
      - 600 by 2020
    » To improve the presenting visual outcome of cataract surgery (> 80% to have visual outcome ≥6/18 after surgery) to conform to standards set by WHO
    » To increase the proportion of IOL surgery to 100% by the year 2010.

Refractive Errors
- Aim – To eliminate visual impairment and blindness due to refractive errors and other causes of low vision
- To provide corrective spectacles to poor people:
  - Screening
  - Refraction
  - Dispensing spectacles
  - Follow-up.

School Eye Screening
- 5 to 7 % of children have refractive errors
- Screening of children aged 10 to 14 years by trained teachers
- Refer children with suspected refractive errors to PMOAs at PHCs for refraction
- Provision of spectacles
- Screen on annual basis.

Low Vision

Retinitis pigmentosa and age related macular degeneration (ARMD):
- Reduction of vision < 6/18 to 6/60 in the better eye
- Affection of fields < 50 degrees
- Causes
  - Adults – Retinitis pigmentosa and ARMD
  - Children – High myopia and nystagmus

Strategies to improve low vision
- Provision of low vision devices at lesser cost
- Development of low vision aid centers at tertiary care level
- Educate eye care professionals regarding low vision aids and about rehabilitation.

Diabetic Retinopathy (DR)
- Incidence of diabetics: 2%
- Diabetic retinopathy: 25%
- Need laser treatment: 30%
- Blind due to DR: 3%

Screening of Diabetics for Retinopathy – Guidelines (by AAO)
- Type I Diabetes – 5 years after onset
- Type II Diabetes – On diagnosis and annually
- Pregnant women with diabetes – First trimester and follow-up every month.

Incidence of Duration of Retinopathy
- 50% after 10 years
- 70% after 20 years
- 90% after 30 years.

Glaucoma
- Criteria for glaucoma
  i. IOP > 21 mm of Hg
  ii. C/D ratio > 0.5
  iii. Visual field defects
- If 1 and 2 are positive refer for field assessment

Glaucoma - Incidence
- 6% above 50 years
- 4% above 35 years.

Corneal Blindness

Prevalence

Adults: 1%
Children: 27%

Causes
- Injury to cornea
- Corneal ulcers
- Vitamin A deficiency:
  - 80% can be cured by corneal transplantation
  - Development of eye banks and eye donation centers
  - Limitation: Lack of good donor corneas
  - Hospital Cornea Retrieval Programme (HCRP) to retrieve good corneas
  - 60 % of donor corneas to be utilized
- Trachoma.

Childhood Blindness

Prevalence 0.5 to 1 per 1,000 children (below 15 years).

Strategies
- Strengthening primary eye care program to eliminate preventable causes
- Developing surgical support for curable blindness.

Activities for Control
- Measles immunization preferably MMR
- Vitamin A supplementation
- Nutrition education to mothers
- Avoidance of harmful traditional practices
- Inclusion of eye care in school textbooks
- Better antenatal care to decrease premature births
- Monitoring use of oxygen in newborn
- Better service facilities to treat
  - Congenital cataract
  - Congenital glaucoma
  - Corneal opacity
  - Retinopathy of prematurity
  - Squint

- Screening of all babies at well baby clinic
- Screening of all children at the age of 3 to 5 years
- Screening of all children in blind schools.

Human Resource Development Strategies
- Eye care team
- Ophthalmologist medical and surgical services
- PMOAs: Primary eye care and refraction
- To make the system cost effective.

Infrastructure Development

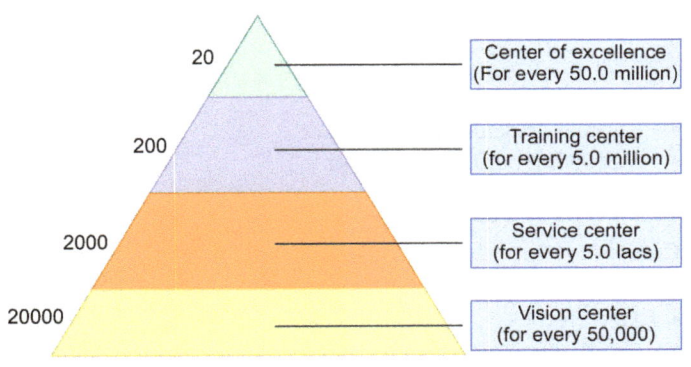

Functions of Various Centers

Centers of Excellence
- Professional leadership
- Strategy development
- Continued medical education (CME)
- Laying of standards and quality assurance
- Research.

Training Centers
- All medical colleges
- Tertiary eye care including retinal surgery, corneal transplantation, glaucoma surgery, etc
- Training and CME.

Service Centers
- Cataract surgery
- Other common eye surgeries
- Facilities for refraction
- Referral services.

Vision Centers
- Refraction and prescription of glasses
- Primary eye care
- School eye screening program
- Screening and referral services.

Conclusion
"Right to See" basic human right motto
- To ensure no citizen goes blind needlessly or being blind does not remain so
- By use of skills and resources, sight can be prevented from deterioration or restored if lost.

Objectives of Vision 2020
- Elimination of avoidable blindness
  - Provision of high quality comprehensive eye care accessible and acceptable to all.

13. Write short notes on rehabilitation of blind.
The methods of rehabilitation are:
- **Braille system of education:** Braille characters are made up of raised dots arranged in two columns of three. Blind schools teach this system of education. Partially blind persons may use large print books
- **Low vision aids:** The term low vision denotes vision between 6/60 and 6/18 with best correction.
  Low vision aids are usually based on the principle of magnification.
    - Ordinary magnifying glass: It is a biconvex circular lens
    - Rectangular magnifying lens: It is more useful for reading
    - Stand magnifier
    - Binocular loupe: This is head band magnifier. Base in prisms are incorporated
    - Jewelers or watch maker's loupe: It provides magnified monocular vision
    - Telescopic (Galilean) system: It provides binocular correction with larger field and greater depth
    - The computer-aided closed circuit television system
    - Non-optical devices like special lamps and large print materials
- Mobility training with the help of a stick and seeing dogs. All blinds should be made to feel that they are equally useful and not inferior to the sighted persons
- Vocational rehabilitation: Blind persons can be trained in book-binding, candle and chalk making, cottage industries and as telephone operators. They need encouragement and job opportunities
- **Job reservations:** All these methods will help them in looking after themselves and facilitate them to earn their livelihood. Rehabilitation of the blind is as important as the prevention and control of blindness.

14. Mention important dates in ophthalmology.
- *National Eye Donation Fortnight* – from August 25th to September 8th. To encourage and create awareness for eye donation.
- *National Eye Donation Day* – September 8th.
- *World Sight Day* – it is observed on the second Thursday of October every year to draw attention on blindness.
- *World Glaucoma Day* – March 12th of every year is observed as Glaucoma day to spread awareness regarding Glaucoma.
- *World Glaucoma Week* – between March 11th to 17th every year to create awareness of Glaucoma.

CHAPTER 23

Clinical Examination

- **Name**
- **Age**
- **Sex**
- **Occupation**
- **Complaints:**
  - Dimness of vision—sudden or gradual
  - Pain in the eyes
  - Redness
  - Watering
  - Itching and foreign body (FB) sensation
  - Headache.

Causes of Sudden Loss of Vision

- **Painful:**
  - Acute congestive glaucoma
  - Acute iridocyclitis
  - Injuries to eyeball—chemical and mechanical.
- **Painless:**
  - Central retinal artery occlusion
  - Massive vitreous hemorrhage
  - Retinal detachment: Involving macula
  - Ischemic central retinal vein occlusion.

Causes of Gradual Loss of Vision

- **Usually painless:**
  - Cataract
  - Primary open angle glaucoma
  - Diabetic retinopathy
  - Toxic amblyopia
  - Uncorrected refractive error.
  - Age related macular degeneration

Types of Watering of Eyes

- **Lacrimation:** Increased secretion of tears:
  - Primary, reflex, or central.
- **Epiphora:**
  - Inadeqate drainage of tears
  - Obstruction in lacrimal passage.

Itching of the Eyes

Causes

- Allergic conjunctivitis
- Blepharitis
- Dry eye

- Topical drug allergy
- Following contact lens wear.

Foreign Body Sensation

Causes

- Blepharitis
- Dry eye
- Trichiasis
- Corneal abrasion
- Corneal foreign body
- Superficial punctate keratitis.

Causes of Headache

- Ophthalmic
- ENT
- Medical
- Neurological
- Psychiatric.

Ophthalmic Causes of Headache

- Refractive errors: Hypermetropia and astigmatism
- Convergence insufficiency
- Contact lens overwear
- Iritis and acute congestive glaucoma
- Herpes zoster, orbital cellulitis and
- Supraorbital fissure syndrome.

Other Complaints

- Halos around light
- Photophobia
- Flashes of light
- Double vision
- Night blindness
- Spots in front of eyes
- Vertigo and giddiness.

Halo's around light

Causes

- Conjunctivitis
- Incipient cataract
- Glaucoma.

Photophobia

Causes

- Corneal abrasion
- Corneal edema

- Anterior uveitis
- Albinism
- Aniridia.

Photopsia (Seeing Flashes of Light) Seen in

- Traction of vitreous on retina
- Retinitis
- Migraine
- Impending retinal detachment
- Posterior vitreous detachment.

Double Vision (Diplopia)

Causes

- *Uniocular diplopia*
  - Keratoconus
  - Double pupil
  - Iridodialysis
  - Incipient cataract
  - Subluxated lens
  - Decentered intraocular lens.
- *Binocular diplopia*
  - High anisometropic glasses (uniocular aphakic glasses)
  - Paralytic squint (3, 4, or 6 nerve palsies)
  - After squint correction when abnormal retinal correspondence is present
  - Myasthenia gravis
  - Thyroid disorder.

Night Blindness (Nyctalopia)

Causes

- Vitamin A deficiency
- Retinitis pigmentosa
- Congenital night blindness
- Pathological myopia
- After pan retinal photocoagulation
- Chorioretinal degenerations
- Siderosis bulbi.

Day Blindness (Hemeralopia)

Causes

- Central corneal opacity
- Central nuclear or polar cataract
- Congenital deficiency of cones.

Spots in Front of Eyes (Floaters): Seen In

- Posterior vitreous detachment
- Posterior uveitis
- Vitreous hemorrhage
- Corneal opacity.

History

- **Past history:** Previous disease, treatment or operations. History of using glasses for distance or near vision.
- **Personal history:** Tobacco, alcohol, hypertension, diabetes, kidney, blood, heart disease, foci of infection.
- **Family history:** Diabetes, hypertension, glaucoma, and congenital cataract.

Clinical Examination

- Acuity of vision
- Inspection:
  - **Head position:** In severe bilateral ptosis, head is elevated with an intention to see clearly.
  - In paralytic squint, the head is turned in the direction of paralysed muscle action.
  - **Orbit:** Protrusion of eyeball—proptosis.
  - **Eyeball:** Prominent in high myopia, Grave's disease, sunken in phthisis bulbi.
  - **Eyelids:** In ptosis, upper eyelid covers more than 2 mm of superior part of cornea.
  - In Grave's disease, sclera above superior limbus is visible due to lid retraction.
  - In Lagophthalmos, the patient is unable to close the lids fully.
  - **Lid margins:** Crusting at lid margins—conjunctivitis due to mucus or pus.
  - Scales at lid margins: Blepharitis.
  - Swelling at lid margin: Stye or marginal chalazion.
  - Inward turning of eyelid margin: Entropion.
  - Outward turning of lid margin: Ectropion.
  - **Lacrimal sac:** Swelling and tenderness
  - Swelling in the sac area near the medial canthus suggests dacryocystitis.
- **Visual acuity:**
  - Distant vision—6/6
  - Near vision—N6
  - Distant vision: Tested at 6 meters since rays coming from it are parallel.
  - If vision is less, to be tested with pinhole. (See Instruments and Lenses chapter)
  - V/A is written as numerator/denominator.
  - Numerator is distance of the patient from the chart.
  - Lesser the denominator, vision is better.
  For example, V/A -6/18 means the patient reads from the distance of 6 meters what a normal person can read from a distance of 18 meters.
- **Head posture:**
  - Normal: Straight and forward
  - Elevation or depression:
    » Vertical muscle palsy
    » Ptosis
  - Turn: Rectus muscle palsy
  - Tilt: Oblique muscle palsy.
- **Lids**
  - Position: Upper lid covers 1 to 2 mm of cornea at 12 o'clock
  - Lower lid tangential to limbus at 6 o'clock
  - Thickness
  - Edema
  - Localized swelling: Chalazion or Stye
  - Lagophthalmos.
- **Palpebral fissure:**
  - Vertical—8 to 9 mm
  - Horizontal—20 to 25 mm
  - Narrow—atrophic bulbi, phthisis bulbi, ptosis, lid edema, microphthalmos
  - Wide—lid retraction, exophthalmos, proptosis.

- **Conjunctiva**
  - Congestion bulbar, palpebral
  - Follicle, papilla
  - Scar if any
  - Abnormal lesions: Pterygium, phlycten, and hemorrhage.
- **Types of congestion.**

Feature	Conjunctival	Ciliary
Site	Marked in fornices	Marked around limbus
Color	Bright red	Purple or dull red
Arrangement of vessels	Superficial and branching	Deep and radiating from limbus
On moving conjunctiva	Congested vessels also move	Congested vessels do not move
Blanching with adrenaline	Blanches	Does not blanch
Causes	Acute conjunctivitis	Acute iridocyclitis, keratitis, acute glaucoma

Limbus—nodule causes
- Congenital: Dermoid
  - Dermolipoma
  - Raised naevus.
- Inflammation: Episcleritis
  - Nodular form of scleritis.
- Allergic: Phlycten
  - Vernal catarrh: Limbal form
  - Ophthalmia nodosa.
- Vascular: Hemangioma
- Traumatic: FB granuloma
  - Implantation cyst
  - Iris prolapse.
- Degenerative: Pinguecula
  - Cystic pterygium.
- Nutritional: Bitot's spot.
- Neoplastic: Papilloma
  - Epithelioma.
- Miscellaneous: Ciliary staphyloma.

Sclera
- Color
- Thickness
- Ectasia.

Cornea
- Size
- Surface: Abrasion, ulcer, scar
- Shape: Keratoconus, after perforation, pseudocornea, anterior staphyloma, transparency, vascularization.
- Corneal sensation: Pressure effect, destruction, scar—no sensation.

Features	Superficial	Deep
Color	Bright red, well defined	Diffuse red, ill defined
Visibility beyond limbus	Can be traced	Cannot be traced
Branching	Arborescent	Runs parallel in brush like fashion
Surface of cornea	Epithelium is raised, corneal surface is uneven	Cornea hazy but smooth
Origin of vessels	From conjunctival vessels	From anterior ciliary arteries
Causes	Trachoma, phlyctenular keratoconjunctivitis, superficial corneal ulcer	Interstitial keratitis, disciform keratitis, sclerosing keratitis, chemical burns

Size
- Vertical: 11 mm
- Horizontal: 12 mm
- Increased: Megalocornea, buphthalmos
- Decreased: Microcornea, microphthalmos.
  Shape
  - Flat: Cornea plana, atrophic bulbi
  - Conical: Keratoconus
  - Globular: Keratoglobus, buphthalmos, anterior staphyloma.
- Surface: Smooth and regular
  - Window reflex
  - Placido disk: Distortion of rings if surface is not smooth
  - Corneal staining with fluorescein will be positive if there is abrasion or ulcer.
- Transparency: Clear in normal cornea
  - Hazy in corneal edema due to keratitis, acute congestive glaucoma, iridocyclitis, and opacity.

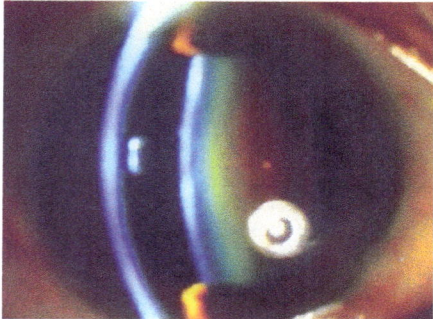

Fig. 23.1: Optical section of cornea.

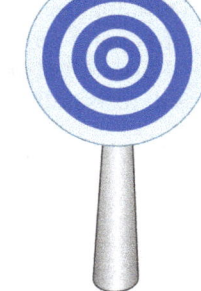

Fig. 23.2: Placido disk.

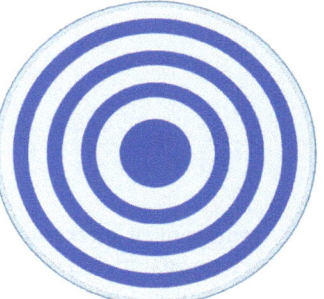

Fig. 23.3: Placido's disc reflex from normal cornea.

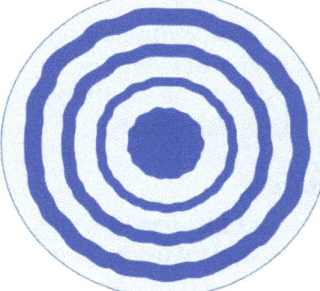

Fig. 23.4: Reflection from irregular cornea.

Corneal Opacity (See Cornea Chapter)

Types
- Nebula
- Macula
- Leukoma
- Adherent leukoma.

Corneal Sensation

Decreased in:
- Contact lens wearers
- Herpes simplex/zoster
- Acute congestive glaucoma
- Absolute glaucoma
- Lesions of 5th nerve, leprosy.

Anterior Chamber

Depth
- Shallow
- Deep
- Irregular
- Contents—6
  i. Aqueous
  ii. Blood
  iii. Pus/pseudohypopyon
  iv. Lens
  v. Vitreous
  vi. Foreign body.

Shallow Anterior Chamber

Causes
- Hypermetropia
- Perforated corneal ulcer
- Postoperative wound leak
- Intumuscent cataract
- Angle closure glaucoma
- Choroidal detachment
- Malignant glaucoma.

Deep Anterior Chamber

Causes
- Myopia
- Aphakia
- Keratoconus
- Acute iridocyclitis
- Total posterior synechiae
- Morgagnian cataract.

Irregular Anterior Chamber

Causes
- Adherent leuckoma
- Iris bombe
- Tilting of lens
  Iris:
  - Color: Brown or black
    » Blue: Patrial albinism
    » Pink: Total albinism
  - Pattern: Moon surface
  - Abnormal adhesion: Synechiae—anterior/posterior, ring, occlusive, and seclusive
    » Nodules
    » Operation marks
    » Movements
    » Vascularization.
- **Pupil**
  - Number
  - Situation
  - Size
  - Shape
  - Color: Black (normal), slightly grey, jet black, glistening, and capsular remnant
  - Reactions to light.

Miosis: Constriction of the pupil
- Iridocyclitis
- Drugs: Parasympathomimetic
- Morphine poisoning
- Horner's syndrome
- Pontine hemorrhage
- Physiological
  » Senile pupil
- During sleep
- Due to strong light.

Mydriasis: Dilatation of the pupil
- Affection of afferent nerve: Optic atrophy
- Affection of efferent nerve
- Drugs: Sympthomimetic or parasympatholytic
- Acute congestive glaucoma
- Absolute glaucoma
- 3rd nerve palsy
- Internal ophthalmoplegia
- Adie's pupil.

Pupillary reactions
- Direct and consensual
- Abnormal reactions
- Total afferent pupillary defect (TAPD): Complete optic nerve lesion
- Relative afferent pupillary defect (RAPD): Incomplete lesion
- Marcus Gunn pupil
- Argyll Robertson pupil
- Adie's pupil.
- **Lens**
  - Color
    » Grey
    » Jet black
    » White
  - Brown/ black
  - Phakodonesis: Tremor of the lens
  - Purkinje-Sanson images:
    » 1, 2, 3 – erect and virtual
    » 4 – inverted and real.

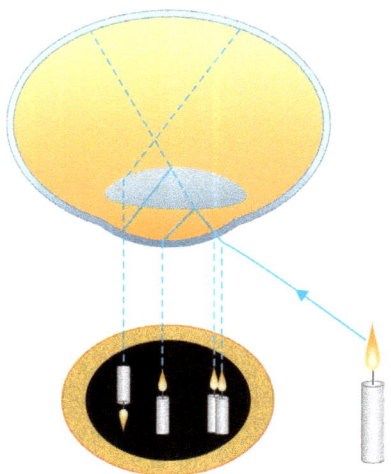

Fig. 23.5: Purkinje-Sanson images.

Seen in dark room with pen torch for the reflected images on reflecting surfaces of eye
- 1st image: Anterior corneal surface
- 2nd image: Posterior corneal surface
- 3rd image: Anterior lens surface
- 4th image: Posterior lens surface—against movement
- Of the four reflecting surfaces, 1st three act like convex mirror and the 4th act as concave mirror
- 1st, 2nd, 3rd images: Move with movement of light
- Mature cataract: 4th image is absent
- Aphakia: 3rd and 4th images are absent.

Difference between immature and mature cataract	Immature cataract	Mature cataract
Vision	> Hand movements to varying degree	Hand movements
Color of lens	Greyish white	White
Iris shadow	Present	Absent
Fundal glow in distant direct ophthalmoscopy	Red glow interrupted by black opacities	Absent

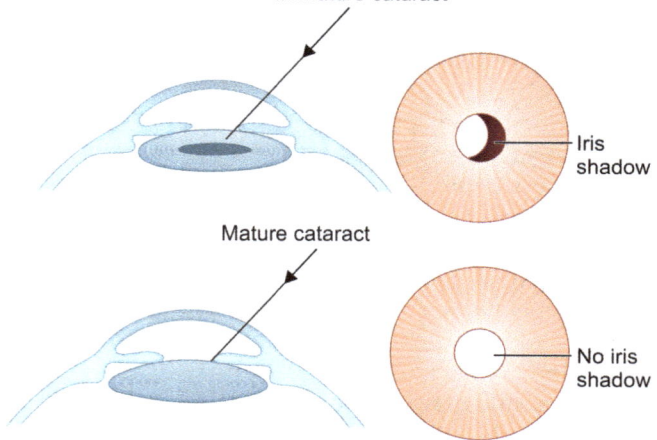

Fig. 23.6: Iris shadow.

- Ocular motility
  - Uniocular
  - Binocular.
- Cover test
- Actions of extraocular muscles (EOM).

Muscle	Primary	Secondary	Tertiary
Medial rectus	Adduction	—	—
Lateral rectus	Abduction	—	—
Superior rectus	Elevation	Intorsion	Adduction
Inferior rectus	Depression	Extorsion	Adduction
Superior oblique	Intorsion	Depression	Abduction
Inferior oblique	Extorsion	Elevation	Abduction

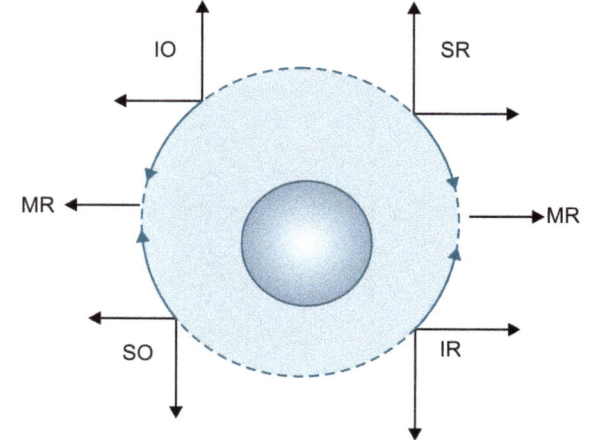

Fig. 23.7: Action of muscles.

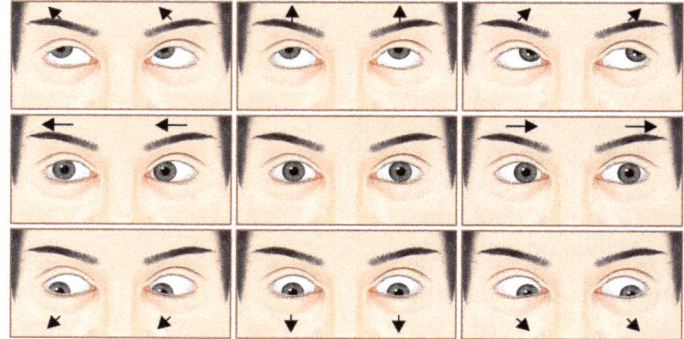

Fig. 23.8: Positions of gaze.

Palpation
- Orbit:
  - Margin
  - Swelling
  - Tenderness.
- Eyeball:
  - Tenderness
  - Pulsation
  - Digital tension
  - Lymph nodes.

Case Sheet-proforma.		
Name	Age	Sex
Occupation		
Chief complaint		
Duration		

Past History
- H/o diabetes, hypertension, or any major illness (RS, CVS)
- H/o previous eye surgery
- H/o using glasses: Distance and near.

Personal History
H/o smoking, alcoholism.

Family History
H/o glaucoma, cataract.

Clinical Examination
- RE
- LE
- Visual acuity (distance and near)
  - with and without glass
  - with pinhole.
- Orbit
  - Swelling
  - Margins – growth
  - Tenderness.
- Eyeball
  - Size
  - Tenderness.
- Eyelids
  - Ptosis
  - Chalazion
  - Entropion
  - Ectropion
  - Blepharitis
  - Trichiasis
  - Lagophthalmos
  - Scars of surgery.
- Palpebral aperture
- Lacrimal apparatus
  - Swelling
  - Redness/tenderness
  - Regurgitation/discharge
  - Fistula
  - Scar.
- Conjunctiva
  - Congestion: Conjunctival/ciliary/localized
  - Papillae, follicles, nodules, concretion
  - Phlycten
  - Pterygium
  - Xerosis/Bitot's spots
  - Symblepharon
  - Scar of surgery.
- Limbus
  - Phlycten
  - Pterygium
  - Pinguecula
  - Herberts pits
  - Scar of surgery (cataract, glaucoma).
- Sclera
  - Color
  - Thickness
  - Ectasia
  - Inflammation (episcleritis/scleritis)
  - Scar of surgery.
- Cornea
  - Size
  - Shape
  - Surface (curvature)
  - Sensation
  - Transparency
  - Vascularization
  - Corneal opacities:
    » Situation
    » Size
    » Shape
    » Density: Nebula, macula, leukoma
    » Iris inclusion
    » Pigmentation
    » Vascularization Ectasia.
- Anterior chamber
  - Depth
  - Content.
- Iris
  - Color
  - Pattern (normal/distorted)
  - Synechiae
  - Iridectomy
  - Iris bombe
  - Prolapse
  - Iris atrophy, nodules, pigmentation, neovascularization
  - Adherent leukoma.
- Pupil
  - Size
  - Situation
  - Shape
  - Color
  - Reaction (direct/consensual)
  - IOL
  - Updrawn pupil.
- Lens
  - Transparency
  - Grey
  - Greyish white
  - White
  - Amber, brown or black
  - Glistening reflex
  - Aphakia.
- Ocular motility
  - Duction, versions, vergences
- Cover test
  - Cover uncover
  - Alternate cover
  - Prism cover.
- Palpation
  - Tenderness
  - Digital tension
  - Orbital margin
  - Preauricular nodes.
- Intraocular pressure (IOP)
- Fundus examination: Direct and indirect ophthalmoscopy
- Slit lamp examination to confirm the above findings.

CHAPTER 24

Instruments and Lenses

Wire Speculum

Wire speculum is used to separate the eyelids during intraocular surgery. Since it is light weight, it hardly exerts any pressure on the eyeball.

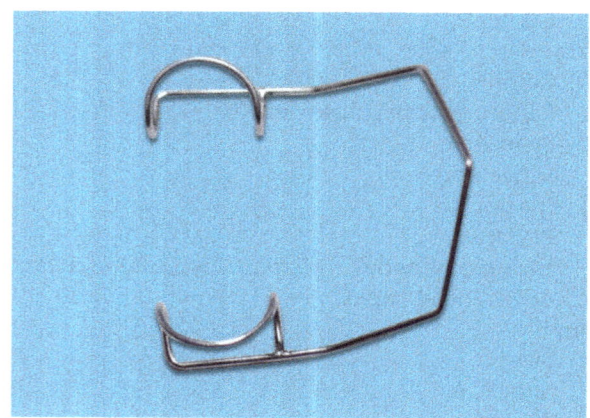

Fig. 24.1: Wire speculum.

Dastoor's Superior Rectus Forceps

Dastoor's superior rectus forceps is used to hold superior rectus muscle for passing bridle suture meant to fix rotate the eyeball in downward gaze in cataract and glaucoma surgery.

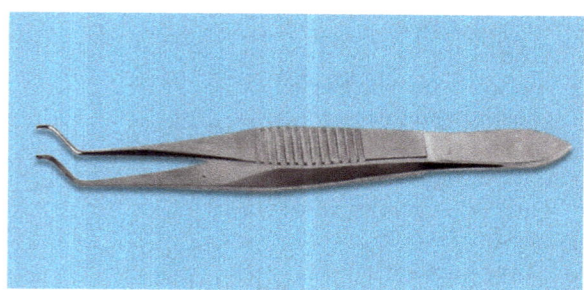

Fig. 24.2: Dastoor's superior rectus forceps.

Plain Forceps

Plain forceps are used to hold the conjunctiva for making limbal or fornix based conjunctival flap.

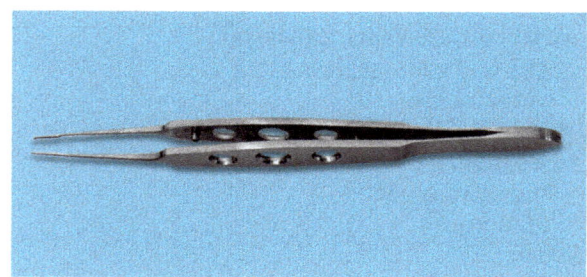

Fig. 24.3: Plain forceps.

Conjunctival Scissors

Conjunctival scissors is used to cut the conjunctiva to make fornix based or limbal based conjunctival flap for cataract and glaucoma surgery. It is also used in pterygium excision. It has sleek and long blades.

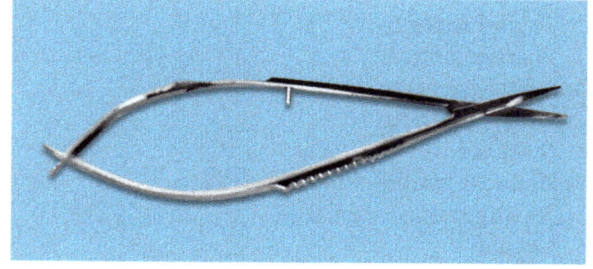

Fig. 24.4: Conjunctival scissors.

Corneal Scissors

Corneal scissors is used to extend the limbal section in conventional extracapsular cataract extraction (ECCE).

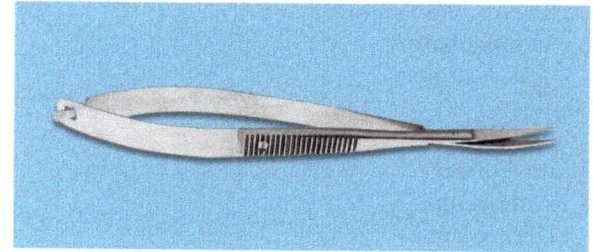

Fig. 24.5: Corneal scissors.

Dewecker's Scissors

Dewecker's scissors has a V-shaped blade at one end. It is used to cut iris in iridectomy.

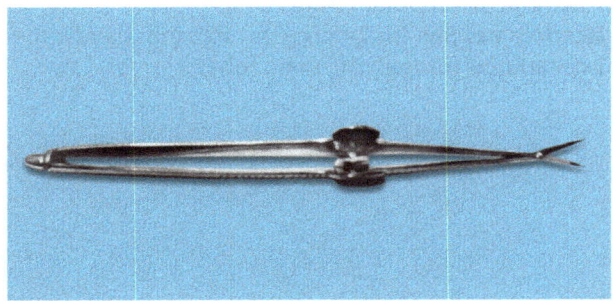

Fig. 24.6: Dewecker's scissors.

Types of Iridectomies

Peripheral, sector or basal and optical
- Peripheral: Is the removal of iris tissue at the periphery in glaucoma surgeries.
- Sector or Basal: To facilitate lens delivery in cataract operation with poor mydriasis, and iris prolapse.
- Optical: To provide vision in central corneal opacities.

Vannas Scissors

Vannas scissors is a fine delicate scissors with sharp edges.

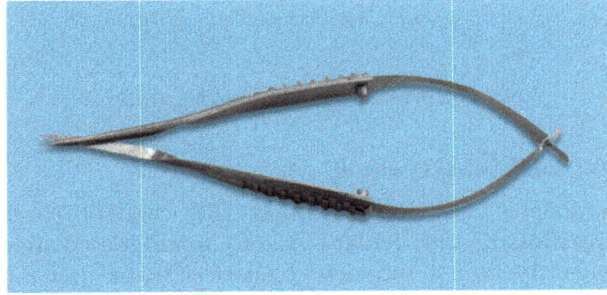

Fig. 24.7: Vannas scissors.

Uses:
- To cut loose or floating capsule in anterior chamber.
- To do anterior vitrectomy.
- To cut corneoscleral suture.
- To do sphincterotomy when pupil is not dilating.

Bard Parker Handle with No.11 and No.15 Blades

The Bard Parker handle number eleven blade has a sharp tip and number fifteen blade has a curved tip.

It is used to make incision groove in cataract surgery and trabeculectomy. It is also used to make skin incision in various extraocular surgeries.

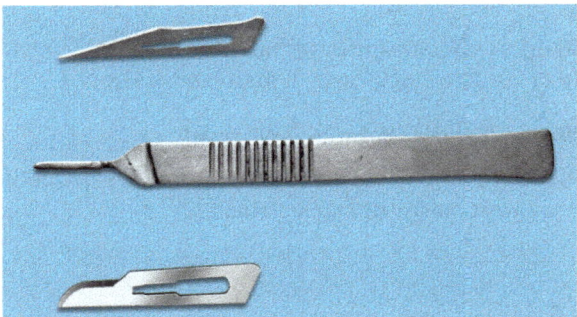

Fig. 24.8: Bard Parker handle with No. 11 and No.15 blades.

Crescent Blade (Tunnel Blade)

Crescent blade is used to make valvular or tunnel incision in the sclera in small-incision cataract surgery (SICS).

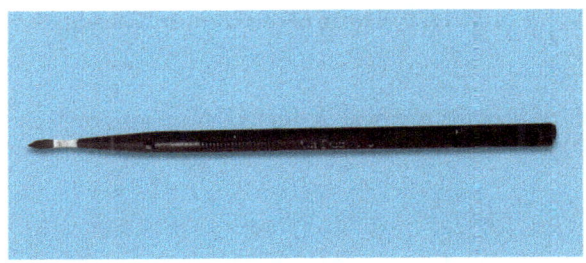

Fig. 24.9: Crescent blade (tunnel blade).

Entry Blade (Keratome)

Entry blade is used to make entry into anterior chamber in SICS. It is also used to do paracentesis.

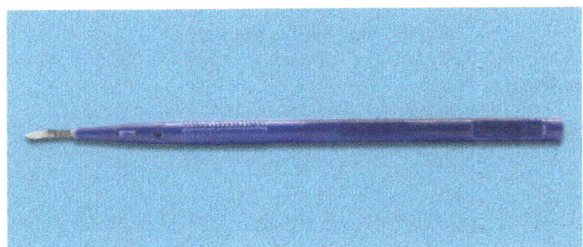

Fig. 24.10: Entry blade (keratome).

Side Port Blade

Side port blade is used to make entry into anterior chamber to pass second instrument during cataract surgery. Only one side of the blade is sharp.

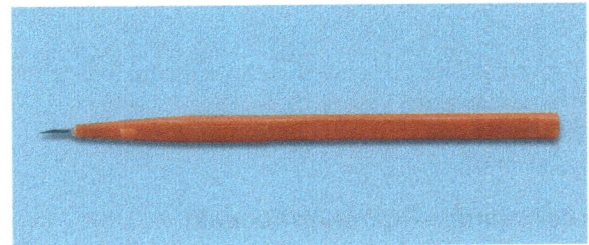

Fig. 24.11: Side port blade.

Uses

- To inject viscoelastic or trypan blue dye.
- To clean 12 o'clock cortical matter with Simcoe.

Cystitome Needle (Bent 26 G Needle)

Cystitome needle is used to incise anterior capsule in can opener capsulotomy or capsulorhexis.

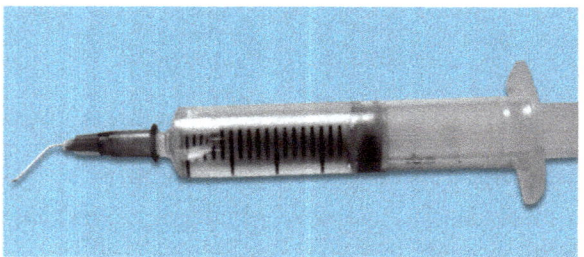

Fig. 24.12: Cystitome needle (Bent 26 G needle).

Vectis

Vectis is used for removal of nucleus from anterior chamber in SICS. It is also useful to deliver subluxated lens.

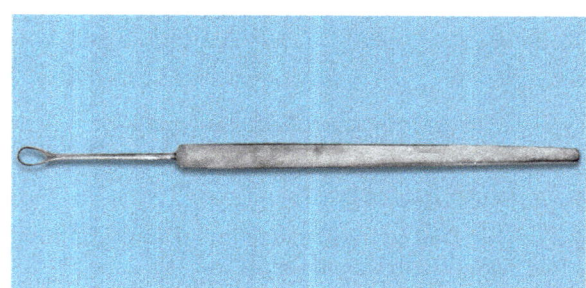

Fig. 24.13: Vectis.

Lens Hook

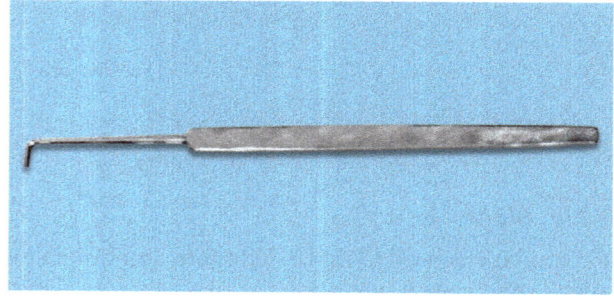

Fig. 24.14: Lens hook.

Uses

- To give counter pressure in delivering the lens in ECCE
- In squint surgery
- Retinal detachment surgery
- Enucleation.

Simcoe Irrigation Aspiration Cannula

Simcoe irrigation aspiration cannula is used for irrigation of anterior chamber and aspiration of cortical matter during ECCE or SICS. It is also used to remove hyphema and viscoelastic from anterior chamber. The regular cannula has irrigation tip on the right side and aspiration on the left while in the reverse type it is vice versa.

- **Direct simcoe**: Aspiration is through silicon tube and irrigation is from main dripset.
- **Reverse simcoe**: Irrigation is through the silicon tube and aspiration is through the main tube.

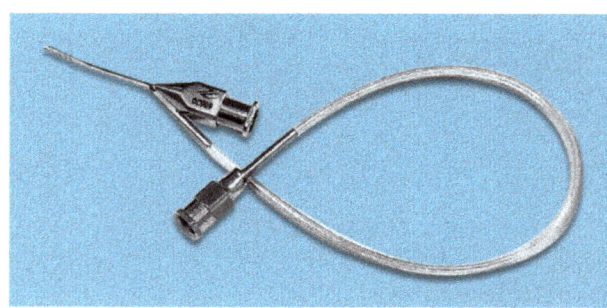

Fig. 24.15: Simcoe irrigation aspiration cannula.

McPherson Lens Holding Forceps

McPherson lens holding forceps is used to hold the intraocular lens during insertion into posterior chamber.

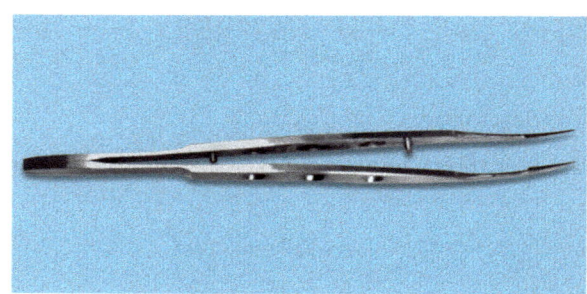

Fig. 24.16: McPherson lens holding forceps.

Lens Dialer (Sinskey Hook)

Lens dialer is a fine stout instrument with a bent tip. It is used for rotating the intraocular lens into horizontal position. It engages the hole in intraocular lenses (IOL) or optic haptic junction.

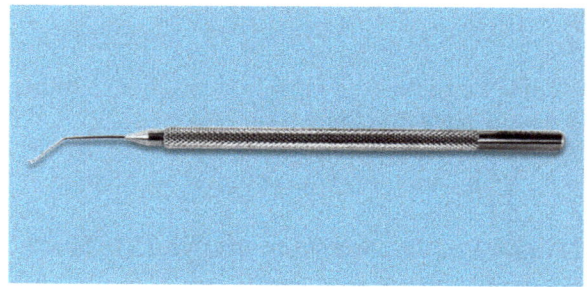

Fig. 24.17: Lens dialer (Sinskey hook).

Uses

- To prolapse the nucleus into anterior chamber in small-incision cataract surgery (SICS)
- To rotate the lens nucleus

- To chop the nucleus in phacoemulsification
- To prolapse the nucleus into anterior chamber in SICS.

Barraquer's Needle Holder: (Curved Tip)

Castroviejo's needle holder has straight tip. They are used to hold the suture needle during suturing.

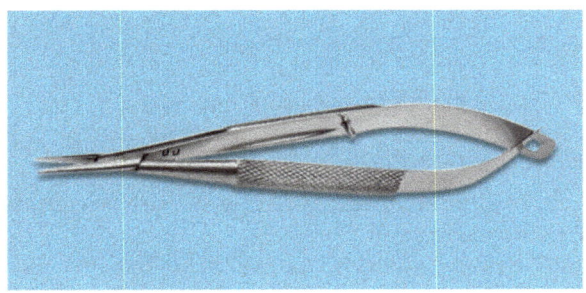

Fig. 24.18: Barraquer's needle holder (curved tip).

St. Martin Forceps

It has fine limbs having 1 × 2 teeth. It is used to hold the cornea or sclera during suturing.

Lim's or Colibri's forceps are also used.

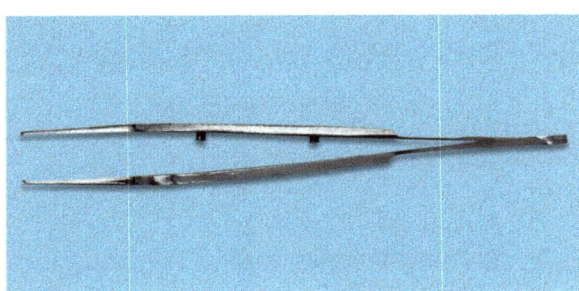

Fig. 24.19: St. Martin forceps.

Castroviejo's Caliper

It is used to obtain measurements in millimetre.

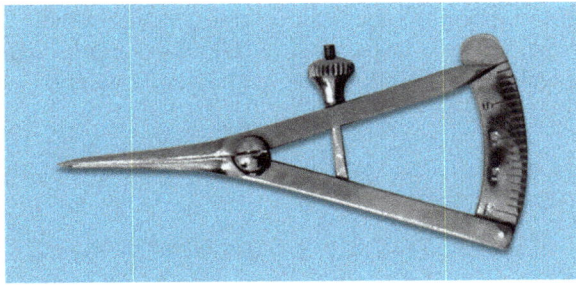

Fig. 24.20: Castroviejo's caliper.

Uses

- In SICS, to mark the length of incision
- In squint surgery, to measure the length of muscle to be resected
- In retinal detachment surgery, to mark the exact site of retinal break
- In ptosis surgery, to measure the length of levator palpebrae superioris (LPS) muscle for resection.
- To measure the corneal diameter.

Lens Spatula and Iris Repositor

The spatulated end (on the left side) is used to give counter pressure during lens delivery in cataract surgery. The flattened end (on the right side) is used to reposit the iris back into anterior chamber in cataract surgery.

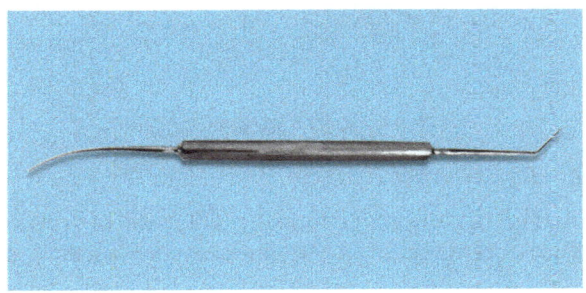

Fig. 24.21: Lens spatula and iris repositor.

Chalazion Clamp

It is a forceps having a screw for fixing the limbs like a clamp. It is self retaining and hemostatic. It is used to fix the chalazion during surgery. The solid disc is applied on skin side of lid at the site of chalazion. The hollow ring is applied on the tarsal conjunctiva. It is used in incision and curettage of chalazion.

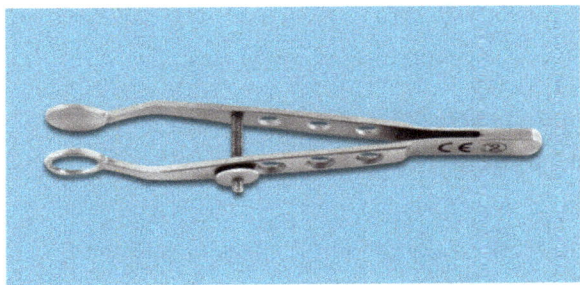

Fig. 24.22: Chalazion clamp.

Chalazion Scoop

It is used to curette contents of chalazion after making vertical incision on the conjunctival side.

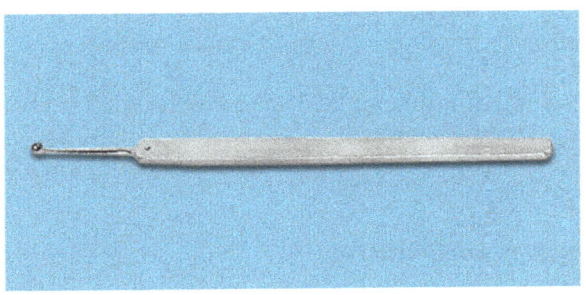

Fig. 24.23: Chalazion scoop.

Muller's Lacrimal Speculum

It is self-retaining and hemostatic. It is used in dacryocystectomy and dacryocystorhinostomy.

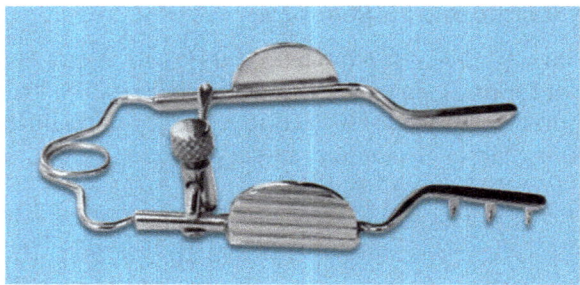

Fig. 24.24: Muller's lacrimal speculum.

Citelli's Bone Punch

It is used for making an opening in medial wall of orbit during dacryocystorhinostomy. It helps in removing bone fragments.

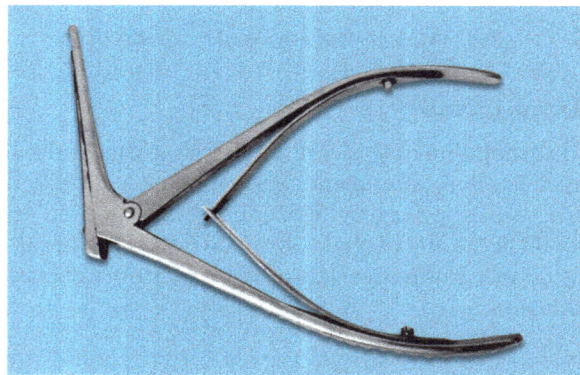

Fig. 24.25: Citelli's bone punch.

Bowman's Lacrimal Probe

It is a long probe with rounded tip.

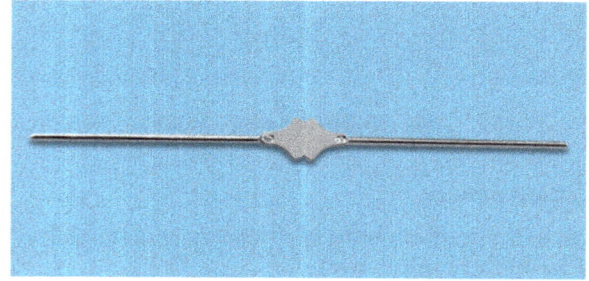

Fig. 24.26: Bowman's lacrimal probe.

Uses
- Probing of nasolacrimal duct to access the site of block in the lacrimal passages
- Probing to open the passages in case of congenital dacryocystitis.

Desmarre's Lid Retractor

It is used to retract the upper lid to examine the eye in children and in uncooperative patients.

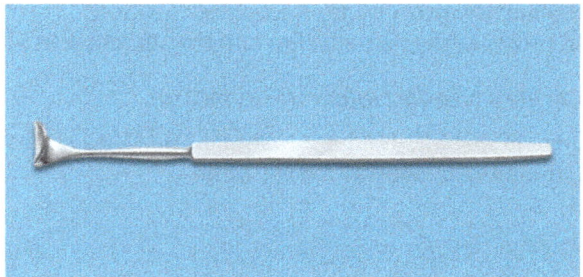

Fig. 24.27: Desmarre's lid retractor.

Enucleation Spoon

It is a curved spoon with the central cleavage to accommodate optic nerve during enucleation.

Enucleation is the surgical removal of the eye ball and a portion of optic nerve from the orbit.

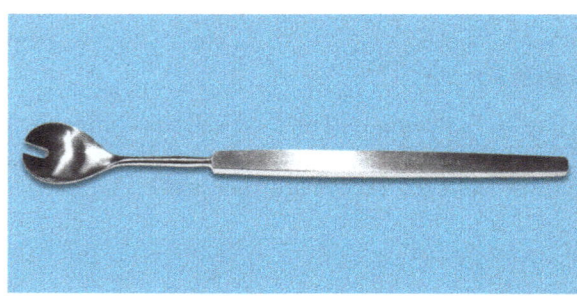

Fig. 24.28: Enucleation spoon.

Indications for Enucleation
- **Absolute:**
    - Eye donation from cadaver.
    - Malignant tumors of eyeball
    - Severely injured eye.
- **Relative:**
    - Painful blind eye
    - Phthisis bulbi
    - Bleeding anterior staphyloma.

Evisceration Spoon

It is broad spoon to scoop out the contents of eyeball.

Evisceration is the scooping out all the contents of the globe leaving behind the sclera and the optic nerve.

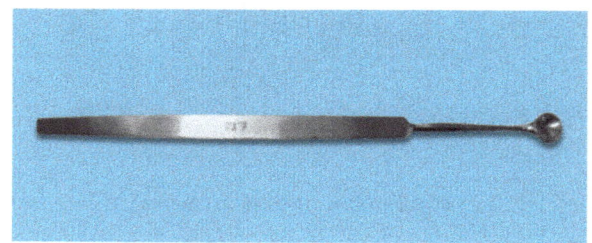

Fig. 24.29: Evisceration spoon.

Indications for Evisceration
- Panophthalmitis
- Expulsive hemorrhage
- Severely bleeding anterior staphyloma.

Lenses Spherical Concave Lens

Objects appear to move in both meridian (horizontal and vertical). Objects appear to move in same direction of movement of the lens. There is minification of object.

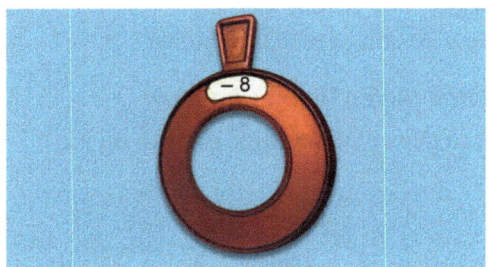

Fig. 24.30: Spherical concave lens.

Uses
- To correct myopia
- Used in direct ophthalmoscope
- Diagnostic
  - Hruby lens (-55D)
  - Malingering test—place high minus in good eye. If the patient reads through the bad eye, he is malingering.

Spherical Convex Lens

Objects appear to move in both meridian (horizontal and vertical). Objects appear to move in opposite direction of movement of the lens. There is magnification of object.

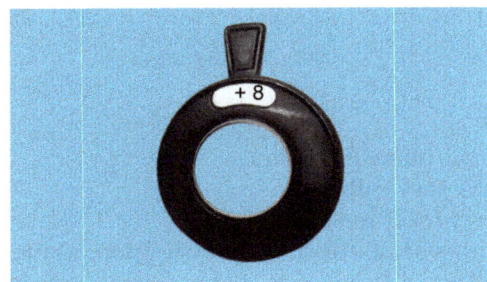

Fig. 24.31: Spherical convex lens.

Uses
- **Therapeutic:**
  - To correct hypermetropia, presbyopia, aphakia
  - Low visual aids.
- **Instrumental:**
  - Direct and indirect ophthalmoscope
  - Microscopes
  - Synoptophore
  - Binocular loupe.
- **Diagnostic:**
  - Condensing lens in indirect ophthalmoscope.
  - +78, +90D lenses to view retina
  - Placido's disc (+3D).

Cylindrical Concave Lens

Objects appear to move in one meridian only in same direction of movement of the lens, i.e., perpendicular to the direction of axis of lens.

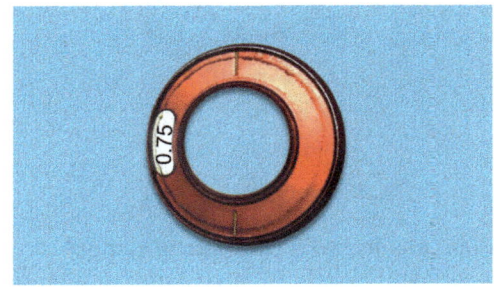

Fig. 24.32: Cylindrical concave lens.

Uses
- Simple myopic astigmatism
- Compound myopic astigmatism
- Mixed astigmatism.

Cylindrical Convex Lens

Objects appears to move in one meridian only and in opposite direction of movement of the lens, i.e., perpendicular to the direction of axis of lens.

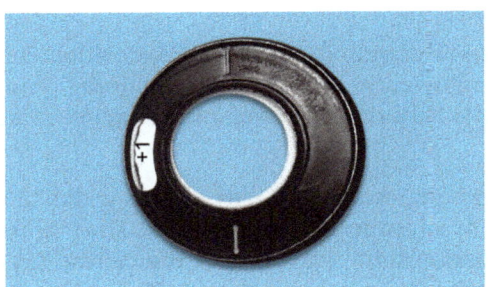

Fig. 24.33: Cylindrical convex lens.

Uses
- Simple hypermetropic astigmatism
- Compound hypermetropic astigmatism
- Mixed astigmatism.

Prism

- Keep the prism in front of the eye and rotate the prism. The object appears to move towards the apex of prism.
- Look a straight line with the prism. The line appears to be broken towards the apex of prism. There is no horizontal or vertical movement of objects.
- Touch the lens. Prism is thicker on one side.
- Thickness depends on the power of prism.
  One Prism dioptre—shift of object by 1 cm situated at the distance of 1 meter. [Uses of prism is given in miscellaneous chapter].

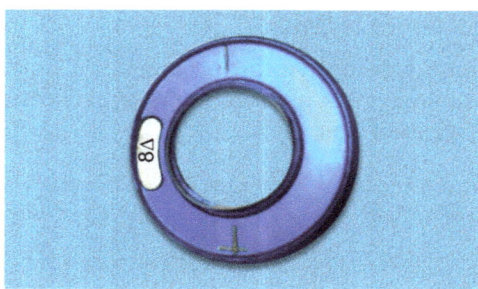

Fig. 24.34: Prism.

Pin Hole

- Black opaque disc with tiny hole in center.
- Diameter of pinhole between 0.5 mm to 1.2 mm.

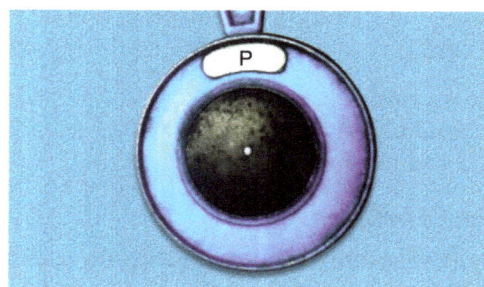

Fig. 24.35: Pin hole.

Principle
Peripheral rays coming to the eyes are occulded. Only central rays are allowed to pass through the nodal point of lens. Central rays fall directly on fovea and a clear image is obtained.

Uses
- To find out whether defective vision is due to refractive error or any other ocular pathology. The vision improves in cases of refractive error as the central rays passing through the pin hole are straight. The vision deteriorates in ocular pathology.
- Two pin hole test—used in macular function test.

Stenopaeic Slit
- It is a black colored opaque disc with a slit in the center.
- Diameter of slit = 1 mm; length = 20 mm.

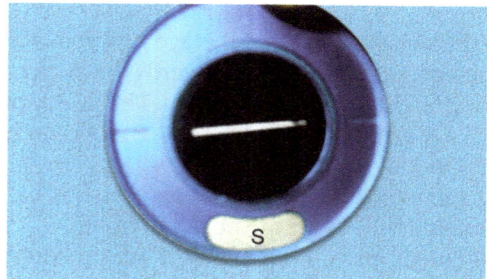

Fig. 24.36: Stenopaeic slit.

Uses
- To determine axis of astigmatism.
- In Finchams test—to differentiate glaucomatous halo from halo due to incipient cataract. The halos are intact in acute congestive glaucoma. They are broken in immature cataract.
- To know axis for optical iridectomy.

Maddox Rod (Refer Squint Chapter)
Red colored glass with multiple grooves on it.

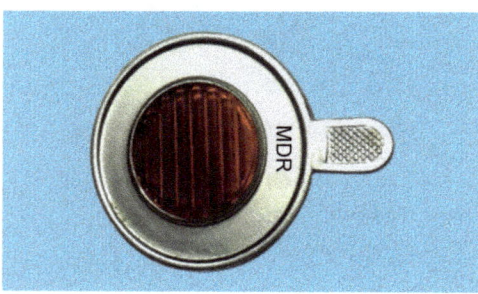

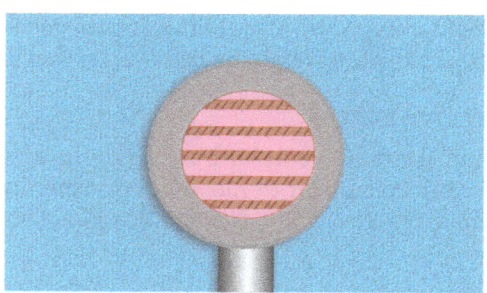

Fig. 24.37: Maddox rod.

Principle
To dissociate binocular vision.
- One eye sees bulb.
- Other eye sees red line.
- Patient is seated with both eyes open. Maddox rod is placed in right trial frame with horizontal grooves. Patient to look at a distant lighted bulb. Patient is asked to say whether red line is running through the centre of it or left or right side of it.

Types of Phoria
- *Orthophoria:* Red line will run through the centre of bulb
- *Exophoria:* Red line will be to left of bulb (crossed)
- *Esophoria:* Red line will be to right of bulb
- *Hyperphoria:* Red line below or above bulb
- *Cyclophoria:* Red line runs obliquely.

Uses
- To test muscle balance for distant vision
- Detects phorias for distance
- Used for macular function test
- For diagnosis of abnormal retinal correspondence.

Miscellaneous

1. Lasers in ophthalmology.

The laser is an acronym of light amplification by stimulated emission of radiation.

The properties of the laser are:
- It is monochromatic: Single wavelength of light
- It is collimated: All photons run parallel
- It is coherent: Always in the same phase
- It is polarized at a high energy level.

Laser effects on ocular tissues are:
- *Photoablation:* Ablation of corneal tissue without thermal damage—LASIK surgery
- *Photodisruption:* Optical breakdown to disrupt tissues by the formation of plasma— NdYAG laser in posterior capsular opacification
- *Photocoagulation:* Controlled burn to tissues and leaking vessels—diabetic retinopathy
  Types of retinal photocoagulation:
  - Focal: 50 µm for 0.1 second
  - Grid: 100 µm for 0.1 second
  - Panretinal photocoagulation (PRP), Sector: 200 µm for 0.2 second
- **Photodynamic Therapy**: Verteporfin (sensitizer dye) and diode laser (690 nm) is used to treat the subretinal neovascular membrane in age-related macular degeneration (ARMD).

Laser	Wavelength in nm	Clinical application
Nd:YAG	1,064	Posterior capsulotomy, iridotomy
Frequency-doubled Nd:YAG	532	Retinal photocoagulation, cyclophotocoagulation
Argon green laser	514	Retinal photocoagulation, trabeculoplasty
Diode laser	800	Retinal photocoagulation
Krypton red	714	Retinal photocoagulation
Excimer (argon fluoride)	193	Laser in situ keratomileusis (LASIK), laser epithelial keratomileusis (LASEK), photorefractive keratectomy (PRK), photorefractive or photherapeutic keratectomy
Femtosecond laser	1,053	Corneal refractive surgery

Indications for Laser
- *Posterior Segment*
  - Retinal tear and lattice degeneration
  - Macular edema (diabetic, CSME, BRVO)
  - Choroidal neovascularisation
  - –CSR
  - Retinal angioma, ocular tumors
  - Intraoperative endolaser treatment
- Anterior segment
  - Glaucoma
    » Argon laser trabeculoplasty
    » Selective laser trabeculoplasty
    » Laser peripheral iridotomy
  - Cataract
    » YAG laser posterior capsulotomy
    » Femtosecond laser cataract surgery
  - Refractive surgery
    » LASIK
    » Phototherapeutic keratectomy.

2. Nystagmus.

Definition
It is rapid, rhythmic, symmetrical, involuntary, oscillatory movement of the eyes which is usually horizontal and bilateral. Nystagmus means 'to nod'.

Causes
It is due to disturbance of sensory, motor apparatus controlling normal binocular position. These may be ocular (sensory deprivation), labyrinthine and vestibular or related to the central nervous system.

Classification
- **Based on etiology:**
  - Physiological:
    » End gaze
    » Optokinetic
    » Vestibulo-ocular reflexes
  - Pathological:
    » Congenital
      a. Infantile manifest:
        ▪ Idiopathic
        ▪ Albinism

- Aniridia
- Leber congenital amaurosis
- Bilateral optic nerve hypoplasia
- Bilateral congenital cataract

b. Infantile latent
c. Infantile manifest latent
d. Nystagmus blockage syndrome

» Acquired:
  a. Secondary to visual loss
  b. Toxic or metabolic
  c. Neurological disorders (tumor, trauma, multiple sclerosis, etc.)

Based on pattern of manifestation:
- Manifest
- Latent
- Manifest latent

Based on direction of movement:
- Horizontal
- Vertical
- Rotatory

Based on pattern of movement:
- Jerky
- Pendular.

Clinical Features

In congenital and infantile nystagmus the vision is very poor. Besides rhythmic ocular movements, the patient may complain of headache, giddiness, photophobia, moving of stationary objects and occasional diplopia.

Treatment

- Correction of refractive error to improve the vision
- Prism therapy: Prisms are used to correct the head position and shifting the image into null point area
- Nystagmus surgery: The surgery improves the visual acuity and broadens the null zone
- Severe disabling nystagmus can be treated with retrobulbar injections of botulinum toxin.

3. Dyes (vital stains) in ophthalmology.

- Fluorescein 2%—stains epithelial defects. It is appreciated better under blue filter as it appears brilliant green due to fluorescence
- Indocyanine green for retinal and choroidal angiography
- Rose Bengal 1%: To stain devitalized tissue in conjunctiva and cornea and mucous strands—useful in diagnosis of dry eye
- Trypan blue (0.06%): To stain anterior capsule.

Fluorescein

- It is a nontoxic indicator dye and weakly acidic.
- It is used as diagnostic agent.
- The solution is reddish-brown in color.
- When diluted it is yellowish-green with UV light it emits green fluorescein.
- The solution is likely to get contaminated with *Pseudomonas* and hence used as sterile strips.

Uses of Fluorescein

- Fluorescein angiography
- Detection of corneal epithelial defects
- Applanation tonometry
- Tear film assessment
- Hard contact lens fitting
- To test lacrimal drainage system patency
- Seidel's test to find out leakage of aqueous from the anterior chamber
- Anterior segment angiography
- Fluorophotometry.

4. Fluorescein angiography.

Principle

- Excitation of fluorescein at 490 nm (blue)
- Fluorescein emission at 530 nm (green)
- Fluorescein remains intravascular within the retina but leaks from the choroidal circulation
- 70–80% of fluorescein is protein bound
- 20–30% is free fluorescein.

Technique

5 mL of 10% fluorescein or 3 mL of 25% fluorescein is injected intravenously into the antecubital vein. Reaches retina within 9 seconds.

Phases

- Preretinal choroidal flesh
- Arterial
- *Capillary:* Capillary filling with venous lamina flow
- *Venous:* Early, mild and late.

Side Effects

Yellowish discoloration of the skin, dark urine, nausea and vomiting, red after image, phlebitis, syncope, and anaphylactic shock.

Hyperfluorescence

- Atrophy of retinal pigment epithelial cells (window defect)
- Dye in subretinal space
- Dye in retinal pigment epithelial detachment
- Dye leakage from retinal vessels
- Dye leakage from choroidal or retinal new vessels
- Dye leakage from optic nerve head in papilledema
- Staining of tissues by dye—drusen.

Hypofluorescence

- Masking by abnormal materials

For example: Blood, melanin or hard exudates

- Retinal ischemia
- Choroidal ischemia
- Atrophy of vascular tissue

For example: Myopia.

5. Uses of prisms in ophthalmology.

- **Diagnostic:**
  - Measurement of angle of strabismus objectively by prism cover test
  - Measurement of strabismus subjectively by Maddox rod
  - Assessment of possible diplopia after proposed strabismus surgery
  - Measurement of fusional reserve
  - Assessment of microtropia (4 prism diopter test)
  - Assessment of simulated blindness (malingering)
- **Instruments:**
  - Slit-lamp/operating microscope
  - Keratometer
  - Pachymeter
  - Applanation tonometer
- **Therapeutic:**
  - To treat convergence insufficiency
  - To relieve diplopia.

Dots in Ophthalmology

- Horner Trantas dots—a collection of eosinophils at the limbus in vernal conjunctivitis
- Gunn's dot—light reflections from internal limiting membrane around disc and macula
  - Mittendorf's dot—Whitish spot at posterior lens surface which is the remnant of the hyaloid artery.

6. Lines in ophthalmology.

- *Arlt's Line:* White conjunctival scar at the junction of lower 1/3rd and upper 2/3rd of the superior tarsus which occurs in trachoma (stage III – cicatrization stage).
- *Stocker's Line:* Pigmented line of iron deposits in the base of corneal epithelium in front of advancing head of the pterygium.
- *Ferry's Line:* Iron deposition at the border of filtering bleb in trabeculectomy
- *Hudson-Stahli Line:* Deposition of iron in (derived from tears) in the epithelium of cornea in old age which occurs in a line corresponding to that of lid closure. It runs horizontally and usually bilateral and symmetrical.
- *Schwalbe's Line:* This is the junction between the angle structure and the cornea – anterior most limit of the angle of the anterior chamber.
- *Sampaolesi's Line:* Pigment deposition anterior to Schwalbe's line seen in pseudoexfoliation syndrome.
- *Khodadoust Line:* Seen in severe endothelial rejection after penetrating keratoplasty—linear arrangement of endothelial precipitates.
- *Paton's Line*: Circumferential retinal folds due to disc edema seen between disc and macula.

7. Striae in ophthalmology.

- *Haab's Striae:* Horizontal or curvilinear line seen in buphthalmos due to breaks in Descemet's membrane—occurs due to stretching of eyeball.
- *Vogt's Striae:* Thin vertical stress lines in deeper stroma seen in keratoconus.

8. Pearls in ophthalmology.

- *Elschnig's Pearls:* Type of after cataract—Subcapsular epithelial cells lining the equatorial region of lens proliferate and develop into large balloon like cells filling the pupillary area.
- *Iris Pearls:* Granulomatous nodules seen on the surface of iris in leprosy. Also called as leprotic nodules.

9. Rings in ophthalmology.

- *Coat's Ring:* It is white ring seen on the cornea following metallic foreign body.
- *Fleischer's Ring:* It is a yellowish-brown to the green ring of pigment hemosiderin surrounding the base of the cone in keratoconus at the level of the base of the epithelium.
- *Kayser-Fleischer Ring:* It is yellowish-brown or greenish ring seen in the peripheral cornea at the level of Descemet's membrane in Wilson's disease due to altered copper metabolism.
- *Wessely's Ring:* Ring of stromal infiltrate in herpetic disciform keratitis—indicates junction between viral antigen and host antibody.
- *Weiss Ring:* This is a ring of glial tissue detached from the margin of optic disc-pathognomonic of posterior vitreous detachment.
- *Soemmering's Ring:* Dense ring formed in the equator of the lens behind the iris (a type of after cataract).

10. Triangle in ophthalmology.

- *Arlt's Triangle:* Keratic precipitates arranged in triangular form with base down on the back of the cornea which is seen in iridocyclitis.

11. Spots in ophthalmology.

- *Bitot's spot:* It is a raised silvery white foamy triangular patch of keratinized epithelium situated on bulbar conjunctiva in the interpalpebral area usually on the temporal side
- *Foster-Fuchs spot:* Small black spot on the fovea in high myope due to macular hemorrhage
- *Roth's spot:* Hemorrhage in the retina with a white center seen in bacterial endocarditis, leukemia, etc.

12. Pseudos in ophthalmology.

- *Pseudophakia:* It is the condition of aphakia when corrected with an artificial intraocular lens implant.
  Signs are:
  - Surgical scar near limbus
  - Anterior chamber slightly deeper than normal (due to difference in thickness between natural and implanted lens)
  - Pupil is black
  - Mild iridodonesis
  - Glistening reflex from IOL
  - Visual status and refraction depends on the power of IOL implanted.
- *Pseudomyopia:* Overaction of accommodation in hypermetropia due to accommodative spasm. Cycloplegic

refraction will reveal this condition. The blurred vision clears when the patient looks through a concave lens.
- *Pseudocornea*: Iris is covered by layers of exudates which are usually covered by fibrous connective tissue and corneal or conjunctival epithelium. It usually follows perforated corneal ulcer or sloughed cornea.
- *Pseudohypopyon:* The collection of materials in the anterior chamber resembling hypopyon is called pseudohypopyon.

Causes: Seedling from intraocular tumors—metastasis, ghost cell glaucoma, lens materials.

- *Pseudoexfoliation:* The deposition of dandruff like material on the anterior lens capsule, the pupillary border, the trabecular meshwork and the other parts of the anterior segment of the eye.
- *Pseudopterygium*: It formed as a result of adhesion of a fold of chemotic conjunctiva with the marginal corneal ulcer. It is of inflammatory origin and it is commonly seen in gonorrheal or diphtheritic conjunctivitis, burns or chemical injuries.
- *Pseudoglioma*: It is also called leukocoria. The conditions which resemble retinoblastoma are called pseudoglioma.

Causes: Retrolental fibroplasia, persistent hyper plastic primary vitreous, cyclitic membrane, endophthalmitis, exudative retinopathy of coats, coloboma of choroid, and congenital cataract.

- *Pseudotumor:* This is an idiopathic inflammatory orbital lesion which produces proptosis due to non-neoplastic mass in the orbit.
- *Pseudoproptosis:* It is an apparent protrusion of eyeball without increase in any orbital contents or mass.

Causes: High myopia, contralateral enophthalmos, and lid retraction.

- *Pseudostrabismus:* It is an apparent squint due to anatomical abnormalities in the absence of true squint.
- *Pseudoesotropia:* It is due to prominent epicanthal skin fold that obscure part of normally visible nasal part of globe.
- *Pseudoexotropia*: It is seen in hypertelorism in which there is an abnormally wide separation of the eyes.
- *Pseudotumor cerebri:* It is often termed as benign intracranial hypertension. It is a disorder associated with raised intracranial pressure in the absence of an intracranial space occupying lesions.
- *Psuedopapilledema*: Resemble papilledema but there is no edema of optic disc. It is usually due to congenital anomalies of disc, drusen of optic disc, high astigmatism, hypermetropia, etc.
- *Pseudomembrane:* It is a coagulum on the surface of the conjunctival epithelium. Its removal leaves intact epithelium and there is no bleeding. It is seen in streptococcal and diphtheritic conjunctivitis.
- *Pseudoptosis:* It is drooping of the upper eyelid due to edema in conjunctivitis or due to fibrosis in trachoma.
- *Pseudo-Argyll Robertson pupil:* Some of the nerve fibers to medial rectus may innervate pupillary sphincter muscles, so that there is more pupillary constrictions during convergence than the response to light.
- *Pseudo Von Graefe's Sign:* Some of nerve fibers to inferior rectus innervate the elevator. The lid retracts when the patient looks down. It is seen in aberrant regeneration of 3rd nerve.
- *Pseudorosette:* It is seen in well differentiated retinoblastoma. Several layers of cells may be seen forming a lumen with blood vessels in the center.
- *Pseudoneuritis:* It is seen in hypermetropic eye where the disc has similar picture like papilledema but there is no disc edema.
- *Pseudoretinitis Pigmentosa:* These are atrophic changes in the choroid following chorioretinitis. They are often associated with pigmentary changes resembling retinitis. pigmentosa. Such pictures are seen in rubella or syphilitic retinopathy, quinine or Phenothiazine toxicity.
- *Pseudogerontoxon:* Resembles arcus senilis. It is due to gelatinous thickening (Cupid's bow) at superior part of limbus which is seen in bulbar form of vernal catarrh.
- *Pseudo-Foster Kennedy syndrome:* It is seen in anterior ischemic optic neuropathy (AION). In one eye, atrophy of edematous disc and in another eye edematous disc is seen. Altitudinal field defect is usually seen in this syndrome.

13. Nodules in ophthalmology.

- *Koeppe's Nodule:* Seen in granulomatous uveitis, situated at pupillary border. It consists of macrophages. It induces posterior synechia.
- *Busacca's Nodule:* Seen in granulomatous uveitis. It is situated away from the pupillary border near collarette. It usually seen in sarcoidosis
- *Lisch Nodule:* Small nodules seen on the iris of prepubertal children in Neurofibromatosis
- *Dalen-Fuchs Nodule:* It is seen in symphathetic ophthalmitis. It consists of epitheloid macrophages which appear as yellowish white spots in the fundus.
- *Leprotic Nodules or Iris Pearls:* These are granulomatous nodules seen in leprosy.

14. Anesthesia in ophthalmic surgeries.

Ophthalmic surgeries are performed usually under local anesthesia unless the patient is uncooperative or child.

Local anesthesia is given as:
- Surface anesthesia
- Regional anesthesia.

Surface Anesthesia:
- 4% lignocaine or 1% amethocaine or 0.5% proparacaine hydrochloride
- For corneal foreign body removal, nasolacrimal duct syringing, tonometry or gonioscopy.

Regional Anesthesia:
- Peribulbar block
- Retrobulbar block
- Facial block.
- *Peribulbar Block:* Injection of local anesthetic is given external to the muscle cone in the orbit. 24G needle is used. The facial block is not required. It is the anesthesia

of choice. Injection of 7–8 mL of anesthetic agent is injected into the peripheral space of orbit. It is usually given through lower eyelid adjacent to orbital margin at the junction of lateral 1/3rd or middle 1/3rd. The second injection can be given through the upper lid at the junction of medial 1/3rd and middle 1/3rd of orbital margin. After injection, bulbar pressure is given on closed lids for 5–10 minutes with the help of fingers or super pinky to reduce intraocular pressure. Anesthetic agent consists of 2% xylocaine with or without adrenaline, 0.5% bupivacaine in the ratio of 3:2. Injection hyaluronidase (1,500 IU) is added to one bottle of 30 mL of 2% xylocaine. Hyaluronidase spreads the anesthesia in the orbit.

Retrobulbar Block
- *Retrobulbar block:* 25 or 27G long needle is inserted into the muscle cone behind the globe. 3–4 mL of local anesthetic is injected.
- *Facial Block:* The anesthetic agent is given in front of the tragus of the ear to block terminal branches of facial nerve.

15. Antivascular endothelial growth factors (Anti-VEGF).

Mode of Action
They act by decreasing the abnormal new blood vessel formation. They also decrease the leakage and swelling of retina. They improve the function of inner blood retinal barrier.

These drugs control the neovascularization:
- Pegaptanib (Macugen): Dose 0.3 mg every 6 weeks intravitreally
- Ranibizumab (Lucentis): Dose 0.5 mg every 4 weeks intravitreally
- Bevacizumab (Avastin): Half-life of this is twice that of ranibizumab and is cost effective. Dose 1.25 mg.
- Aflibercept (Eylea): It has higher potency.

Indications:
- Wet age-related macular degeneration
- Diabetic macular edema
- Proliferative diabetic retinopathy
- Retinopathy of prematurity (ROP)
- Macular edema in central retinal vein occlusion (CRVO).

16. Computer vision syndrome.

Eyestrain with symptoms of headache, blurred near vision, burning sensation in the eyes, neck, shoulder, and back pain in persons working for long hours with computers are known as computer vision syndrome.

Causes
Characters on the computer screen do not have their contrast or well-defined edges. These characters (pixels) are brightest at the center and diminished in intensity towards the edges. This makes it difficult for our eyes to maintain focus and remain fixed on to these images.

Treatment
- Correct even small refractive errors
- Increase blink rate
- Proper blinking
- Eliminate bright source of light from the field of vision
- Pre-presbyopes (35–40 years) also need glasses due to poor accommodative facility or decreased amplitude of accommodation
- Single vision lens or progressive lens for computer distance are needed.

Remedial Measures
- Proper optical correction
- Proper viewing distance (24 inches)
- Downward viewing angle (15–29°)
- Proper room lighting
- Blink frequently and take breaks
- Use antiglare screen
- Lubricating eye drops
- 20-20-20 Rule. Take short breaks for your eyes every 20 minutes for 20 seconds and look at objects situated 20 feet away.

The solution to computer vision syndrome is simply a combination of good basic eye care, good visual workstation ergonomics, a good optical correction and controlled environmental factors.

Annexure

List of cases kept in practical examination for Undergraduates in Ophthalmology

Long Cases
1. Immature cataract (Pg: 78, 182)
2. Mature cataract (Pg: 78, 182)
3. Traumatic cataract (Pg: 81)
4. Aphakia (Pg: 81)
5. Pseudophakia (Pg: 193)
6. After cataract (Pg: 81)
7. Subluxation (Pg: 82)
8. Complicated cataract (Pg: 82)

Short Cases

Eyelids
1. Chalazion (Pg: 127)
2. Stye (Pg: 126)
3. Blepharitis (Pg: 125–126)
4. Trichiasis (Pg: 127)
5. Entropion (Pg: 128–129)
6. Ectropion (Pg: 129)
7. Hordolum internum (Pg: 127)

Conjunctiva
1. Phylecten (Pg: 39)
2. Pinguecula (Pg: 40)
3. Pterygium (Pg: 40–41)
4. Bitot's spots (Pg: 42)
5. Symblepharon (Pg: 130)
6. Subconjunctival hemorrhage (Pg: 41)
7. Nodule at the limbus (Pg: 41)

Cornea
1. Corneal ulcer (Pg: 45–47)
2. Corneal opacities (Pg: 57)
3. Adherent leukoma (Pg: 57)
4. Anterior staphyloma (Pg: 55)
5. Bullous keratopathy (pg: 58)

Sclera
1. Episcleritis (Pg: 60)
2. Scleritis (Pg: 61)

Iris
1. Acute iridocyclitis (Pg: 65–70)

Glaucoma
1. Acute congestive glaucoma (Pg: 69)
2. Phacomorphic glaucoma (Pg: 95)
3. Phacolytic glaucoma (Pg: 95)

Lacrimal apparatus
1. Acute dacryocystitis (Pg: 134–135)
2. Chronic dacryocystitis (Pg: 135–136)
3. Lacrimal fistula (Pg: 134–135)
4. Mucocele of sac (Pg: 135)

Eyeball
1. Phthisis bulbi (Pg: 56)
2. Panophthalmitis (Pg: 74–75)
3. Lagophthalmos (Pg: 131)
4. Bell's palsy (Pg: 131)

Index

Page numbers followed by *f* refer to figure.

A

Abrasion 46
Abscess, corneal 55
Acanthamoeba keratitis 49
Accommodation 7
    mechanism of 7*f*
    reflex 153
Acidic injuries 140
Acute dacryocystitis 134*f*
    clinical features of 134
    complications of 134
    etiology of 134
    treatment of 134
Acute iridocyclitis 69
    clinical features of 65
    complications of 65
    differential diagnosis of 65
    management of 65
Acute membranous conjunctivitis
    clinical features of 36
    differential diagnosis of 36
    etiology of 36
    treatment of 36
Acute mucopurulent conjunctivitis 34
    clinical features of 33
    etiology of 33
    treatment of 33
Acute purulent conjunctivitis
    clinical features of 34
    complications of 34
    etiology of 34
    treatment of 34
Adenovirus 33, 36
Adherent leukoma 57
    treatment for 58
Adie's pupil 154
Adrenaline 21
Adrenergic
    drugs 22
    inhibitors 22
    stimulators 22
Adult cornea, dimensions of 2
Adult eyeball, dimensions of 1
Advanced diabetes eye disease 107
Age-related macular degeneration 117
    treatment of 117
Alkaline injuries 140
Alpha-2 adrenergic receptor agonists 92
Alternate cover test 165
Altitudinal field defects 18
Amblyopia 168
American Thyroid Association, classification of 148
Amikacin 21
Aminoglycosides 21
Amoeboid ulcer 52
Amsler grid 117*f*
Amyloidosis 98
Anesthesia, regional 194
Angiospasm, stage of 110
Anisocoria 155
Anisometropia 30
    compound 30
    mixed 30
    simple 30
Anterior chamber 142, 181, 183
    angle of 8, 9*f*, 88
    deep 181
    irregular 181
    lens 85*f*
    peripheral 86
    shallow 181
    signs 66
    structures forming angle of 2
Anterior segment 1*f*
    lesions 170
Antiallergic drugs, role of 19
Antibiotics 37
Antibodies, serum 69
Anticholinesterases 22
Antifibrotics 19
Antiglaucoma drugs 19, 22
Antihistaminics 19
Anti-inflammatory agents 19
Antimicrobial agents 19
Antivascular endothelial growth factors 195
Anton's sign 17
Aphakia 30, 81, 96
    correction of 81
Aphakic glasses, disadvantages of 81
Applanation tonometry 87
Aqueous
    cells 66
    deficiency 136
    flare 66
    functions of 8
    humor, components of 8
    outflow, pathway for 8
    secretion of 9
    study of 69
Arcuate scotoma 18, 92*f*
Arcus juvenilis 56
Arcus senilis 56
Argon laser trabeculoplasty 93
Argyll Robertson pupil 154
Arlt's line 193
Arlt's triangle 193
Arteries, posterior communicating 17*f*
Arterioles, silver wiring of 110*f*
Arteritis, nonspecific 61
Arthritis, rheumatoid 61
Artificial drainage shunts 93
Artificial tears 21
A-scan 80*f*
Asteroid hyalosis 98
Astigmatic lens 29*f*
Astigmatism 23, 29, 29*f*
    asymmetrical 29
    clinical features of 28
    compound hypermetropic 28*f*
    compound myopic 28*f*
    corneal 28
    etiology of 28
    forms of 28
    irregular 28
    lenticular 28
    mixed 28*f*
    regular 28
    simple
        hypermetropic 23*f*
        myopic 28*f*
    treatment of 28
    types of 28, 30
Atherosclerotic changes 108
Atrophic papilledema 158*f*
Atropine 20
    action of 20
    side effects of 20
    uses of 20

Autonomic nerves 5
Axial hypermetropia, pathological causes of 26

B

Bacillus subtilis 74
Bagolini striated glasses test 10, 167, 167f
Band keratopathy 56, 68, 68f
Bard Parker handle 185, 185f
Barraquer's needle holder 187, 187f
Basal cell carcinoma 132
Bell's palsy 131, 138f
Bell's phenomenon 131
Bent 26 g needle 186
Berlin's edema 143f
Beta-adrenergic receptor antagonists 92
Beta-blockers 92
Bicarbonate 21
Binasal field defect 18
Binocular diplopia 179
Binocular vision 10
    grades of 10
    tests for 10, 166
Birth hypoxia 173
Bitemporal occipital disease 18
Bitot's spot 42, 42f, 193
Bjerrum's scotoma 14, 15, 15f, 92f
Bjerrum's screen 13f, 89, 89f
Blepharitis 125
    posterior 126
    squamous 125, 125f, 126
    ulcerative 125, 125f, 126
Blind
    spot 13
        normal 14
    rehabilitation of 177
    spot enlargement 14, 18
Blindness 172
    absolute 172
    avoidable 172, 173
    childhood 173, 176
    control of 174, 175f
    day 179
    economic 172
    prevalence of 172, 173
    sea of 13f
    social 172
    statistics 173
    types of 172
Blood
    aqueous barrier 8
    retinal barrier 120
    sugar 69
    tests 84
    uric acid 69
Blunt injuries 141
    clinical features of 141
Bowman's lacrimal probe 188, 188f
Bowman's membrane 44
Braille system of education 177
Branch retinal vein occlusion 112
    features of 113
    types of 113
Broad-spectrum antibiotic eye drops 34
B-scan 84
    ultrasonography 80
Bulbar conjunctiva 130f
Bullous keratopathy 58
Buphthalmos 90f, 91
Bupivacaine 21
Busacca's nodule 67, 194

C

Calcarine lesion, anterior 17f
Canalicular block 139
Canaliculi 138
Carbachol 20
Carbonic anhydrase inhibitors 22, 93
Carboxymethyl cellulose 21
Carotids, internal 17f
Castroviejo's caliper 187, 187f
Cataract 77, 81
    complicated 68, 82
    control 176
    coralliform 83f
    coronary 83f
    cortical 77
        immature 78
    diabetic 82
    hypermature 78, 78f
    intumescent 79f
    mature 78, 78f, 182
    metabolic 82
    posterior subcapsular 79
    sunflower 144f
    surgery
        complications of 81
        indication for 80
    sutural 84f
    traumatic 81
    types of 82
    unilateral 84
Catarrhal form 135
Cavernous sinus 147f
    communications of 148
    thrombosis 147, 148f
Cecocentral scotoma 15, 15f
Ceftriaxone 21
Cellulitis
    orbital 148, 150, 150f
    preseptal 149, 149f, 150
    stage of 134
Central retinal artery occlusion 18
    causes of 111
    clinical features of 111
    complications of 111
    differential diagnosis of 111
    treatment of 111, 112
Central retinal vein occlusion
    clinical features of 112
    complications of 112
    pathogenesis of 112
    treatment of 112
    types of 112
Central serous retinopathy 118, 118f
    differential diagnosis of 118
    signs of 118
    symptoms of 118
    treatment of 118
Cephalosporins 21
Chalazion 127, 127f
    clamp 187, 187f
    scoop 187, 187f

Chalcosis 144
Chemical injury 140f
    treatment of 140
Cherry-red spot 111f
    causes of 112
Chiasma 12f, 18
    central 12f
    lateral 12f
Chiasmal lesions, lateral 13
Chlamydia trachomatis 36
Chloroquine amblyopia 161
Cholinergic agents 137
Cholinergic drugs 22
Cholinesterase inhibitors, irreversible 22
Chorioretinal atrophy 24f, 91f
Chorioretinitis 68
Chorioretinopathy, central serous 120
Choroid 64, 121, 143
    blood supply of 64
    circumscribed malignant melanoma of 123f
    coloboma of 122
    layers of 3
    malignant melanoma of 123
    structure of 64, 64f
Choroidal detachment 115, 115f
Choroidal rupture 143, 143f
Choroiditis 71
    central 14
    healed 71
Chronic dacryocystitis
    clinical features of 135
    complications of 135
    etiology of 135
    management of 135
Cicatricial entropion 129
Cicatrization, stage of 46
Ciliary band 88
Ciliary body 3, 3f, 64, 121, 142
    anteromedial surface of 88
    functions of 64
    stroma of 64
    structure of 64
Citelli's bone punch 188, 188f
City University test 10
Clostridium welchii 74
Coat's ring 193
Cocaine 21
Color blindness 10
Color vision tests 10, 103
Comitant squint 162, 163
    management of 168
Computed tomography scan 17
Computer vision syndrome 195
Concomitant squint management 168
Cones, types of 54
Congenital cataract 122, 173
    etiology of 83
    management of 83
    types of 83
Congenital dacryocystitis
    clinical features of 133
    differential diagnosis of 133
    etiology of 133
    treatment of 133
Congenital glaucoma 86

clinical features of 90
etiology of 90
treatment of 90
Congestion
ciliary 41
circumcorneal 66
conjunctival 41
types of 180
Conjunctiva 33, 142, 180, 183
catarrhal inflammation of 34
degenerative conditions of 39
glandular tissues of 33
normal flora of 33
Conjunctival scissors 184, 184f
Conjunctivitis 33
acute 69
follicular 36
angular 35, 35f
classification of 33
giant papillary 38
membranous 36
pseudomembranous 36
Contact lenses 29, 31, 102
advantages of 32
indications for 32
Conventional extracapsular cataract extraction 80
Convex lens 27, 28f
Cornea 2, 44, 56, 128f, 142, 170, 180, 183
blood
staining of 142f
supply of 2
diseases of 45
ectatic conditions of 53
inflammation of 45
irregular 180f
nerve supply of 2
normal 180f
nutrition of 45
optical section of 180f
principal meridians of 28
structure of 44f
totally opaque 140f
Corneal blindness 176
causes of 174
Corneal edema 58
causes of 58
Corneal endothelium 44f
features of 2
Corneal light reflex 165
Corneal opacity 90f, 181
clinical features of 57
etiology of 57
management of 57
sequela of 58
trachomatous 37
types of 57
Corneal reflection tests 165
Corneal ulcer 42f, 45
bacterial 48
complications of 47
differential diagnosis of 46
management of 46
nonhealing 49
types of 46
uncomplicated 45

Cortical blindness 17
clinical features of 156
Corticosteroids 19
Corynebacterium
diphtheriae 36
xerosis 33, 42
Cotton wool spots 104
Cover test 183
Cover-uncover test 165
Crescent blade 185, 185f
Cryopreservation 59
Cryotherapy 124
Crypts of Henle 33
Crystalline lens 83f
Cuneiform cataract 78f, 79
Cupuliform cataract 78f
Cyclitic membrane 68, 122
Cyclopentolate 20
Cyclophoria 190
Cycloplegics 19, 20, 47, 70
relative action of 20
Cylindrical concave lens 189, 189f
Cylindrical convex lens 189, 189f
Cystitome needle 186, 186f
Cystoid macular edema 118, 119f
etiology of 119
Cysts 132
Cytomegalovirus
complement fixation test 69
retinitis 171

D

Dacryocystectomy 136
Dacryocystitis 133
acute suppurative 134
Dacryocystography 139
Dacryocystorhinostomy 136
contraindications for 136
Dalen-Fuchs nodule 71, 72f, 194
Dark adaptometry 103
Dastoor's superior rectus forceps 184, 184f
Degeneration, corneal 56, 57
Dendritic ulcer 51, 52f
Denominator 8
Dermatomyositis 61
Descemet's membrane 44
Descemetocele 55, 55f
Desmarre's lid retractor 188, 188f
Deuteranopia 10
Dewecker's scissors 185, 185f
Dexamethasone phosphate 19
Dextroelevation 164
Dextroversion 164
Diabetes mellitus 170
ocular manifestations in 170
Diabetic Control and Complication Trial 107
Diabetic retinopathy 108, 176
classification of 104
clinical features of 104
management of 104
pathogenesis of 104, 104f
risk factors of 104
screening 108
study 107
treatment of 107
Diphtheroids 33

Diplopia 167f, 179
Direct ophthalmoscope 101, 101f
Disk edema 110f
District Blindness Control Society 174
features of 174
formation of 174
functions of 174
Donor cornea, excision of 59
Donor eyes, preservation of 59
Down's syndrome 82
Drainage, order of 5
Dry eye 136
drugs used for 21
etiology of 136
investigations for 136
tests for 137
treatment of 136
Dystrophies 57
corneal 57

E

Early treatment diabetic retinopathy study 107
classification 105
Ectatic cicatrix 48f
Ectoderm, surface 6, 6f
Ectopia lentis 82
Ectropion 129, 129f
pupillae 68
Edema, macular 106f
Edridge-green lantern test 10
Electroencephalography 18
Electrooculogram 103
Electroretinography 102, 103f
Elschnig's pearls 193
Elschnig's spots 110
Emmetropia 23
Encysted mucocele 135
Endocrine exophthalmos 151
Endolaser photocoagulation 108f
Endophthalmitis 122
bacterial 73
clinical features of 73
etiology of 73
following penetrating injury 74f
infective 73
management of 73
noninfective 73
postoperative posterior 74f
vitrectomy study 74
Endothelium 44
Entropion 128, 128f
congenital 129
Enucleation 75, 124
indications for 188
spoon 188, 188f
Epikeratophakia 26, 31
Epiphora 178
causes of 138
Epiretinal membrane 98
Episcleritis 39, 60, 60f
simple 60
Epithelioma, malignant 40
Epithelium 44
Erythrocyte sedimentation rate 69
Esophoria 190

Esotropia 163, 167
    types of 167
Ethambutol amblyopia 161
Ethyl alcohol amblyopia 160
Eva Kohner's classification 105
Evisceration 75
    indications for 188
    spoon 188
Exenteration 124
    indications for 124
Exophoria 190
Exophthalmos 152
    thyrotoxic 149f
    thyrotropic 149f
Exotropia 163
    types of 168
External lacrimal fistula, stage of 134f
Extorsion 164
Extraocular extension 122
    stage of 124
Extraocular muscles 4, 76f, 164
    action of 4, 164
    anatomy of 4f
    field of action of 164f
    origin of 164
    palsy, pathological sequelae of 168
Exudative detachment 114
    clinical features of 114
    treatment of 115
Exudative retinal detachment 113
Eye
    anatomy of 1, 1f
    bank 59
    blood supply of 5
    care
        education 175
        service delivery, levels of 175
    collection
        contraindications for 59
        procedure for 59
    development of 5
    drops 19
    emmetropic 25f, 27f
    hypermetropic 27f
    injuries to 140
    itching of 178
    myopic 25f
    nerve supply of 5
    normal 7
    physiology of 7
    reflecting surfaces of 182
    signs 149
    spots in front of 179
    watering of 178
Eyeball 1, 27, 179, 183
    axial length of 80f
    coats of 1
    cutting optic nerve and removal of 76f
Eyelashes 128f
Eyelid 170, 179, 183
    function, impaired 136
    glands of 4
    layers of 4, 125
    margin, outward turning of 129f

F

Facial
    block 195
    cleanliness 37
Farnsworth-Munsell 100 hue test 10
Ferry's line 193
Festooned pupil 68f
Fiber arrangement 12f
Fibrin-platelet emboli 111
Field testing methods 14f
Fistula
    corneal 47f, 55
    stage of 134
Flare, grades of 66
Fleischer's ring 54f, 193
Florid stage 51
Flower petal appearance 119f
Fluorescein 192
    angiogram 113
    angiography 69, 102, 192
    dye disappearance test 138
    uses of 192
Fluorometholone 19
Fluoroquinolones 21
Foldable posterior chamber lens 85f
Follicles 39, 39f
Follicular conjunctivitis 36
Foramina, orbital 5
Foster-Fuchs spot 193
Foster-Kennedy syndrome 157, 157f
Fourth nerve palsy, clinical features of 169
Foveal electroretinogram 80
Frisby stereo test 10
Fuchs spot 24f
Fundus 27, 160
    camera 88
    changes 23
    fluorescein angiography 118f, 119f
    normal 100f
Fungal
    corneal ulcer, treatment of 47
    endophthalmitis 73, 74
    organisms affecting eye 21
    ulcer 49
Fusion 10

G

Galactosemia 82
Galactosemic cataract 82
Geniculate body, lateral 11, 13, 18
Geniculate hemianopia 16
Geographic ulcer 52f
Ghost cell
    arteritis 111
    glaucoma 97
Glands, mucin-secreting 33
Glaucoma 18, 86, 96, 173, 176
    acute congestive 69
    ciliary block 96
    classification of 86
    flecken 94f
    hemolytic 97
    hemosiderotic 97
    malignant 96
    management of 93
    neovascular 96, 96f
    phacolytic 95f
    phacomorphic 95f
    pigmentary 95
    steroid-induced 96
    treatment of 92
Glaucomatous stage 122, 124
Goblet cells 33
Goldmann applanation tonometer 87f
Goldmann bowl perimetry 89
Goldmann three-mirror lens 102
Gonioscopic lenses, types of 88
Gonioscopy 88
Graves' disease 149
    signs of 148
Graves' ophthalmopathy 148

H

Haab's striae 193
Haemophilus aegyptius 33, 34
Halo's around light 178
Harada's disease 62
Hard exudates 104, 106f
Hard lens 32
Head posture 179
Headache
    causes of 178
    ophthalmic causes of 178
Hemangioma 132
Hemeralopia 179
Hemianopia 16
    altitudinal 17
    binasal 17
    bitemporal 17, 17f, 18
    heteronymous 17
    homonymous 16, 18
    incongruous left homonymous 16f
    inferior altitudinal 18f
    left homonymous 16f, 17f
    occipital lobe 17
    right homonymous 17f
    superior altitudinal 18f
    types of 16
Hemibranch retinal artery 18
Hemiretinal vein occlusion 113
Hemorrhage 106f
    choroidal 143
    deep retinal 104
    intraocular 97
    macular 14
    retinal 104
    subconjunctival 41, 141f, 142
    superficial retinal 104
Herpes simplex 33, 52
    keratitis 51
Herpes zoster 52, 61
    ophthalmicus
        clinical features of 52
        etiology of 52
        management of 52
Herring's law 164
Heterophoria 162
    management of 168
Heterotropia 162
    management of 168

Hirschberg's test 165, 165f
Histamine 19
Holmgren's wool test 10
Homatropine 20
Hordeolum externum 126, 127
Hordeolum internum 127
Horner syndrome 154
Horner-Trantas spots 38
Horseshoe tear 114f
Hudson-Stahli line 193
Human immunodeficiency virus retinopathy 171
Hutchinson's pupil 154
Hydroxyethyl 21
Hydroxypropylmethyl cellulose 21
Hyperemia 34
Hyperfluorescence 192
Hyperlacrimation
    causes of 138
    central 138
    primary 138
Hypermetropia 23, 27
    clinical features of 26
    components of 26
    etiology of 26
    latent 26
    total 26
    treatment of 26
    types of 26
Hyperosmotic 22
    agents 93
Hyperphoria 190
Hyperpigmentation 91f
Hypertensive retinopathy 109f, 110f
    classification of 108
    clinical features of 108
    complications of 108, 110
    management of 110
    pathogenesis of 108
Hyphema 142f
    traumatic 142
Hypofluorescence 192
Hypoparathyroidism 82
Hypopigmentation 91f
Hypopyon 48, 67
    inverse 48
    mechanism of 48
    ulcer 48, 48f
        clinical features of 48

I

Imidazoles 21
Immature cataract 78, 78f, 182
    differential diagnosis of 78
Indocyanine green angiography 102
Infarction, bilateral occipital 17
Infection
    control of 46
    modes of 45
    orbital 171
    Inflammations orbital 62, 149
Injuries
    causes of 141
    clinical features of 141
    mechanical 141
    perforating 143
    treatment of 141
Ink-blot appearance 118
Interstitial keratitis
    clinical features of 50
    etiology of 50
    treatment of 50
Intorsion 164
Intracranial pressure, generalized raised 157f
Intraepithelial neoplasia, conjunctival 40
Intraocular lenses 84
    indication for 85
    parts of 85
    power of 80, 85
    types of 84, 85f
Intravitreal injections 19, 107, 115
Iridectomise, types of 185
Iridodialysis 142f
Iris 3f, 63, 72f, 121, 142, 170, 181, 183
    anterior surface of 3f, 63f
    atrophic patches 94f
    atrophy 68
    color 67
    layers of 63
    neovascularization of 68
    nodules 67, 67f
    pearls 193, 194
    prolapse 47f, 144, 144f
    repositor 187, 187f
    root of 88
    shadow 78f, 182f
    signs 67
    stroma 63
    structure of 2
Irradiation 124
Ishihara pseudoisochromatic plate test 10
Isopter 13

J

Jones dye tests 139, 139f

K

Kaposi's sarcoma 170
Kayser-Fleischer ring 193
Keith-Wagner-Barker classification 109
Keratectomy, photorefractive 26, 26f
Keratic precipitates 66, 66f
Keratitis
    acute epithelial 51
    classification of 45
    exposure 45, 50
    neuroparalytic 50
    neurotrophic 45, 50
    nonpurulent 45
    sclerosing 68
    superficial 45
    types of 45, 51
Keratocele 55
Keratoconus 53, 54
Keratoglobus 54
Keratomalacia 43f
Keratome 185, 185f
Keratometry 80f
Keratopathy 38, 68
    climatic droplet 56
Keratophakia 31
Keratoplasty 58
Khodadoust line 193
Kinetic perimetry 13
Koch-weeks bacillus 33, 34
Koeppe's nodule 67, 194
Krause glands 33
Krimsky's test 165
    uses of 165
Kuhnt-Szymanowski's procedure, Byron Smith modification of 129f

L

Lacquer cracks 24f
Lacrimal abscess 134f
    stage of 134
Lacrimal apparatus 133, 133f, 183
    anatomy of 133
Lacrimal gland 133
    accessory 33, 137
Lacrimal pump mechanism 137f
Lacrimal puncta 133
Lacrimal sac 133, 138, 179
Lacrimal syringing test 138
Lacrimation 65, 178
Lagophthalmos 131, 131f
Lamellar keratoplasty, types of 58
Lang's two-pencil test 10
Laser
    assisted in situ keratomileusis 26, 26f
    indications for 191
    interferometry 80
    therapy 93
    trabeculoplasty, selective 93
Latanoprost 22
Lead
    amblyopia 161
    poisoning 14
Leber's optic atrophy 14
Legal blindness 172, 173
Lens 6f, 68, 77, 142, 181, 183
    anatomy of 77
    bulging of anterior surface of 7f
    capsule 77
    dialer 186, 186f
    dimensions of 2
    epithelium 77
    fibers 77
    hook 186, 186f
    inferior subluxation of 85f
    material of 85
    metabolism of 10
    non-contact 102
    particle glaucoma 95
    spatula 187, 187f
    spherical concave lens 189
    structure of 2
    superior subluxation of 85f
    transparency 2
Leprosy 171
    ocular manifestations in 171
Leprotic nodules 194
Lesions
    causes of 12
    chiasmal 18

macular 18
types of 11
Leukocoria, causes of 122
Leukoma 57
Lidocaine 21
Lids 125, 179
cross section of 125f
ecchymosis of 141f
edema 66
margin rolls inwards 128f
margins 179
stickiness of 34
tumors 132
Light
near dissociation 154
rays, refraction of 9
reflex 153
pathway 153f
Limbus 180, 183
Lipid deficiency 136
Lisch nodule 194
Lister's perimeter 88f
Long sightedness 23
Loteprednol etabonate 19
Low vision 172, 176, 177
Lowe's syndrome 82
Lymphangioma 132

M

MacCallan's classification 37
Macrolides 21
Macula 57, 100
disciform degeneration of 14
Macular degeneration
dry age related 117
wet age-related 117
Macular edema, clinically significant 106f
Macular function tests 79
Macular hole 14, 103, 103f
Macular retinal detachment 14
Macular sparing 18
Macular splitting 16f, 17f
Macular star 109f
Maculopathy 106
Maddox rod 190, 190f
test 79f, 166, 166f
Maddox wing 166
Magnetic resonance imaging 17
Malnutrition 173
Manz glands 33
Marcus Gunn
jaw-winking phenomenon 131
pupil 154
Mass, orbital 62
Mast cell stabilizers 19, 38
McPherson lens holding forceps 186, 186f
Measles 33
Megalocornea 90f, 91
Meibomian cyst 127f
Mesoderm 6
Metastasis, stage of 124
Methyl alcohol amblyopia 160
Methyl cellulose 21
Methylprednisolone 19
Meyer's loop 12
Microaneurysms 105f

Microvascular leakage 105
Miosis 181
Miotics 92
role of 20
Molluscum contagiosum 33, 127, 170
Mooren's ulcer 53, 53f
Morgagnian cataract 79, 79f
Motor nerves 5
Mucin deficiency 136
Mucocele, lacrimal 135f
Mucolytics, topical 137
Muller's cells 100
Muller's lacrimal speculum 188, 188f
Mumps 33
Munson's sign 54, 54f
Muscles 182
action of 182f
ciliary 64
insertion of 164
pair of 164
Mycobacterial infection 171
Mycotic hypopyon ulcer 48
Mydriatics 19, 70
Myelinated nerve fibers 18
Myopia 23
clinical features of 23
congenital 23
etiology of 23
high 14
pathological 23
simple 23
treatment of 23
types of 23
Myopic disk 18
Myotonia dystrophy 82
Myxovirus 33

N

Nasolacrimal duct 133, 138
block 139
National Eye Donation Day 177
National Eye Donation Fortnight 177
National Program for Control of Blindness 172, 174
Near reflex 153
Nebula 57
Neisseria gonorrhoeae 33, 36
Neisseria meningitidis 33
Neural ectoderm 6
Neuralgia 61
Neurofibromatosis 132
Neuro-ophthalmic infections 171
Neuro-ophthalmology 153
Neuroprotective drugs 93
Neuroretinitis 156, 156f
Nevus 132
Newcastle virus 33
Night blindness 179
Nodular episcleritis 60
Noninfectious systemic diseases 65
Nonproliferative diabetic retinopathy 105f, 106f
Nonsteroidal anti-inflammatory drugs 19, 70
uses of 19
Nuclear cataract 78, 79, 79f
Nuclear hardness, grades of 80

Nuclear sclerosis 78
Nuclei, types of 83f
Nutritional deficiency 171
ocular manifestations in 171
Nyctalopia 179
Nystagmus 191

O

Obstruction, cilioretinal 111
Occlusio pupillae 68
Ocular chemical injury severity 140
Ocular disease 34
Ocular movements 131
Ocular pharmacology 19
Ocular surgery 61
Ocular toxicity 20
Ocular trauma 173
Ocular viscosurgical devices 21
Oculomotor nerve 5
Oil droplet reflex 54f
Opacity 46
clearing of 58
Opaque nerve fibers 14
Open globe eye injuries 141
Open sky technique 99
Ophthalmia neonatorum 35f, 173
clinical features of 35
differential diagnosis of 35
etiology of 35
management of 35
Ophthalmic surgeries, anesthesia in 194
Ophthalmology 19, 20, 177, 193
community 172
dots in 193
indirect 101, 101f
lasers in 191
lines in 193
nodules in 194
rings in 193
spots in 193
triangle in 193
Optic atrophy 18, 157f
clinical features of 159
consecutive 159, 159f
differential diagnosis of 159, 160
etiology of 159
glaucomatous 92, 160
ischemic 160
management of 159
primary 92, 159, 159f, 160
secondary 159, 159f, 160
vascular 160
Optic canal 146
Optic chiasma 11
Optic cup, formation of 6f
Optic disk 18
coloboma of 14
drusen 18
Optic groove, formation of 6f
Optic nerve 11, 12f, 18, 143, 157f
blood flow 88
coloboma 18
dimensions of 4
drusen 18
head analysis 88
inflammation of 155

lesions 11
    proximal part of 12, 12f
Optic neuritis 14, 18, 62
    clinical features of 155
    differential diagnosis of 155
    etiology of 155
    management of 155
Optic neuropathy, ischemic 18, 156
Optic radiation 11
    hemianopia 16
    middle part of 13
    part of 12f
    upper part of 13
Optic tract 11, 12f, 18
    lesion 13
Optic vesicle 6f
    formation of 6f
Optical coherence tomography 88, 103, 104f
Oral contraceptives 161
Orbit 146, 179, 183
    anatomy of 4, 146
    blowout fractures of 152
    cysts of 151
    surgical spaces of 147, 147f
    tumors of 151
Orbital fissure
    inferior 146
    superior 146, 146f
Orbitotomy 152
Organ culture method 59
Organic material injury, reaction of 145
Orthophoria 162, 167f, 190
Osteopathies 151

P

Pain 65
Palpation 183
Palpebral fissure 179
Pannus 37
Panophthalmitis 74, 75f, 148
Papillae 39, 39f
Papilledema 14, 18, 156, 157f, 158
    chronic 158f
    clinical features of 157, 158
    differential diagnosis of 157
    early 158, 158f
    end stage 158f
    established 158f
    etiology of 157
    late 158f
    management of 157
    pathogenesis of 157
Papillitis 68, 155, 156
Papillomacular bundle, interruption of 14f
Paracentesis 49, 69
Paracentral scotoma 15, 15f, 91f
Paralytic ectropion 129
Paramyxovirus 33
Paranasal sinuses, mucocele of 151
Parasympathomimetics 22, 92
Parietal lobe lesion 18
Parinaud's syndrome 154
Pars plana
    approach 99
    vitrectomy 108, 115
        indications for 99

Pars planitis 70
Paton's line 193
Pellucid marginal degeneration 56
Penicillin G 21
Periarteritis 111
Peribulbar block 194
Peribulbar injections 19
Pericystitis, acute suppurative 135
Perimetry 88
Persistent hyperplastic primary vitreous 99, 122
Phacoemulsification 80
    advantages of 80
    principle of 80
Phenylephrine 20
    side effects of 20
    uses of 20
Phlyctenular conjunctivitis 39
    clinical features of 39
    differential diagnosis of 39
    etiology of 39
    treatment of 39
Phoria, types of 190
Photoablation 191
Photocoagulation 124, 191
    bilateral panretinal 18
Photodynamic therapy 118, 191
Photophobia 65, 178
Photophthalmia 141
Photopsia 179
Photoretinitis 119
Photostress test 80
Phthisis bulbi 56, 68
    causes of 56
Picornavirus 33
Pigment dispersion, causes of 56
Pigment epithelial detachment 120
Pilocarpine 20
    side effects of 20
Pin hole 190, 190f
Pinguecula 40, 40f
Placido's disc 54, 180f
    reflex 180f
Plain forceps 184, 184f
Plexiform neuroma 132
Polyarteritis nodosa 61
Polychondritis 61
Polyenes 21
Polypeptides 21
Polyvinylpyrrolidone 21
Positron emission tomography 17
Posterior segment 2, 191
    lesions 170
Postneuritic optic atrophy 159, 159f
Povidone 21
Prednisolone 19
    acetate 19
Pregnancy, retinopathy of toxemia of 110
Presbyopia 30
Pressure, intraocular 9, 86, 183
Primary angle closure glaucoma 86, 93
    acute congestive phase of 94f
    clinical features of 93
    stages of 93
    treatment of 93
Primary open angle glaucoma 86
    clinical features of 91

investigations of 91
    treatment of 91
Prism 189, 190f
    cover test 165, 166, 166f
    glasses expand peripheral field 17
    over fixing eye 165f
    uses of 193
Proliferative diabetic retinopathy 105, 106, 106f, 107f
Proparacaine 21
Propionibacterium epidermidis 33
Proptosis 150, 152
    acute 151
    bilateral 151
    causes of 150
    intermittent 151
    investigations of 150
    treatment of 150
    unilateral 151
Propyl cellulose 21
Prostaglandin analogues 93
Protanopia 10
Pseudo von Graefe's sign 194
Pseudo-Argyll Robertson pupil 194
Pseudocornea 48f, 55, 194
Pseudoesotropia 194
Pseudoexfoliation 96f, 194
    glaucoma 96
Pseudoexotropia 194
Pseudo-Foster Kennedy syndrome 194
Pseudogerontoxon 38f, 194
Pseudoglioma 122, 194
Pseudohypopyon 48, 194
Pseudomembrane 194
Pseudomyopia 193
Pseudoneuritis 156, 194
Pseudophakia 96, 193
Pseudoproptosis 194
Pseudopterygium 40, 41, 194
Pseudoptosis 194
Pseudoretinitis pigmentosa 194
Pseudostrabismus 194
Pseudotumor 194
    cerebri 194
Psuedopapilledema 194
Psychosensory reflex 153
Pterygium 40, 40f, 41
    clinical features of 40
    differential diagnosis of 40
    etiology of 40
    parts of 40
    treatment of 40
Ptosis 130, 130f
    evaluation of 130
    mild 131
    moderate-to-severe 131
    treatment of 130
    types of 130
Pulsating proptosis, causes of 151
Punctate epithelial
    erosion 38
    keratitis 51
Pupil 181, 183
    abnormal 154
Pupillary reaction 68, 181
    abnormal 153
Pupillary reflex 153

Purkinje-Sanson images 182f
Purulent keratitis 45

Q

Quadrantanopia
    inferior 16, 16f
    superior 16f
Quiescent stage 122, 123
Quinine amblyopia 161

R

Radial keratotomy 25f
Radionuclide dacryocystography 139
Red cell glaucoma 97
Red eye, differential diagnosis of 41
Reflex hyperlacrimation 138
Refraction, errors of 23
Refractive error 32, 174, 176
    amount of 31
Refractive power 7
Refractive status 85
Refractive surgery 32
    principle of 32
Regression, stage of 46, 51
Regurgitation test 138, 139
Retina 3, 100, 121, 143
    examination of 101
    functions of 100, 101
    layers of 100
    nerve fiber pattern of 14f
    peripheral 100
    structure of 3, 4f, 100, 100f
Retinal artery occlusion 111
Retinal break 143
    diagnostic of 114
Retinal detachment 62, 114f, 115
    clinical features of 113
    differential diagnosis of 113
    pathogenesis of 113
    treatment of 113
    types of 116
Retinal disease 18
    bitemporal 18
Retinal fibers 11
Retinal function, investigations of 102
Retinal necrosis
    acute 171
    progressive outer 171
Retinal nerve fiber layer 86
    assessment, method of 103
Retinal vascular lesions 11
Retinal vein occlusion 111
    types of 112
Retinal vessels, obstruction of 111
Retinitis pigmentosa
    clinical features of 116
    differential diagnosis of 116
    inheritance of 116
    pathogenesis of 116
    treatment of 116
Retinoblastoma 121, 122
    clinical features of 121
    differential diagnosis of 121
    genetics of 121
    management of 121
    pathology of 121
    undifferentiated 121
Retinopathy
    coats exudative 122
    of prematurity 122
    phases of 108
    preproliferative 105
    stage of 110
Retinoscope, end point in 31
Retinoscopy 31
Retrobulbar block 195
Retrobulbar injections 19
Retrobulbar neuritis 156
    differential diagnosis of 156
    treatment of 156
Reversible cholinesterase inhibitors 22
Rhegmatogenous detachment 113, 115
    mechanism of 113, 113f
Rhegmatogenous retinal detachment 113
    treatment of 115
Rho kinase inhibitor 93
Riddoch's phenomenon 17
Rings scotoma 116f
Rodent ulcer 132
Rose Bengal staining 137
Roth's spot 193
Rubella, congenital 173
Rubeosis iridis 68, 72, 73f

S

Salus' sign 110f
Salzmann's nodular degeneration 56
Sampaolesi's line 193
Scanning laser
    ophthalmoscope 88
    polarimetry 88
Scar, corneal 174
Scheie's classification 109
Schiotz indentation tonometer 87f
Schirmer's test 137
Schlemm's canal 88
School eye screening 176
    program 175
Schwalbe's line 88, 193
Sclera 142, 60, 180, 183
    functions of 60
    inflammation of 60
    thickness of 2
Scleral buckling 115
    types of 115f
Scleral fixation lens 85f
Scleral spur 88
Scleritis 60, 61
    anterior 61
        necrotizing 61, 62
    investigations for 62
    necrotizing 61
    non-necrotizing 61
    posterior 61, 62
Scleromalacia perforans 62
Sclerosis, stage of 110
Sclerotic phase 109
    complications of 109
Scotoma 14
    absolute 14
    central 14, 15, 15f, 18
        bitemporal 14, 15, 15f
        suppression 167f
    junctional 14, 15, 15f
    negative 14
    positive 14
    relative 14
    types of 14, 14f
Secondary glaucoma 55, 68, 86
    clinical features of 95
    features of 95
    treatment of 95
    types of 95
Sectoral retinitis pigmentosa 18
Seidel's scotoma 14, 15, 15f
Seidel's sign 91f
Senile cataract
    clinical features of 77
    investigations of 77
    stages of 77
    treatment of 77
    types of 77, 77f
Senile ectropion 129
Senile entropion 128
Sensory nerve 5
Shaffer's grading 88
Sherrington's law 164
Short sightedness 23
Siderosis bulbi 144, 144f
Siegrist's streaks 110
Simcoe irrigation aspiration cannula 186, 186f
Sinskey hook 186, 186f
Sixth nerve palsy, clinical features of 169
Skull
    base of 42
    developmental anomalies of 151
Slit-lamp
    appearance 95f
    biomicroscopy 102f
    examination 54, 82
Small incision cataract surgery 80
Smokestack appearance 118
Snellen distant visual acuity chart 8f
Sodium perborate 21
Soemmering's ring 193
Soft exudates 104, 105f
Spaeth's grading 88
Spastic entropion 128
Special lenses 102f
Spectacles 31
Specular microscope 44f
Spherical concave lens 24, 189f
Spherical convex lens 189, 189f
Sphincter pupillae 64
Squamous cell carcinoma 132
Squint 162
    convergent 163
    divergent 163
    incidence of 162
    incomitant 163, 168
    paralytic 168
    right convergent 165f
    surgery, principle of 168

types of 163f
vertical 163
St. Martin forceps 187, 187f
Staphylococcus aureus 33, 34, 36
Staphylococcus epidermidis 33
Staphyloma 62
    anterior 55, 55f
    posterior 24f
    treatment of 62
    types of 62f
Static perimetry 13
Stenopaeic slit 190, 190f
Stereopsis 10
    tests for 167
Steroid 19, 70
    side effects of 19
    therapy 74
    topical 38, 40, 142
Stocker's line 40, 193
Streptococcus haemolyticus 36
Streptococcus pneumoniae 33, 36
Streptococcus pyogenes 33
Stroma 44, 64
Stromal keratitis 51
Sturm's conoid 29
Stye 126f
Subconjunctival injections 19
Sub-Tenon's injections 19
Sub-Tenon's space 147
Sunrise syndrome 85f
Sunset syndrome 85f
Superficial artery deflects 110f
Superotemporal branch retinal vein occlusion 113f
Supportive therapy 74
Surgery 37, 108
    indications for 84
Symblepharon 130, 130f
Sympathetic ophthalmitis
    clinical features of 71
    etiology of 71
    management of 71
Sympathomimetics 22, 92
Synchysis 98
    scintillans 98
Synechia, posterior 67, 67f, 68
Synergists 164
Syneresis 98
Synoptophore 166, 166f, 167
Syphilis 171
    ocular manifestations in 171
Systemic diseases 82
    ocular manifestations of 170
Systemic lupus erythematosus 61

T

Tarsorrhaphy
    indications for 131
    lateral 131
    method of 131
Tear
    conservatives 137
    elimination of 137
    film 136
        break up time 137
    secretion of 137
    substitutes 137
Temporal crescentic scotoma 17f
Temporal lobe 12f
    lesion 13, 16f, 18
Terrien's marginal degeneration 53, 56
Thermal injuries, management of 140
Third cranial nerve, branches of 5
Third nerve palsy, clinical features of 169
Thrombosis, atherosclerosis related 111
Tissue biopsy 69
Titmus fly test 10
TNO random dot test 10
Tobacco amblyopia 160
Tonometry, types of 87
Toxic amblyopia
    clinical features of 160
    differential diagnosis of 160
    etiology of 160
    management of 160
    types of 160
Toxoplasmic retinochoroiditis 171
Trabecular meshwork 88
Trabeculectomy 93
Trachoma 36, 38
    clinical features of 36
    differential diagnosis of 36
    etiology of 36
    management of 36
Trachomatous follicular inflammation 37
Trachomatous intense inflammation 37
Trachomatous scarring 37, 37f
Tractional retinal detachment 113
    treatment of 115
Translucid scotoma 14
Trichiasis 127
    trachomatous 37
Trigeminal nerve, ophthalmic division of 33
Tritanopia 10
Tropicamide 20
Tuberculosis 171
    ocular manifestations in 171
Tumors 151
    choroidal 62
    common orbital 152
    intraocular 96, 121
    malignant 132
    orbital 152
    stages of 123
Tunnel blade 185, 185f

U

Ulcer 46
    bacterial 49
    perforated 55
    stages of 45
Ulcus serpens 48
Ultrasonic pachymetry 54
Ultrasonography 102
    principle of 102
Uncover test 165
Uniocular diplopia 179
United Kingdom Prospective Diabetes Study 107
Upper lid
    conjunctiva 37f
    excursion 130
Urine tests 84
Uvea 63
    anatomy of 63
    blood supply of 63
Uveitis 64, 65
    allergic 65
    granulomatous 69
    hypersensitivity 65
    infective 65
    intermediate 70
    nongranulomatous 69
    posterior 69, 71
    toxic 65
    traumatic 65
Uveoscleral outflow 9

V

Van Herick's sign 86
Van Herick's slit lamp grading 86
Vancomycin 21
Vannas scissors 185, 185f
Vectis 186, 186f
Vein occlusion 18
Venous drainage 5, 64, 101
Vernal catarrh
    clinical features of 37
    differential diagnosis of 37
    etiology of 37
    treatment of 37
Vertical fissure height 130
Virus, drugs affecting DNA of 22
Viscoelastics 19, 21
Vision
    2020 175
        goal of 175
        objectives of 177
        program, role of 174
    blurred 70
    centers 177
    defective 58, 66
    double 179
    field of 13
    gradual loss of 178
    island of 13f
    mild-to-moderate loss of 117
    near 7
    neurology of 11
    physiology of 9
    sudden loss of 111, 178
    tubular 92f
Visual acuity 7, 179, 183
Visual disability, categories of 173
Visual field 11
    defects 11
    normal 13
Visual loss
    causes of 107
    functional 18
Visual pathway 4, 11, 12
    lesions of 11
    levels of 12f
    three neurons of 11

Visual system 11f
Visually evoked response 18
Vitamin A
    deficiency 43, 173
        ocular manifestations of 42
        pathology of 42
        prophylaxis of 43
        treatment of 42
    foods rich in 43, 43f
Vitrectomy 74, 99
Vitreous 68, 98, 143
    anatomy of 98
    aspiration 69
    degenerations of 98
    degenerative opacities of 98
    detachment, posterior 99
    diseases of 98
    hemorrhage 99
    traction 103
Vogt's striae 193
Vogt's triad 94, 94f
Vossius ring 142f
V-Y operation 129f

W

Watering eyes
    causes of 138
    investigations of 138
Wegener's granulomatosis 61
Weiss ring 193
Wernicke's hemianopic pupil 16, 154
Wessely's ring 193
Wilson's disease 82
Wire speculum 184, 184f
World Glaucoma Day 177
World Glaucoma Week 177
World Health Organization Definition of Blindness 172
World Sight Day 177
Worth 4 dot test 10, 167, 167f

X

Xanthoma 132
Xerophthalmia 42, 43
    types of 42
Xerosis 42, 42f

Y

Yoke muscles 164f

Z

Zeis gland 126f

EU GSPR Authorised Reprsentative
Logos Europe, 9 rue Nicolas Poussin
1700, La Rochelle, France
Phone: +33 (0) 6 67 93 73 78
E-mail: contact@logoseurope.eu

www.ingramcontent.com/pod-product-compliance
Ingram Content Group UK Ltd.
Pitfield, Milton Keynes, MK11 3LW, UK
UKHW050254040725
460398UK00006B/67